RADIOIMMUNOTHERAPY
of CANCER

RADIOIMMUNOTHERAPY of CANCER

edited by
Paul G. Abrams
Alan R. Fritzberg

NeoRx Corporation
Seattle, Washington

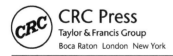

CRC Press
Taylor & Francis Group
Boca Raton London New York

CRC Press is an imprint of the
Taylor & Francis Group, an **informa** business

CRC Press
Taylor & Francis Group
6000 Broken Sound Parkway NW, Suite 300
Boca Raton, FL 33487-2742

First issued in paperback 2019

© 2000 by Taylor & Francis Group, LLC
CRC Press is an imprint of Taylor & Francis Group, an Informa business

No claim to original U.S. Government works

ISBN-13: 978-0-367-39836-1

**Visit the Taylor & Francis Web site at
http://www.taylorandfrancis.com**

**and the CRC Press Web site at
http://www.crcpress.com**

Foreword

The past two decades have provided an opportunity for investigators to explore the capacity of monoclonal antibodies and other targeting molecules to deliver therapeutic doses of radiation via radioisotope conjugates. This book assembles a strong cast of these investigators to review the progress that has been made and to clarify the challenges that remain.

The field of radioimmunotherapy has required the talents of basic scientists in radiation biology, chemistry, physics, and immunology. The clinical trials have involved physician scientists from nuclear medicine, radiation therapy, surgery, gynecology, and medical oncology/hematology. These interdisciplinary translational research efforts have provided a solid scientific basis for both the preclinical and clinical research efforts discussed in each of the chapters. The choice of isotope, the conjugation procedure, and the selection of tumor-displayed target antigen were early issues that persist, but currently with much better insight. The array of targeting molecules now available allows selection of reagents that may already have antitumor activity or may alter the radiation sensitivity of tumor cells (e.g., anti-CD20 and anti-EGFR reagents).

The issues of monoclonal antibody immunogenicity and the need for novel antibody constructs to enhance delivery and distribution of targeting molecules in metastatic tumor deposits have been approached with modern recombinant DNA technology. These reagents may allow repetitive treatments and circumvent many of the tumor vasculature impediments to therapy.

The need to enhance radioisotope delivery to a tumor while reducing radiation exposure to the bone marrow is a basic requirement of future studies. In addition to novel targeting constructs and isotope selection, the use of extracorporeal techniques and regional delivery of therapy (intraperitoneal, intrathecal, etc.)

have provided improved results. The use of pretargeting strategies to enhance antibody deposition in tumors while utilizing small molecule isotope conjugates to limit marrow radiation has undergone considerable progress with impressive tumor dosimetry estimates and antitumor efficacy. The pretargeting strategy emphasizes the continuing need for new tumor cell target antigens (molecules) that are not shared with normal tissues because the enhanced radiation delivery will occur at all sites of pretargeting.

Although several challenges remain in bringing radioimmunotherapy into the mainstream of cancer therapy, the progress described in the chapters of this book provides strong evidence of its success. Indeed, in the first year of this millennium, it is very likely that one or more radiolabeled antibodies will be approved by the FDA for the therapy of non-Hodgkin's lymphoma. This will undoubtedly lead to stronger industry/academic investigator efforts to accomplish similar approvals for one or more of the solid tumors. The combination of antitumor efficacy and high ''quality of life'' treatment regimens represents an important and achievable goal.

Albert F. LoBuglio, M.D.
Director, Comprehensive Cancer Center
Associate Dean, School of Medicine
Evalina B. Spencer Professor of Oncology
University of Alabama at Birmingham
Birmingham, Alabama

Preface

Radioimmunotherapy is the use of antibodies to deliver radiotherapy to cells bearing antigens to which they bind. This modality possesses the potential to improve cancer therapy by increasing the amount of cytotoxic radiation at tumors while reducing the radiation exposure of normal tissues. The concept of radioimmunotherapy goes back to 1956, when a patient was treated with radioiodinated polyclonal antiserum raised against his own melanoma. The advent of monoclonal antibodies in 1975, based on the work of Kohler and Milstein, launched a large effort to use these reagent monoclonal antibodies to selectively deliver cytotoxic reagents, including radiation to tumors. Despite that large effort, radioimmunotherapeutic products for the treatment of the first indication—non-Hodgkin's lymphoma—are only now close to approval and general availability. Progress in solid tumors is at an earlier stage, but encouraging results are being reported.

Despite the extended period of development in radioimmunotherapy over the last 20 or so years, much progress has been made. Some of the many advances include improved tumor antigen selection for antibody specificity, higher-affinity antibodies, protein engineering to create novel forms of antibodies for improved targeting and reduced immunogenicity, choice of radionuclide and linking chemistry, and novel approaches for tumor targeting, such as pretargeting that overcomes the mismatch of short-lived radioactivity with the slow pharmacokinetics of antibody tumor targeting.

This book provides a comprehensive set of chapters that detail the state of the field in radioimmunotherapy. Included are chapters reviewing the technology, aspects of tumor architecture affecting radiotherapy delivery, and clinical applications in the various cancer types that have had significant study.

We wish to thank all the authors who contributed to the book, as well as Dr. Wil B. Nelp, Professor Emeritus of Radiology and Nuclear Medicine, University of Washington, who provided external review of the chapters.

Paul G. Abrams
Alan R. Fritzberg

Contents

Contributors

Paul G. Abrams, M.D., J.D.   CEO, NeoRx Corporation, Seattle, Washington

Donald B. Axworthy   Senior Scientist, Pharmacology, NeoRx Corporation, Seattle, Washington

Paul L. Beaumier, Ph.D.   Scientist, Toxicology Department, Shin Nippon Biomedical Sciences USA, Everett, Washington

Ruud H. Brakenhoff, Ph.D.   Assistant Professor, Department of Otolaryngology/Head and Neck Surgery, Free University Hospital, Amsterdam, The Netherlands

Hazel B. Breitz, M.D.   Research Affiliate, Nuclear Medicine Section, Virginia Mason Medical Center, Seattle, Washington

Øyvind S. Bruland, M.D., Ph.D.   Professor and Consultant Oncologist, Departments of Medical Oncology and Radiotherapy, Norwegian Radium Hospital, Oslo, Norway

Donald J. Buchsbaum, Ph.D.   Professor and Director of Radiation Biology, Department of Radiation Oncology, University of Alabama at Birmingham, Birmingham, Alabama

JianQing Chen, Ph.D.* Department of Radiation Physics, Jubileum Institute, Lund University, Lund, Sweden

Marco Chinol, Ph.D. Chief Radiochemist, Division of Nuclear Medicine, European Institute of Oncology, Milan, Italy

Marta Cremonesi, Ph.D. Physicist, Division of Medical Physics, European Institute of Oncology, Milan, Italy

Remco de Bree, M.D., Ph.D. E.N.T. Surgeon, Department of Otolaryngology/Head and Neck Surgery, Free University Hospital, Amsterdam, The Netherlands

G. L. DeNardo, M.D. Professor Emeritus, Internal Medicine, Radiology and Pathology, University of California, Davis, California

Ann M. Dvorak, M.D. Department of Pathology, Beth Israel Deaconess Medical Center, and Professor of Pathology, Harvard Medical School, Boston, Massachusetts

Harold F. Dvorak, M.D. Chief, Department of Pathology, Beth Israel Deaconess Medical Center, and Mallinckrodt Professor of Pathology, Harvard Medical School, Boston, Massachusetts

Agamemnon A. Epenetos, Ph.D., F.R.C.P. Chief Scientific Officer, Antisoma Research Laboratories, St. George's Hospital Medical School, London, England

Dian Feng, Ph.D. Department of Pathology, Beth Israel Deaconess Medical Center, and Instructor in Pathology, Harvard Medical School, Boston, Massachusetts

Alan R. Fritzberg, Ph.D. Chief Scientist, NeoRx Corporation, Seattle, Washington

Michael Garkavij, M.D., Ph.D. Consultant Oncologist, Department of Oncology, Lund University Hospital, Lund, Sweden

---

* *Current affiliation*: Department of Biochemistry, University of Missouri, Columbia, Missouri.

Roberto Gennari, M.D.   Attending Surgeon, Division of Surgical Oncology, Department of Surgery, European Institute of Oncology, Milan, Italy

J. G. Geraghty   Division of Surgical Oncology, Department of Surgery, European Institute of Oncology, Milan, Italy

Chiara Grana, M.D.   Assistant, Division of Nuclear Medicine, European Institute of Oncology, Milan, Italy

John W. Greiner, Ph.D.   Laboratory of Tumor Immunology and Biology, National Cancer Institute, National Institutes of Health, Bethesda, Maryland

Patricia Horan Hand, Ph.D.*   Laboratory of Tumor Immunology and Biology, National Cancer Institute, National Institutes of Health, Bethesda, Maryland

Cecilia Hindorf, M.Sc.   Department of Radiation Physics, Jubileum Institute, Lund University, Lund, Sweden

Cornelis A. Hoefnagel, M.D., Ph.D.   Department of Nuclear Medicine, Netherlands Cancer Institute, Amsterdam, The Netherlands

Susan J. Knox, M.D., Ph.D.   Associate Professor, Department of Radiation Oncology, Stanford University, Stanford, California

Monica S. Krieger   Corixa Corporation, Seattle, Washington

Claude F. Meares, Ph.D.   Professor and Chairman, Department of Chemistry, University of California, Davis, California

Ruby F. Meredith, M.D., Ph.D.   Professor, Department of Radiation Oncology, University of Alabama at Birmingham, Birmingham, Alabama

Janice A. Nagy, Ph.D.   Department of Pathology, Beth Israel Deaconess Medical Center, and Senior Research Associate, Harvard Medical School, Boston, Massachusetts

Rune Nilsson, Ph.D.   Mitra Medical Technology AB, Lund, Sweden

* *Current affiliation*: Oncological Sciences Initial Review Group, Center for Scientific Review, National Institutes of Health, Bethesda, Maryland.

Joseph A. O'Donoghue, Ph.D.   Assistant Attending Physicist, Department of Medical Physics, Memorial Sloan-Kettering Cancer Center, New York, New York

Giovanni Paganelli, M.D.   Division Director, Division of Nuclear Medicine, European Institute of Oncology, Milan, Italy

Alexander Pihl, M.D., Ph.D.   Professor Emeritus, Department of Biochemistry, Norwegian Radium Hospital, Oslo, Norway

O. Press, M.D., Ph.D.   Professor in Medicine and Biological Structures, University of Washington, and Member, Fred Hutchinson Cancer Research Center, Seattle, Washington

Jasper J. Quak, M.D., Ph.D.   Department of Otolaryngology/Head and Neck Surgery, Free University Hospital, Amsterdam, The Netherlands

Bengt E. B. Sandberg   Mitra Medical Technology AB, Lund, Sweden

Jody E. Schultz, Ph.D.   Research Manager, Molecular Biology, NeoRx Corporation, Seattle, Washington

Hans-Olov Sjögren, M.D., Ph.D.   Department of Tumorimmunology, Lund University, Lund, Sweden

Dale C. Slavin-Chiorini, Ph.D.   Laboratory of Tumor Immunology and Biology, National Cancer Institute, National Institutes of Health, Bethesda, Maryland

Gordon B. Snow, M.D., Ph.D.   Professor and Chairman, Department of Otolaryngology/Head and Neck Surgery, Free University Hospital, Amsterdam, The Netherlands

Sven-Erik Strand, M.B., Ph.D.   Professor, Radiation Physics, Jubileum Institute, Lund University, Lund, Sweden

Konstantinos N. Syrigos, M.D., Ph.D.   Associate Professor of Medical Oncology and Consultant, Third Department of Medicine, University of Athens Medical School, Athens, Greece

Jan G. Tennvall, M.D., Ph.D.   Consultant Oncologist and Nuclear Medicine Physician, Department of Oncology, Lund University Hospital, Lund, Sweden

Louis J. Theodore, Ph.D.   Senior Scientist, Chemistry, NeoRx Corporation, Seattle, Washington

Guus A. M. S. van Dongen, Ph.D.   Department of Otolaryngology/Head and Neck Surgery, Free University Hospital, Amsterdam, The Netherlands

Frank B. van Gog, Ph.D.   Department of Otolaryngology/Head and Neck Surgery, Free University Hospital, Amsterdam, The Netherlands

Gerard W. M. Visser, Ph.D.   Radio Nuclide Center, Free University Hospital, Amsterdam, The Netherlands

Paul L. Weiden, M.D.   Medical Director, Cancer Clinical Research Unit, Virginia Mason Medical Center, Seattle, Washington

Michael R. Zalutsky, Ph.D.   Professor, Department of Radiology, Duke University Medical Center, Durham, North Carolina

1
Dosimetric Principles of Targeted Radiotherapy

Joseph A. O'Donoghue
Memorial Sloan-Kettering Cancer Center, New York, New York

I. INTRODUCTION

For disseminated or diffuse malignant disease a systemic approach to treatment is required. To achieve selective and systemic therapy simultaneously has been a longstanding objective of cancer research (1). This goal cannot be achieved by physical means and requires exploitation of the biological differences between cancerous and noncancerous cells.

Biologically targeted radiotherapy is the selective irradiation of tumors using radioactive isotopes attached to molecular vectors that have some degree of biological specificity for the tumor target. Radioimmunotherapy (2–5) involves the use of antibodies and their fragments. Metabolic targeting, such as with meta-iodobenzylguanidine (mIBG) for the treatment of neuroblastoma (6,7) or pheochromocytoma (8), is based on a unique molecular transport and storage pathway. Other potentially exploitable biological differences include the numbers of hormone or growth factor receptors (9,10) and differences in DNA sequence (11,12). In principle, these also could provide bases for biologically targeted radiotherapy.

At present radionuclides that emit beta particles are by far the most commonly used, and these will be discussed in this chapter. However, there is interest in the use of α-emitting radionuclides for therapy (13–15), and there is at least one ongoing clinical trial featuring [213]Bi-labeled antibody therapy of leukemia (16). In cases where the targeting vector is localized to the nucleus and is in contact with the DNA, the most appropriate radionuclides may be those emitting ultra-low-energy Auger electrons (17–21). Potential targeting molecules for Auger emitters include nucleoside analogs (22,23), steroid hormones (10,24–

1

26), and synthetic oligonucleotides (27). Irrespective of the radionuclides and biological mechanisms involved it is useful to classify targeting agents in the context of four categories:

1. Specificity. There remains a lack of truly tumor-specific targets. Almost all antibodies crossreact with normal cells to some degree. Depending on whether intact antibodies or fragments are used, there is typically some degree of nonspecific hepatic or renal concentration of radionuclide. Non-antibody-targeting molecules also show enhanced uptake in certain normal tissues. For example mIBG is concentrated in the adrenal glands and myocardium.

2. Heterogeneity. Tumor targeting is characteristically heterogeneous. Even with the best available antibodies, tumor regions which express the requisite antigen can be inaccessible to antibody (28). This may be due to elevated interstitial fluid pressure (29) within tumors or the existence of a "binding site barrier" (30). Other possible factors include phenotypic heterogeneity, antigen modulation (31), and anatomical sanctuary sites, as are found for chemotherapy. Heterogeneity in radionuclide distribution gives rise to a corresponding heterogeneity in absorbed dose. The degree of correspondence will be determined by the emission range of the radionuclide (32,33).

3. Potency. The therapeutic potency of targeted radiotherapy is influenced by a number of factors. These include the emission characteristics of the radionuclide, the physical conformation and radiosensitivity of the tumor target, and the degree of heterogeneity of the radiation dose.

4. Range. The ionizing particles emitted as a consequence of nuclear decay have a finite range. This has the advantage that radionuclides do not have to be internalized or in contact with a particular tumor cell in order to sterilize it. Individual tumor cells that have not been targeted may still be sterilized by "crossfire" radiation bound to neighboring cells. The amount of crossfire irradiation depends on the spatial configuration of tumor cells and the emission range of the radionuclide (34,35).

The categories described above are intimately related. For example, using a radionuclide with a longer emission range will improve radiation homogeneity, perhaps worsen the radiation specificity, and affect the therapeutic potency. In addition, the nature of the disease itself is of vital importance. The tumor target may be radiosensitive or resistant; microscopic, macroscopic, or both; systemic or regional. It is the combination and interaction of all these various aspects of treatment and disease that will determine the clinical utility of targeted radiotherapy in any particular instance.

The main theoretical advantage of targeted radiotherapy is that radiation can be delivered *selectively* to tumor deposits that are too small to be detected or treated locally. In these cases, its systemic and selective nature has advantages compared to the alternatives of chemotherapy or total body irradiation, which are systemic but not particularly selective. Given the typically low levels of tumor uptake currently achieved, it is unlikely that targeted radionuclide therapy by itself will be able to achieve local control of bulk solid tumors. However, it could provide a useful "boost" dose to local disease that is being treated by conventional radiotherapy (36,37) or deliver radiation dose to regions of local dissemination near gross disease boundaries.

II. ABSORBED DOSE RATES AND RADIOBIOLOGICAL RESPONSE

There are a large number of beta-emitting radionuclides that have potential clinical application (34,36,38,39), although the number that have actually been used is small. From a dosimetric point of view the most important parameters are the energy emission spectrum and the half-life, $T_{1/2}$. If the number of radionuclide atoms per unit mass is N and the energy emitted per disintegration is E, then the absorbed dose rate is proportional to $NE/T_{1/2}$ for conditions of electronic equilibrium. The ratio $E/T_{1/2}$ is thus a useful indicator of the intrinsic radiotherapeutic potency of the radionuclide.

Absorbed dose rate profiles produced by targeted radiotherapy are complex in both tumors and normal organs. This is caused by biological processes of accumulation and clearance superimposed on a background of physical decay. Many of the radiobiological consequences of these complex time-varying dose rates can be illustrated using the simpler description of a mono-exponentially decreasing dose rate. Consider a simple hypothetical system where the surviving fraction of cells is exponentially related to absorbed dose. This would correspond to a straight line relationship on a semi-log plot, as shown in Figure 1. Radiobiologically, this would be a reasonable assumption for the low absorbed dose rates commonly found in targeted radiotherapy (21,37,40). The slope of the survival curve is a measure of the radiosensitivity of the cells and is characterized by the parameter α. It has been observed that a correlation exists between the in vitro radiosensitivity of tumor cells and the in-vivo radioresponsiveness of tumors of the same type (41,42). For in vitro tumor cell culture, an α value around 0.35 Gy^{-1} is average, 0.5 Gy^{-1} is sensitive, and 0.2 Gy^{-1} is resistant (41). If a nonproliferating cell population characterized by an exponential survival curve is irradiated by a varying dose rate, the time profile of the logarithm of surviving fraction will have the same shape as the time profile of the dose rate. Such a scenario is shown in Figure 2 for a total absorbed dose of 15 Gy delivered by an exponentially decaying dose rate with a half-time of 2 days. The α value used here is 0.35 Gy^{-1}, corresponding to average radiosensitivity.

If the cells are proliferating exponentially, the overall survival is due to a combination of proliferation and radiation-induced sterilization. Such a survival curve is shown in Figure 3 for a cell population doubling time of 4 days. Obvi-

4

O'Donoghue

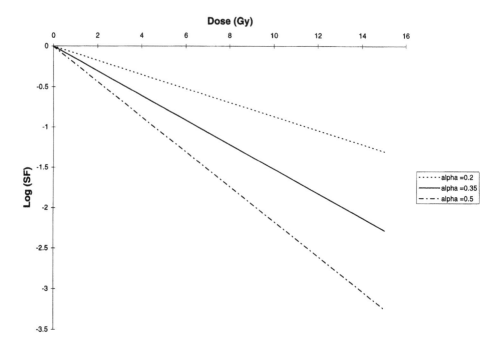

Figure 1 For very low dose rates, the LQ model predicts that radiation survival curves reduce to the simple form of an exponential relationship between surviving fraction and absorbed dose. On a semilog plot this corresponds to a straight line. The slope of the survival curve (α) represents the radiosensitivity of the cell population. For tumor cells grown in vitro, an α value of 0.2 Gy^{-1} is resistant, 0.5 Gy^{-1} is sensitive and 0.35 Gy^{-1} is average.

ously this has a different shape than before. If the initial dose rate is greater than a certain critical value (ln $2/\alpha T_D$, where T_D is the doubling time [37,40,42a], the cell population will decrease until the dose rate falls to this value. At the critical dose rate the rates of proliferation and sterilization are in balance and the treatment is effectively over. This is because the remainder of the dose is delivered at too low a dose rate to reduce the population any further. The nadir of surviving fraction represents the maximum effect of treatment. For a fixed value of absorbed dose the factors that influence the depth of the nadir include the radiosensitivity (shallower for less radiosensitive tumor cells), the proliferation rate (shallower for faster proliferation), and the effective radionuclide half-life (shallower for slower decay). The nadir value of surviving fraction may be used to define an effective dose by comparison to the survival curves of Figure 1. This is the dose that would produce the same biological effect if proliferation was not oc-

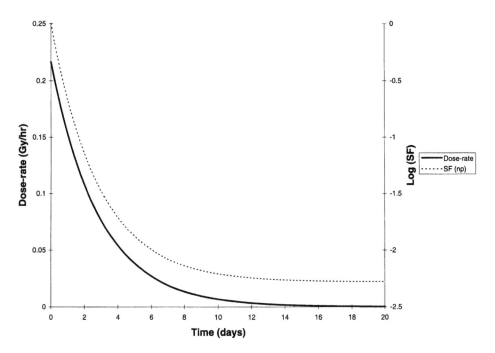

Figure 2 Irradiation of a nonproliferating cell population by an exponentially decaying dose rate. The total dose is 15 Gy, the effective half-life is 2 days, and the radiosensitivity parameter (α) is 0.35 Gy^{-1}. The time profile of surviving fraction has the same shape as the time profile of the dose rate.

curring. Figure 4 shows how, in this example, the effective dose depends on the population doubling time and also the radiosensitivity. Its dependency on radionuclide half-life is not shown in this graph.

Technical note: For a mono-exponentially decaying dose rate the time when the nadir of surviving fraction occurs, T_{eff}, can be calculated as

$$T_{eff} = \frac{T_{1/2}}{\ln 2} \ln\left(\frac{\alpha\, r_0 T_D}{\ln 2}\right)$$

where $T_{1/2}$ is the radionuclide half-life and r_0 is the initial dose rate. The minimum surviving fraction, S_{eff}, is then given by the equation

$$S_{eff} = \exp\left\{-\alpha D_\infty\left(1 - \exp\left(-\ln 2 \frac{T_{eff}}{T_{1/2}}\right)\right) + \ln 2 \frac{T_{eff}}{T_D}\right\}$$

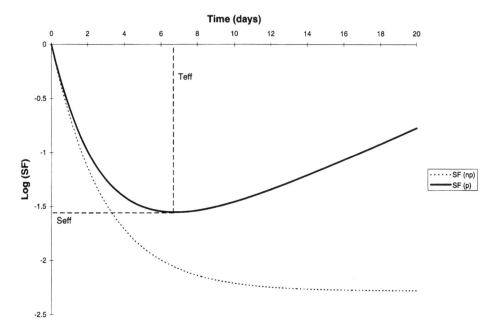

Figure 3   Similar to Figure 2 but this time the cells are proliferating exponentially with a doubling time of 4 days. There is a nadir in surviving fraction, S_{eff}, which occurs at a time, T_{eff}. At this point the rates of proliferation and radiation-induced sterilization are in balance. The effective dose is defined as that which would produce a surviving fraction S_{eff} in the absence of proliferation.

By analogy to an exponential survival curve, where $S = \exp(-\alpha D)$, the effective dose may be defined as

$$D_{eff} = D_\infty \left(1 - \exp\left(-\ln 2 \frac{T_{eff}}{T_{1/2}} \right) \right) - \ln 2 \frac{T_{eff}}{\alpha T_D}$$

This indicates that D_{eff} can be split into three parts. The first part (D_∞) is just the total dose—which would be the effective dose if there was no proliferation. The second part

$$D_\infty \exp\left(-\ln 2 \frac{T_{eff}}{T_{1/2}} \right)$$

is the dose that is ineffective because it is delivered when the dose rate is too low to reduce the cell number. The third part

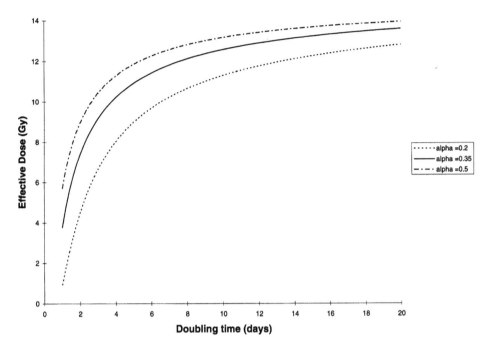

Figure 4 This illustrates how the effective dose is dependent on the population doubling time and the radiosensitivity. For all these curves the total absorbed dose remains constant at 15 Gy. Faster proliferation or greater radioresistance causes a larger proportion of the absorbed dose to be ineffectual.

$$\ln 2 \frac{T_{\text{eff}}}{\alpha T_D}$$

is the dose which is ineffectual because it balances the proliferation that takes place before the effective treatment time occurs.

The therapeutic efficiency may be defined as the ratio of effective to total dose and is given by the equation

$$E = 1 - \frac{\ln 2}{\alpha r_0 T_D}\left(1 - \ln\left(\frac{\ln 2}{\alpha r_0 T_D}\right)\right)$$

All these equations are based on the assumption that the initial dose rate $r_0 > \ln 2/\alpha T_D$. If $r_0 < \ln 2/\alpha T_D$, the therapeutic efficiency is zero and the radiation dose does not reduce the cell population at all.

The intrinsic radiosensitivity of cells and their proliferation rate are thus important determinants of response. Simplistically, radiosensitivity determines how the response depends on absorbed dose while proliferation rate determines how it depends on treatment time. In general, greater doses and shorter treatment times correspond to an increase in the intensity of therapy and a consequently greater response. If the cells are proliferating faster or are more radioresistant, then a greater proportion of the absorbed dose is ineffectual. Dose-for-dose, radionuclides with longer half-lives are less effective than those with shorter values.

These findings are applicable to both proliferating tumor cells and proliferating normal cells such as those found in the gastrointestinal epithelium and the bone marrow. With targeted radiotherapy, tumor to nontumor ratios usually increase with time. The downside to this is that the most favorable differential usually occurs when the absorbed dose rates are very low and thus largely ineffectual. In some circumstances it may be advantageous to use a radionuclide with a shorter half-life to increase the dose rate at earlier times. This may be appropriate when tumor localization is particularly rapid and/or the number of accessible binding sites is restricted. In other cases a longer half-life may be better. The therapeutic effectiveness of radionuclides with excessively long half-lives will be restricted by the number of accessible binding sites per cell.

III. EFFECTS OF EMISSION RANGE ON RESPONSE

The range of a beta particle depends on its energy such that higher energy particles have longer ranges. The range of emissions therefore varies from one radionuclide to another depending on the energy spectrum. This affects the manner in which energy is deposited in the vicinity of radioactive sources. In this section the relationship between tumor size, absorbed dose, and curability are discussed.

If we consider the very simple situation of a spherical volume containing a uniform distribution of activity, it is possible to calculate the absorbed fraction of the energy emitted by the radionuclides (34,43,44). This quantity is the ratio of absorbed energy to emitted energy. It depends on the size of the sphere and the emission spectrum of the radionuclide. If the sphere is large in comparison to the emission range, most of the emitted energy is absorbed and the absorbed fraction will be close to one. If the sphere is small in comparison to the range, a significant proportion of the emitted energy will escape and the absorbed fraction will be less than 1. Figure 5 shows calculated (43) values of the absorbed fraction (ϕ) as a function of sphere diameter for four radionuclides with differing emission spectra. These, together with similar data for 18 other radionuclides, were used in a mathematical modeling study (42) that examined tumor cure probability as a function of size. It was assumed, for each radionuclide, that the activ-

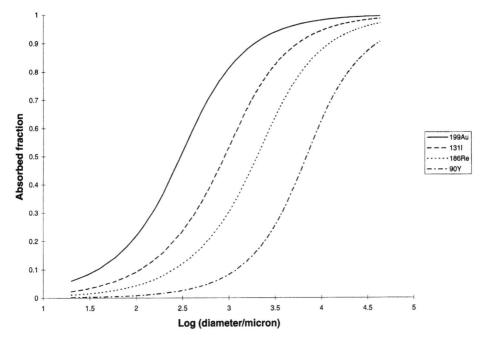

Figure 5 Calculated values of the absorbed fraction (ϕ) as a function of sphere diameter for four radionuclides with differing emission spectra. (From Ref. 43.)

ity per gram was independent of tumor size. Figure 6 shows the calculated relationship between tumor cure probability and tumor size for the radionuclide [131]I. Each curve corresponds to a different value of initial activity per gram of tumor with higher values toward the top. This shows there is a peak of tumor curability which occurs at around 3.4 mm diameter. The relationship between curability and size has the same general shape for all the other radionuclides, differing only in the position of the maximum value. Tumor sizes for maximum curability for a selection of radionuclides are shown in Table 1. These optima occur due to a balance between cell number and energy absorption and differ between radionuclides according to their emission characteristics. In situations where the assumption of size-independent uptake is valid, experimental evidence supports the prediction that smaller tumors can be more difficult to eradicate than larger ones (45,46). However, if smaller tumors have systematically greater specific uptakes than larger tumors, the size-dependent loss of absorption would be countered by a size-dependent increase in uptake and the optimal sizes would be less.

Perhaps the most important point to note from this is that a high-energy

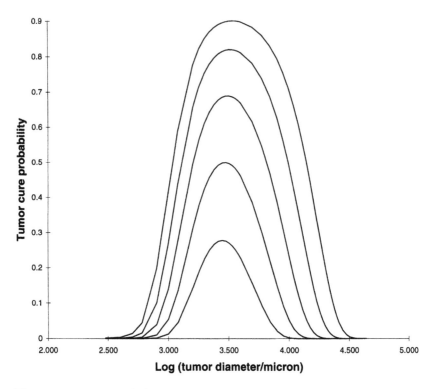

Figure 6 Calculated relationship between tumor cure probability and tumor size for the radionuclide ^{131}I. Each curve corresponds to a different value of initial activity per gram of tumor with higher values toward the top. There is a peak of tumor curability at around 3.4 mm diameter.

long-range emitter will be worse than a lower-energy short-range emitter for therapy of microscopic disease. Conversely, a low-energy short-range emitter will be suboptimal where there are tumor regions devoid of radionuclide uptake. This is because of a reduction in crossfire irradiation from the surrounding regions (34). In this case, higher-energy long-range emitters will produce a greater degree of crossfire irradiation and give a more uniform distribution of dose. As it is likely that both cold spots and microscopic disease will be present simultaneously in patients, there is a rationale for combining short-range and long-range emitting radionuclides in clinical protocols. Figure 7 illustrates the principle of a combined treatment with the long-range emitting radionuclide ^{90}Y together with the short-range emitter ^{199}Au. By a suitable choice of activities it may be possible to extend the range of optimal effectiveness.

Table 1 Optimal Tumor Size Ranges for 22
Radionuclides of Potential Use for Targeted
Radiotherapy

Radionuclide	$T_{1/2}$ (day)	$E/T_{1/2}$ (keV/day)[a]	Optimal size range (mm)
^{32}P	14.3	49	18–30
^{33}P	25.4	3	<0.2–1.0
^{47}Sc	3.35	49	2.0–3.8
^{67}Cu	2.58	60	1.6–2.8
^{77}As	1.62	140	3.6–6.0
^{90}Y	2.67	352	28–42
^{105}Rh	1.47	104	2.0–3.6
^{109}Pd	0.56	780	6–9
^{111}Ag	7.45	47	7–13
^{121}Sn	1.13	101	1.0–2.0
^{131}I	8.02	24	2.6–5.0
^{142}Pr	0.80	1012	24–34
^{143}Pr	13.6	23	6–11
^{149}Pm	2.21	162	8–12
^{153}Sm	1.95	138	2.8–5.0
^{159}Gd	0.77	403	6–9
^{166}Ho	1.12	620	18–25
^{177}Lu	6.71	22	1.2–3.0
^{186}Re	3.78	90	7–12
^{188}Re	0.71	1096	23–32
^{194}Ir	0.80	1003	24–34
^{199}Au	3.14	45	0.4–1.2

[a] For a fixed number of radionuclide atoms, the ratio $E/T_{1/2}$ is proportional to the absorbed dose rate in conditions of electronic equilibrium.

IV. EFFECTS OF HETEROGENEOUS DOSE DISTRIBUTIONS ON RESPONSE

In targeted radiotherapy absorbed dose distributions are characteristically nonuniform. Consider the situation shown in the first panel of Figure 8. The distribution of absorbed dose to a tumor cell population is represented by a normal distribution with a mean of 40 Gy and a standard deviation of 5 Gy, corresponding to a fractional standard deviation of 0.125. The amount of tumor cell sterilization will be determined by the absorbed dose experienced. It is assumed that the relationship between dose and surviving fraction is exponential with an α value of 0.35

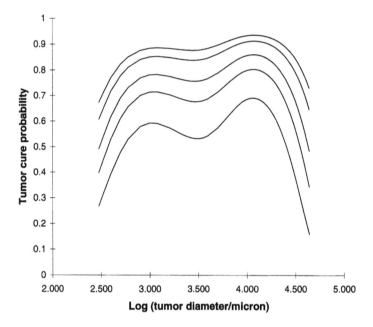

Figure 7 A hypothetical treatment consisting of a combination of the long-range emitting radionuclide ^{90}Y and the short-range emitter ^{199}Au. By a suitable choice of activities it may be possible to extend the range of optimal effectiveness.

Gy^{-1}. For each value of dose the probability of survival is given by multiplying the initial probability by the corresponding surviving fraction. The resulting distribution of survival probability is shown in the second panel. It is apparent that this distribution is displaced to the left compared to the initial distribution. This indicates that the cells most likely to survive are the ones that experience the lowest dose. In contrast, tumor cells that experience a much higher dose than the rest are "overkilled." This means that their number has become insignificant in comparison to the total number of survivors. The total survival probability is the area under the curve of panel b. (Because the survival curve is exponential, this corresponds to a Laplace transform of the original distribution.) It turns out that a uniform dose of 35.6 Gy would have the same biological effect as a dose distribution of mean 40 Gy and standard deviation 5. This illustrates that one of the consequences of heterogeneity is that the effective dose will be less than the mean dose.

What happens as the amount of heterogeneity changes? Figure 9 again represents the dose experienced by a population of tumor cells as a normal distribution with a mean value of 40 Gy. Variation in the degree of heterogeneity is simulated by changing the fractional standard deviation. A fractional standard

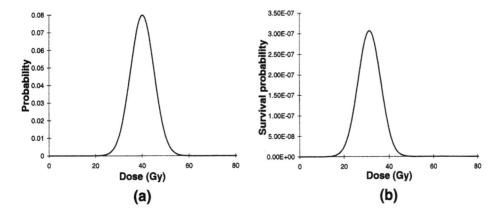

Figure 8 (a) A heterogeneous distribution of absorbed dose to a tumor cell population is represented by a normal probability distribution with mean 40 Gy and standard deviation 5 Gy. (b) The resulting distribution of survival probability is displaced to the left compared to panel (a). The cells most likely to survive are those that experience the least dose. Cells that experience higher doses may be "overkilled." Total survival probability is the area under the curve. In this case a uniform dose of 35.6 Gy would produce the same surviving fraction as the heterogeneous dose distribution.

deviation of zero represents a uniform dose distribution. For non-zero standard deviations, surviving fractions may be calculated using the areas under the survival probability curve as before. This enables the derivation of the corresponding equivalent uniform dose (EUD) that would produce the same surviving fraction. Figure 10 shows the EUD as a function of the fractional standard deviation of the dose distribution. This illustrates that as the heterogeneity increases the EUD, and thus the therapeutic effect, decreases. All these values of EUD correspond to the same mean dose.

These considerations indicate that the most efficient way of sterilizing a tumor cell population is by delivering a uniform dose. Heterogeneous dose distributions are characterized by the "underdosing" of one subpopulation and the "overkill" of another. The implication is that therapeutic strategies should attempt, as far as possible, to reduce the adverse impact of dosimetric heterogeneity on tumor response.

V. THEORETICAL STRATEGIES TO REDUCE DOSIMETRIC HETEROGENEITY

One possible way to reduce heterogeneity is the use of "cocktails" of radionuclides and targeting vectors. This may enable a wider range of effectively targeted

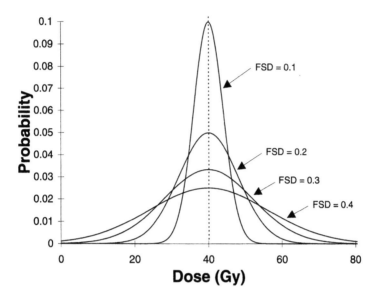

Figure 9 Heterogeneity variation is simulated by changing the fractional standard deviation of the normal distribution (mean 40 Gy). A fractional standard deviation of zero
corresponds to a uniform dose distribution. Surviving fractions may be calculated using
the areas under the corresponding survival probability curves.

tumor cells and, if the targeting agents are not crossreactive, could also allow an
increase in the intensity of therapy. The use of combined modality therapy is
another interesting possibility. Animal model studies have shown that combining
radioimmunotherapy with fractionated external beam radiotherapy can increase
the therapeutic effect without increasing normal tissue toxicity (47–49).

It has also been shown that therapeutic responses in animal models can be
increased by splitting a large single administration of radiolabeled antibody into
a number of smaller administrations (50,51). Given the availability of engineered
molecular vectors with reduced immunogenicity, "fractionation" of targeted radiotherapy may result in reduced dosimetric heterogeneity. This possibility is
considered below using a simplified mathematical model.

Figure 8 represents a large single administration of 40 Gy with a fractional
standard deviation of 0.125. For this example, the surviving fraction, based on
taking the area under the survival probability curve, comes to 3.8×10^{-6}. However, for a uniform dose of 40 Gy, the surviving fraction using the same radiosensitivity parameter would be the smaller value of 8.3×10^{-7}. The difference between the homogeneous and the heterogeneous case corresponds to a factor of
around 4.6 or 0.67 logs of cell kill. Now consider, as an arbitrary example, 10

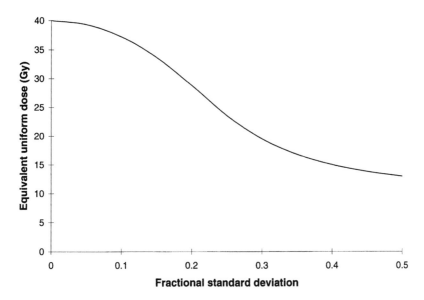

Figure 10   The equivalent uniform dose (EUD) as a function of the fractional standard deviation of the dose distribution. As the heterogeneity increases, the EUD and the therapeutic effect, decreases. All these values of EUD correspond to the same mean dose (40 Gy).

separate administrations, each of which produces a mean dose one-tenth as great (i.e., 4 Gy) and has an identical fractional standard deviation (0.125). Each individual dose with a mean of 4 Gy produces a surviving fraction of 0.25. If we make the assumption that this scenario is repeated for all ten administrations, the resultant surviving fraction would be $(0.25)^{10}$ or 9.7×10^{-7}. Comparing this with a uniform single dose of 40 Gy, the difference in survival is only a factor of 1.2 or 0.067 logs of cell kill. If we now compare the large single administration with the fractionated treatment, the loss of effectiveness is greater for the single dose. In this example, the difference is 0.6 logs of cell kill. This represents a therapeutic gain caused by fractionation.

The magnitude of the possible gain depends on the degree of heterogeneity and the number of fractions. This is illustrated in Figure 11 which shows that the therapeutic gain in terms of additional logs of cell kill increases with the number of fractions and also with increasing heterogeneity. For all of the points on this surface, the mean dose is exactly the same (40 Gy). Figure 11 suggests that the potential gain due to fractionation may be substantial. For this reasoning to be valid, it is necessary that each individual fraction produce a similar biological effect. This would not be the case if the same subpopulation of tumor cells

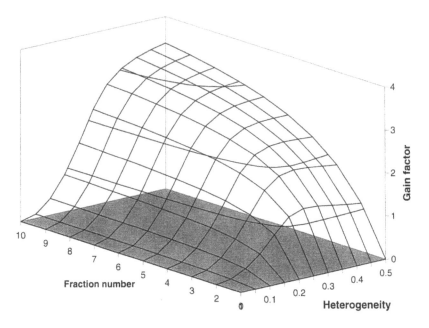

Figure 11   The magnitude of the potential therapeutic gain due to fractionation increases with the number of fractions and increasing heterogeneity. The mean dose is 40 Gy for all points on this surface.

was being targeted over and over again. It is therefore necessary that the spatial distribution of uptake should vary significantly from one fraction to another. In such circumstances the loss of effectiveness will be greater for a large single administration than for a series of smaller fractions.

In contrast to this mechanism, a fractionated therapy is likely to deliver a lower average dose rate to tumor cells. Also, because it entails protraction of treatment, more time will be available for tumor cell proliferation. These characteristics would be expected to reduce its therapeutic effectiveness. For situations of homogeneous uptake or if a fractionated treatment continually targets the same subpopulation, there would not be a therapeutic gain. The implication is that, in these circumstances, fractionation would be worse than a large single administration.

VI. SUMMARY

The most logical primary role of targeted radiotherapy is in the treatment of diffuse or occult disease. Here it has advantages over alternative systemic treatments due to its specificity. It may have a secondary role in the treatment of local disease, particularly in support of local treatments such as surgery or local external beam radiotherapy. Based on the preceding discussions there are several aspects of targeted radiotherapy that should be considered when designing rational treatment strategies.

The therapeutic effectiveness of targeted radiotherapy will be limited by cell proliferation, radioresistance, and low dose rates. It is important to choose a radionuclide that is appropriate for the pharmacokinetic behavior of the targeting vector. Radionuclides should be selected on the basis of maximizing the effective dose to the tumor while remaining below the effective dose that corresponds to the tolerance of the bone marrow. Tumors small in comparison to the radionuclide emission range absorb energy inefficiently. In some circumstances, smaller tumors can be harder to cure than larger ones and there will be a range of tumor sizes where a radionuclide is most effective. This size range will be determined by the emission characteristics of the radionuclide. It is therefore important to also try to match radionuclides to the size spectrum of disease. The clinical reality is that there will probably be a range of tumor sizes and the existence of intratumoral regions devoid of radionuclide. This implies that therapeutic designs which use more than one radionuclide are likely to be better. Heterogeneity in absorbed dose reduces the therapeutic effectiveness. The more heterogeneity, the bigger the loss in effectiveness. Tumor cells that experience the least dose are most likely to act as foci of recurrence and treatment failure. The implication is that strategies should be designed to minimize the impact of dosimetric heterogeneity on tumor response. The use of ''cocktails'' of radionuclides and targeting vectors, combined modality therapy, and, possibly, fractionation of targeted radiotherapy may be useful strategies for clinical investigation.

ACKNOWLEDGMENT

This work was supported in part by NIH/NCI program project PO1-Ca-33049.

REFERENCES

1. Ehrlich P. Collected Studies on Immunity. New York: John Wiley and Sons, 1906.
2. Bruland OS. Cancer therapy with radiolabeled antibodies. An overview. Acta Oncol 1995; 34:1085–1094.
3. Jurcic JG, Scheinberg DA. Radioimmunotherapy of hematological cancer: problems and progress. Clin Cancer Res 1995; 1:1439–1446.
4. Kairemo KJ. Radioimmunotherapy of solid cancers: a review. Acta Oncol 1996; 35: 343–355.

5. Wilder RB, DeNardo GL, DeNardo SJ. Radioimmunotherapy: recent results and future directions. J Clin Oncol 1996; 14:1383–1400.

6. Lashford LS, Lewis IJ, Fielding SL, Flower MA, Meller S, Kemshead JT, Ackery D. Phase I/II study of iodine-131 metaiodobenzylguanidine in chemoresistant neuroblastoma: a United Kingdom Children's Cancer Study Group investigation. J Clin Oncol 1992; 10:1889–1896.

7. van Hasselt EJ, Heij HA, de Kraker J, Vos A, Voute PA. Pretreatment with [^{131}I] metaiodobenzylguanidine and surgical resection of advanced neuroblastoma. Eur J Pediatr Surg 1996; 6:155–158.

8. Sakahara H, Endo K, Saga T, Hosono M, Kobayashi H, Konishi J. ^{131}I-metaiodobenzylguanidine therapy for malignant pheochromocytoma. Ann Nucl Med 1994; 8: 133–137.

9. Ozawa S, Ueda M, Ando N, Abe O, Minoshima S, Shimzu N. Selective killing of squamous carcinoma cells by an immunotoxin that recognizes the EGF receptor. Int J Cancer 1989; 43:152–159.

10. deSombre ER, Shafii B, Hanson RN, Kuivanen PC, Hughes A. Estrogen receptor-directed radiotoxicity with Auger electrons—specificity and mean lethal dose. Cancer Res 1992; 52:5752–5758.

11. Hélène C. The anti-gene strategy: control of gene expression by triplex-forming-oligonucleotides. Anti-cancer drug design 1991; 6:569–584.

12. Cho JY, Parks ME, Dervan PB. Cyclic polyamides for recognition in the minor groove of DNA. Proc Natl Acad Sci USA 1995; 92:10389–10392.

13. Link EM, Michalowski AS, Rosch F. ^{211}At-methylene blue for targeted radiotherapy of disseminated melanoma: microscopic analysis of tumour versus normal tissue damage. Eur J Cancer 1996; 32A:1986–1994.

14. Vaidyanathan G, Larsen RH, Zalutsky MR. 5-[^{211}At] astato-2′-deoxyuridine, an alpha particle-emitting endoradiotherapeutic agent undergoing DNA incorporation. Cancer Res 1996; 56:1204–1209.

15. Strickland DK, Vaidyanathan G, Friedman HS, Zalutsky MR. Meta-[^{131}I]iodobenzylguanidine uptake and meta-[^{211}At]astatobenzylguanidine treatment in human medulloblastoma cell lines. J Neuro-Oncol 1995; 25:9–17.

16. Sgouros G, Erdi YE, Humm JL, Mehta B, McDevitt MR, Finn RD, Jurcic JG, Larson SM, Scheinberg DA. Pharmacokinetics and dosimetry of an alpha-particle emitter labeled anti-CD33 antibody([213Bi]HuM195) in patients with leukemia. J Nucl Med 1997; 38:231P. Abstract.

17. Sastry, KSR. Biological effects of the Auger emitter iodine-125: a review. Report No. 1 of AAPM Nuclear Medicine Task Group No. 6. Med Phys 1992; 19:1361–1370.

18. Howell RW. Radiation spectra for Auger-electron emitting radionuclides: report No. 2 of AAPM Nuclear Medicine Task Group No. 6. Med Phys 1992; 19:1371–1383.

19. Adelstein SJ. The Auger process: a therapeutic promise? AJR 1993; 160:707–713.

20. Humm JL, Howell RW, Rao DV. Dosimetry of Auger-electron-emitting radionuclides. Report No. 3 of AAPM Nuclear Medicine Task Group No. 6. Med Phys 1994; 21:1901–1915.

21. Wheldon TE, O'Donoghue JA. The radiobiology of targeted radiotherapy. Int J Radiat Biol 1990; 58:1–21.
22. Kassis AI, Van den Abbeele AD, Wen PYC, Baranowska-Kortylewicz J, Aaronson RA, DeSisto WC, Lampson LA, Black PM, Adelstein SJ. Specific uptake of the Auger electron-emitting thymidine analogue 5-[123I/125I] iodo-2'-deoxyuridine in rat brain tumors: diagnostic and therapeutic implications in humans. Cancer Res 1990; 50:5199–5203.
23. Mariani G, Cei A, Collecchi P, Baranowska-Kortylewicz J, Van den Abbeele AD, Di Luca L, Di Stefano R, Viacava P, Ferdeghini EM, Di Sacco S, Salvadori PA, Bevilacqua G, Adelstein SJ, Mosca F, Kassis AI. Tumor targeting in vivo and metabolic fate of 5-[iodine-125]iodo-2'-deoxyuridine following intratumoral injection in patients with colorectal cancer. J Nucl Med 1993; 34:1175–1183.
24. Holt JA, Scharl A, Kullander S, Beckman MW. Intracellular actions of steroid hormones and their therapeutic value, including the potential of radiohalosteroids against ovarian cancer. Acta Obstet Gyn Scand 1992; 155(suppl):39–53.
25. Beckmann MW, Schnarl A, Rosinsky BJ, Holt JA. Breaks in DNA accompany estrogen-receptor-mediated cytotoxicity from 16 alpha [^{125}I] iodo-17-beta-estradiol. J Cancer Res Clin Oncol 1993; 119:207–214.
26. Hughes A, Gatley SJ, deSombre ER. Comparison of the distribution of radioiodinated-E-17 alpha-iodovinyl-11 beta-methoxyestradiol and 2-iodo-1,1-bis (4-hydroxyphenyl)-phenylethylene estrogens in the immature rat. J Nucl Med 1993; 34:272–280.
27. Panyutin IG, Neumann RD. Sequence-specific DNA double strand breaks induced by triplex forming ^{125}I labelled oligonucleotides. Nucl Acids Res 1994; 22:4979–4982.
28. Oosterwijk E, Bander NH, Divgi CR, Welt S, Wakka JC, Finn RD, Carswell EA, Larson SM, Warnaar SO, Fleuren GJ, Oettgen HF, Old LJ. Antibody localization in human renal cell carcinoma: a phase I study of monoclonal antibody G250. J Clin Oncol 1993; 11:738–750.
29. Jain RK. Delivery of novel therapeutic agents in tumors: physiological barriers and strategies. J Natl Cancer Inst 1989; 81:1–7.
30. Juweid M, Neumann R, Paik C, Perez-Bacete MJ, Sato J, van Osdol W, Weinstein JN. Micropharmacology of monoclonal antibodies in solid tumors: direct experimental evidence for a binding site barrier. Cancer Res 1992; 52:5144–5153.
31. Old LJ, Stockert E, Boyse EA, Kim JH. Antigenic modulation: loss of TL antigen from cells exposed to TL antibody. J Exp Med 1968; 127:523–539.
32. Yorke ED, Williams LE, Demidecki AJ, Heidorn DB, Roberson PL, Wessels BW. Multicellular dosimetry for beta-emitting radionuclides: autoradiography, thermoluminescent dosimetry and three-dimensional dose calculations. Med Phys 1993; 20: 543–550.
33. Humm JL, Macklis RM, Lu, XO, Yang Y, Bump K, Beresford B, Chin LM. The spatial accuracy of cellular dose estimates obtained from 3D reconstructed serial tissue autoradiographs. Phys Med Biol 1995; 40:163–180.
34. Humm JL. Dosimetric aspects of radiolabelled antibodies for tumor therapy. J Nucl Med 1986; 27:1490–1497.

35. Goddu SM, Rao DV, Howell RW. Multicellular dosimetry for micrometastases: dependence of self-dose versus cross-dose to cell nuclei on type and energy of radiation and subcellular distribution of radionuclides. J Nucl Med 1994; 35:521–530.

36. Wessels BW, Rogus RD. Radionuclide selection and model absorbed dose calculations for radiolabeled tumor associated antibodies. Med Phys 1984; 11:638–645.

37. Fowler JF. Radiobiological aspects of low dose rates in radioimmunotherapy. Int J Radiat Oncol Biol Phys 1990; 18:1261–1269.

38. Mausner LF, Srivastava SC. Selection of radionuclides for radioimmunotherapy. Med Phys 1993; 20:503–509.

39. Zweit J. Radionuclides and carrier molecules for therapy. Phys Med Biol 1996; 41: 1905–1914.

40. Dale RG. Dose-rate effects in targeted radiotherapy. Phys Med Biol 1996; 41:1871–1884.

41. Fertil B, Malaise EP. Intrinsic radiosensitivity of human cell lines is correlated with radioresponsiveness of human tumors: analysis of 101 published survival curves. Int J Radiat Oncol Biol Phys 1985; 11:1699–1707.

42. Deacon JM, Peckham MJ, Steel GG. The radioresponsiveness of human tumours and the initial slope of the cell survival curve. Radiother Oncol 1984; 2:317–323.

42a. O'Donoghue JA. The impact of tumor cell proliferation in radioimmunotherapy. Cancer 1994; 73(suppl):974S–980S.

43. Bardiès M, Chatal JF. Absorbed doses for internal radiotherapy from 22 beta-emitting radionuclides: beta dosimetry of small spheres. Phys Med Biol 1994; 39:961–981.

44. Siegel JA, Stabin MG. Absorbed fractions for electrons and beta particles in spheres of various sizes. J Nucl Med 1994; 35:152–156.

45. Gaze MN, Mairs RJ, Boyack SM, Wheldon TE, Barrett A. ^{131}I-meta-iodobenzylguanidine therapy in neuroblastoma spheroids of different sizes. Br J Cancer 1992; 66: 1048–1052.

46. Weber W, Weber J, Senekowitsch-Schmidtke R. Therapeutic effect of m-[I-131]iodobenzylguanidine and m-[I-125]iodobenzylguanidine on neuroblastoma multicellular tumor spheroids of different sizes. Cancer Res 1996; 56:5428–5434.

47. Buchegger F, Rojas A, Delaloye AB, Vogel CA, Mirimanoff RO, Coucke P, Sun LQ, Raimondi S, Denekamp J, Pelgrin A, Delaloye B, Mach JP. Combined radioimmunotherapy and radiotherapy of human colon carcinoma grafted in nude mice. Cancer Res 1995; 55:83–89.

48. Vogel CA, Galmiche MC, Buchegger F. Radioimmunotherapy and fractionated radiotherapy of human colon cancer liver metastases in nude mice. Cancer Res 1997; 57:447–453.

49. Sun LQ, Vogel CA, Mirimanoff RO, Coucke P, Slosman DO, Mach JP, Buchegger F. Timing effects of combined radioimmunotherapy and radiotherapy on a human solid tumor in nude mice. Cancer Res 1997; 57:1312–1319.

50. Schlom J, Molinolo A, Simpson JF, Siler K, Roselli M, Hinkle G, Houchens DP, Colcher D. Advantage of dose fractionation in monoclonal antibody-targeted radioimmunotherapy. J Natl Cancer Inst 1990; 82:763–771.

51. Buchsbaum D, Khazaeli MB, Liu T, Bright S, Richardson K, Jones M, Meredith R. Fractionated radioimmunotherapy of human colon carcinoma xenografts with 131I-labeled monoclonal antibody CC49. Cancer Res 1995; 55(suppl):5881s–5887s.

2
Radionuclide Dosimetry and Radioimmunotherapy of Cancer

Ruby F. Meredith and Donald J. Buchsbaum
University of Alabama at Birmingham, Birmingham, Alabama

Susan J. Knox
Stanford University, Stanford, California

I. CLINICAL ASPECTS OF RADIOIMMUNOTHERAPY

A. Antibodies

The development of radiolabeled antibodies that bind to tumor-associated antigens for effective radioimmunotherapy (RIT) of malignancy has been very challenging (1–4). Although murine antibodies have been the most widely used for RIT studies, the problems related to immunogenicity have resulted in numerous modifications involving the reengineering of antibodies. One of the simplest approaches has been enzymatic cleavage to form fragments. They generally have more utility for imaging than RIT because of lower tumor uptake, whereas products from recombinant DNA technology have resulted in a variety of types of constructs with applicability to RIT. Advantages of more humanized constructs (mouse-human chimeric, complementarity-determining region-grafted, minibodies) include less immunogenicity, which may allow for repeated dosing, longer effective half-life, which may produce a higher uptake and radiation absorbed dose in tumor, and the potential for larger amounts of antibody to be tolerated without adverse effects. The technologic advancements have allowed for the development of constructs that are not only humanized but may have specific binding sites for a radiolabel, drug, toxin, or effector function.

21

B. Determinants of Radioimmunotherapy Effects and Approaches to Improve the Therapeutic Ratio (19)

There are a number of pathologic and physiologic factors that have challenged the development of effective RIT (5–10). These have generally resulted in poor tumor uptake, limiting the delivery of radiolabeled antibody to tumor and often resulting in an unsatisfactory therapeutic ratio.

The distribution of systemically administered radiolabeled antibodies has often been unfavorable in lymphoma patients with splenomegaly and/or bulky disease with large tumor burdens, resulting in similar localization of antibody in normal organs and targeted tumor. Important determinants of radiolabeled monoclonal antibody (MAb) biodistribution in patients with lymphoma include spleen size (11,12), tumor burden (11,13) and the preinfusion or coinfusion of unlabeled MAb (13,14). Press et al. (11,12) have reported that favorable biodistributions in patients with non-Hodgkin's lymphoma (NHL) were obtained in 100% of splenectomized patients, 77% of patients with normal-size spleens, and only 12.5% of patients with splenomegaly. In high-dose RIT studies the Seattle group has not treated patients with splenomegaly or treated such patients only after splenectomy which improved the distribution of ^{131}I-anti-B1 antibody. In contrast, the DeNardo group found no clear evidence to exclude patients with splenomegaly from ^{131}I-Lym-1 therapy for B-cell lymphoma, although splenomegaly was associated with decreased radiation dose to the spleen and, in some cases, to other tumor sites (15). Shen et al. (15) reported that splenomegaly was associated with decreased tumor doses only in patients with extraordinarily large spleens, and that there was no clear relationship between spleen volume and tumor doses, although tumor doses were low in five patients with spleen volumes $\geq$970 mL. There was also no apparent relationship between spleen volume and therapeutic response to ^{131}I-Lym-1 since two of five patients with spleen volumes $\geq$970 mL responded to treatment and two of six splenectomized patients did not respond to treatment. Press et al. (11,13) also estimated tumor burden using computed tomography and found that only 1 of 12 patients with >500 cc of tumor had a favorable ^{131}I-MAb biodistribution, whereas 23 of 31 patients with $\leq$500 cc of tumor had favorable biodistributions ($p < .001$).

Preloading with unlabeled antibody before injection of radiolabeled MAb has been useful for improving the subsequent distribution of radiolabeled antibody in several studies and has become widespread practice (16). Several studies have shown marked effects of different masses of unlabeled MAb on the biodistribution and pharmacokinetics of radiolabeled MAb (13,14,17). Improvements in biodistribution of radiolabeled MAb following preadministration or coadministration of unlabeled MAb are presumably secondary, in part, to decreased nonspecific uptake of intact MAb molecules by cells with Fc receptors within the reticuloendothelial system and binding to normal B-cells in lymphoid tissue.

In addition to predosing, various avenues of research have been pursued for the purpose of improving the therapeutic ratio over that achieved with simple intravenous (IV) administration of radiolabeled intact IgG antibodies (18,19). In addition to the genetic engineering aspects of antibody construct production, other modifications include improved chelator chemistry; multistep pretargeting strategies (20); hyperthermia, external beam radiation, and other mechanisms that may increase tumor blood flow and vascular permeability; adjuvant use of radio-sensitizers or protectors, growth factors, cytokines, and hypoxic cytotoxins; and integration with gene therapy in a manner that may amplify tumor targeting. An area showing particular promise in preclinical studies is the use of adjuvant interferon (21,22). Recently, interferon has been demonstrated to increase tumor antigen expression in human biopsies (23,24) and improved therapeutic efficacy of interferon in combination with RIT in clinical trials has been reported (25).

C. Radioimmunotherapy Effects on Normal Tissues

Acute symptoms after initial systemic RIT have generally been infrequent, mild, and consistent with that expected of a minor allergic reaction. When present, these symptoms often respond to antihistamines and acetaminophen. Rarely, more severe symptoms occur such as laryngeal edema or bronchospasm, which have quickly responded to agents used for a more severe allergic reaction including steroids, epinephrine, oxygen, and antihistamines. A serum-sickness-type phenomenon including joint aches and fever can occur about 2 weeks after therapy. This has been common after intraperitoneal RIT but not after RIT using other routes of administration. CNS administration has resulted in signs and symptoms generally consistent with local edema and inflammation which have responded to steroids.

Normal organ dose tolerances for RIT (with exponentially decreasing low dose rate irradiation) are not well defined and appear to be higher than the $TD_{5/5}$ for fractionated (high dose rate) external beam radiation. This is expected based on dose rate effects. Therefore, most organs should be less sensitive to the lower dose rate irradiation from RIT than high dose rate external beam irradiation.

The dose limiting toxicity for systemic and intraperitoneal (IP) RIT not followed by hematologic rescue has been bone marrow suppression. The use of cytokines and other manipulations that have decreased marrow toxicity in preclinical studies has not had sufficient effects in human trials to allow substantial dose escalation without preparation for hematologic reconstitution (26,27). In high-dose RIT studies to date, cardiopulmonary (12) and hepatic (28–30) toxicity may become dose limiting when the limitations of hematologic toxicity are bypassed by using bone marrow or peripheral blood stem cell reinfusion.

The relatively frequent late toxicity that has been observed after high-dose systemic RIT with ^{131}I-labeled antibodies (12) has been abnormal thyroid function. Patients treated with high-dose RIT continue to be followed for the development of late effects. Late bowel toxicity has not been associated with RIT as it has been with IP instillation of non-tumor-specific phosphorous-32 (^{32}P) radionuclide therapy.

II. SUMMARY OF CLINICAL RESULTS AND RADIATION DOSES

The selection of radionuclides for RIT has been reviewed elsewhere (31–35). Sequential imaging studies following administration of MAb labeled with small quantities of radionuclides (e.g., 5 mCi) allow for study of the biodistribution of the radiolabeled MAb before therapy and estimation of anticipated absorbed radiation doses in normal tissues and tumors from a therapeutic dose of RIT. When possible, imaging studies use MAb labeled with the same radionuclide that will be used for therapy. This requires that the emission(s) from the radionuclide be well imaged by gamma cameras. The absence of photon emission makes imaging with yttrium-90 (^{90}Y) difficult. Therefore, indium-111 (^{111}In)-labeled MAb have commonly been used for imaging before administration of therapeutic doses of ^{90}Y-labeled MAb. ^{111}In has a chemistry similar to ^{90}Y with gamma emissions of 173 and 247 keV. Optimal imaging of known sites of disease generally occurs at 3 to 6 days after antibody administration. In a recent study by DeNardo et al. (36), the validity of using tracer studies to predict radiation absorbed doses from therapeutic doses of the same radiolabeled MAb was studied. Radiation doses to tissues and tumors were reliably predicted from tracer studies with R $\geq$ 0.95 for bone marrow and tumor doses. In a recent review of imaging studies in 173 patients with hematologic malignancies (37), the rate of tumor visualization was 72%. Excellent results have also been reported by Goldenberg et al. (38) with imaging of 49/60 known sites of disease and detection of 41 occult tumor sites. In addition, Kaminski et al. (16) have reported imaging of all known disease sites >2 cm with ^{131}I-anti-CD20 MAb. The effective biological half-life of radiolabeled murine MAb is variable, and depends, in part, on the particular antibody, its antigenic specificity, and the method utilized for radiolabeling the MAb. For many antibodies, it has been reported to be in the range of 1.5 to 3.0 days.

Selected studies have been summarized in tabular form for expediency, with no intention to misrepresent results. However, it is often difficult to fully categorize the data as reported since selected patients may have received several treatments, or because details are inconsistent or unclear. For instance, outcome description does not always correspond to the total number of patients treated, and clinical response results are sometimes uncertain, such as finding no evidence of disease on posttreatment laparotomy but not being able to assess the area of previous known disease. There is the possibility of some overlap when investigators provide an update with more than the original number of patients and do not specify that the total number of patients includes some for whom results were previously reported. Clinical and dosimetry results may be combined that were separately reported and may not reflect the exact same patient group. Although the units included in the tables do not all conform to current standard international units, mCi has been primarily used to specify the amount of radioactivity administered since this unit is more frequently reported in the literature (1 mCi = 37 MBq).

A. Central Nervous System Tumors

There has been more variety in the treatment of central nervous system (CNS) disease than most other malignancies in terms of using several antibodies, radionuclides, and routes of administration as summarized in Table 1. Therapy has also been studied in the adjuvant setting as well as with gross recurrent disease after multiple prior conventional treatments. Frequently the therapy has been for nonbulky residual disease. Responses in this setting may be difficult to measure radiographically or by other means. Thus, end points for efficacy measurements have included quality of life and length of disease-free interval or survival. When given in the adjuvant setting such as the trial conducted by Brady and colleagues (39,40), these criteria were used and compared to similar patients treated in national cooperative group clinical trials to show a benefit of RIT.

CNS disease can be divided into patients with a leptomeningeal spread pattern that receive intrathecal therapy or those with intracranial disease that can be treated with intralesional or intracavity directed therapy. Compared to most RIT, bone marrow toxicity has not usually been the dose-limiting toxicity for treating CNS disease with RIT. This is expected since therapy has often been given by a nonsystemic route. Local toxicity consisting of cerebral edema and its secondary effects have been frequent but generally transient among patients receiving RIT for CNS disease. A nonacute change noted after RIT with ^{131}I-81C6 has been evidence of leptomeningeal fibrosis with an increased protein level in the CSF (41). For leptomeningeal disease, doses have usually not been calculated but theoretical considerations of dose distribution and marrow dose from irradiation near the vertebral bodies have been published. Richardson et al. (42) reported 33 to 58 Gy to meningeal surfaces in the thoracic and lumbar spine areas while the brain meninges received 0 to 6 Gy from intrathecal administration of ^{131}I antibodies. The dose to the whole body calculated from urinary measurements ranged from 0.00054 to 0.0008 cGy/mCi. Dosimetry and clinical results reported from studies of CNS disease are summarized in Table 1. As expected, estimated tumor doses following local/regional administration were greater than

Table 1 Radioimmunotherapy Dosimetry and Clinical Results of CNS Disease Using Various Antibody Conjugates and Administration Routes

Antibody conjugate (reference)	Tumor origin (route)	Dose infusion (mCi)	Tumor dose (Gy)	Uptake	Disease effect	Comments
[125]I-425 (39)	Glioblastoma 60 pt; (most IV, some IA)	50 weekly × 3	—	—	Surv. comparable to best reported with standard Rx	[125]I-425 was given as adjuvant after 1° resection + RT
[131]I-anti-EGFr (113)	Recurrent gliomas (IV or IA)	40–140	12.5 maximum	Bx ratio Tumor/ Nl brain = .004/.0015 %ID/g ratio range 0.24– 23.89	6/10 improved 1 in remission at 3 years	Scans with Bx of specific and nonspecific Ab. Similar blood clearance for all Ab with ^{125}I, or ^{123}I, ^{131}I labeling
^{131}I-BC-2 and/or BC-4 (114,115)	Recurrent gliomas, 24 pt (intratumor)	15–57 × 1–5	202–769 $\bar{X}$ tumor dose 0.98 cGy/mCi	Tumor/back-ground 16.6 at 24 h 2.4% ID/g at 24 h	3/17 CR 3/17 PR 5/17 S, median 9 mo.	No toxicity reported
^{90}Y-MUC2-63 (116)	Glioma 10 high grade 3 relapsed low grade (intratumor [2 pt] or IV)	3.9–22.7 total = 37.8 IV 2.2–142 intratumor	Intratumor = 264–619 IV = 0.03–0.47	% uptake of dose = 100% for intratumor IV = 0.01–.3%	Tumor necrosis after intratumor infusion; 2 IV pt. had clinical improvement	One intratumor pt had Prog at other site

^{131}I-BC-2 (117)	Recurrent glioblastoma (intratumor, multiple injections)	3–31 $\overline{X} = 14.9$	70–440 [0.98 cGy/mCi] cumulative	Tumor 4.9% ID/g 24 h $\overline{X}$ tumor/background = 16.7	3/10 stable 2/10 PR 1/10 CR 4/10 no response	Dosimetry and pharmacokinetics were done from tracer with repeat imaging 1–240 h.
^{131}I-BC-4 (118)	Glioma (intratumor)	1–6 × 49.5	>300/cycle	—	49% response rate (66% for small vol) med surv. 23 mo.	^{131}I-BC-4 was given as part of initial Rx for 31 of 59 pt.
^{131}I-81C6 (41)	Glioma leptomeningeal (CSF)	40–100	14.4–34	—	1/31 PR radiographic 13/31 S radiographic	Pt. had received prior multi-modality therapy, marrow dose: 11.8–28 cGy

Abbreviations used in tables: Ab, antibody; Bx, biopsy; CR, complete response; CLR, clinical clearance of disease; CSF, cerebrospinal fluid; Cy, cyclophosphamide; est, estimated; FU, follow up; Gr, grade; HAMA, human antimouse antibody; IA, intra-arterial; ID, injected dose; IP, intraperitoneal; IT, intratumor; IV, intravenous; med, median; mo, months; MR, minor response of >25% but <50% tumor regression; MTD, maximum tolerated dose; NED, no evidence of disease; nl, normal; PR, partial response of >50% tumor regression; Prog, progression; pt, patient; RT, external beam radiation therapy; Rx, treatment; S, stable; SCCa, squamous cell carcinoma; surv, survival; TBI, total body irradiation.
Also please note that units used do not necessarily conform with SI convention; however, they are used in the manner most frequently reported.

those achieved with IV administration. Antitumor effects were noted in most trials using local/regional administration of radiolabeled antibodies among patients who were refractory to conventional therapy.

B.   Intraperitoneal Radioimmunotherapy

In general, IP administration of RIT has resulted in higher response rates and higher tumor doses than RIT administered IV as summarized in Table 2. The majority of IP RIT trials have been in ovarian cancer, whereas IV therapy has been performed less frequently (43). In addition to the emphasis on clinical outcome noted in Table 2, dosimetry to tumor and normal organs for IP RIT has been characterized as discussed in the next section.

C.   Dosimetry Consideration for the Intraperitoneal Route of Administration

Some nontherapy studies also allow for comparison of routes of administration for similar patients or agents. For instance, although most therapy has been performed with intraperitoneal administration for ovarian cancer, prelaparotomy studies allow subsequent biopsies to be analyzed for tumor uptake. When ^{131}I-Mov-18 was given intravenously, tumor uptake was $4.2 \pm 1.0\%$ injected dose (ID)/kg with normal tissue uptake of $1.8 \pm 0.5\%$ ID/kg. This ratio is on the order of that demonstrated by other antibodies administered IV whereas IP administration generally provides a higher tumor/normal ratio (44). Larson and colleagues also reported the tendency for higher antibody uptake after IP as compared to IV administration. They studied 10 patients following IP administration of ^{131}I-B72.3 antibody 4 to 14 days before laparotomy. Biopsy samples analyzed for tumor uptake showed a range of 0.1% to 270% ID/kg, with one patient having a cumulative uptake of a total of 40% of the injected dose. Similarly, other investigators performing biopsy sampling for uptake analysis after IP administration also tended to find a wide variance of tumor uptake and an average uptake higher than that achieved with IV administration (45).

The total tumor dose delivered in the Larson study was calculated to range from 10 to 117 cGy/mCi, while the marrow dose was estimated to be 0.99 to 1.2 cGy/mCi, which gives a tumor to marrow ratio as high as 96. Larson noted that reports of average marrow doses from the Hammersmith group from IP administration of ^{131}I antibody were about 25% higher than those calculated for Larson's study (46). This discrepancy is probably due to the different fraction of cumulative activity assigned to the red marrow in these studies.

Data included in the dosimetry Table 2 and other reports show considerable variability in radiation absorbed doses that can be substantial even for biopsy samples from the same patient. This variability is higher than has been reported

Table 2   Clinical Results and Dosimetry of Selected IP Radioimmunotherapy Trials

Antibody conjugate (reference)	Dose/infusion (mCi)	Tumor dose (Gy)	Disease effect	Peritoneal dose cGy/mCi (total)	Normal organ dose (cGy/mCi)	Comments
^{131}I-HMFG1 ^{131}I-AUA1 (46,91,92)	20–205 1–4 Rx	80	9/16 CLR <2 cm 3/6 CR for microscopic 8/8 Prog. >2 cm	(147–443)	Whole body dose 0.44 ± 1.29 Intestine dose 2.54–15.98 Spleen dose 6.1–52.8	GI complaints Mild myelotoxicity
^{131}I-B72.3 + others (115)	21–150	7.7–46	2/15 CR; 2/15 PR; 3/15 S Surv. 5–>28 mo	—		Grade 1 various toxicities
^{131}I-2G3 (90)	15–150	6–60 to serosa	3/4 ↓ ascites ≥ 50 mCi		—	Uptake .02–.0002 % ID/g, no specific uptake in 3/5
^{90}Y-HMFG1 (119)	5–30	21.7 cGy/mCi nonspecific dose to peritoneum	1/6 CR of small nodules 3/5 ↓ ascites 12/13 Rx as adjuvant NED ≤20 mo	27.1		Myelotoxicity ≥15 mCi Myelotoxicity decreased with EDTA
^{90}Y-OC125 (120) ^{186}Re-NR LU-10 (121–123)	3–21 25–100/m²	1.5–10.5 2–36 cGy/mCi to peritoneal surface	1/12 PR 13/17 Prog. ↓ tumor 4/17 ≤5 mm nodules	17.0 ± 8.8 Range 2–36	Whole body 0.68 ± 0.28	— Alternate techniques were used for some dose estimates.
^{177}Lu-CC49 (124–126)	16.5–92.2 (10–45/m²)	21.7–46.6	1/13 PR gross disease 9/9 ≤1 cm nodules Prog 1.5–21 mo 4/5 microscopic NED >6–35 mo	30.6 ± 12.6	Whole body 0.4–0.9	Tumor dose for 3 pt; others imaged, but dose not determined. Tumor:marrow dose ratio = 58–139:1

from imaging studies, and is limited by the relatively small number of tumors studied and the inherent inhomogeneity of antibody and dose distribution within tumors. It has been shown in animal studies that antibody uptake varies with tumor mass (47), and this may be a contributing factor (48,49). Dosimetry for tumors and normal organs varied moderately for nonbiopsy methods also as indicated by data summarized in Table 2. Some of the variance between studies reflects alternate dosimetry methods for dose estimation.

D. Systemic Radioimmunotherapy for Solid Tumors

Results of treatment with RIT alone for GI malignancies have poor response rates as shown in Table 3. For some other adenocarcinomas, such as breast and prostate, the responses are somewhat improved and appear to increase with aggressive therapy including the use of hematologic rescue. The best results in solid tumors have been reported in early trials for hepatomas and cholangiocarcinomas that were treated with RIT as a component of multimodality therapy. Although Table 3 provides tumor and normal organ dosimetry estimates from various trials of IV or IA administration of radiolabeled antibodies for solid tumors, a study of leukemic patients (50) is also included for comparison of marrow doses since the marrow is targeted in leukemic patients due to disease involvement. Among these patients the marrow dose was generally greater than 100-fold over that in patients with solid tumors not known to have marrow involvement. Even the relatively low marrow doses reported for the solid-tumor patients resulted in dose-limiting marrow suppression. The dose to other normal organs has usually been higher than that to marrow but has not resulted in clinically significant toxicity. Comparisons can be made in Table 3 for use of the same antibody by different groups such as ^{90}Y-CYT-356, different tumors treated with the same antibody conjugate such as ^{131}I-CC49, and the same patients studied for biodistribution of different antibodies as for ^{131}I-chB72.3 versus ^{131}I-ch17-1A.

E. Radioimmunotherapy of Non-Hodgkin's Lymphoma

Results of clinical studies using RIT to treat patients with NHL have been encouraging with relatively high response rates and durable responses. Table 4 summarizes tumor dosimetry and response rates for selected clinical RIT trials in NHL. Mean tumor doses and ranges of tumor doses expressed as cGy/mCi and cGy are shown for six different studies along with the corresponding overall response rates. As can be seen, there was a wide range of estimated tumor doses (cGy/mCi) in different patients in the reported studies. Part of the variability in tumor doses (cGy) is due to dose escalation during the studies which resulted in patients receiving variable doses (mCi/infusion) of radiolabeled antibody. Nevertheless, there was a suggestion of a dose response relationship with the highest tumor doses occurring in patients (13) treated in a study with the highest response rate and relatively low tumor doses observed in the study with the lowest response rate (38).

Table 5 shows individual patient dosimetry and clinical response data for patients treated with ^{90}Y-anti-CD20 MAb. Again, the wide variability in tumor doses can be appreciated with the suggestion of a dose response relationship. In this study, the mean tumor dose for patients with a complete response was 617.1 cGy (range 149.9 to 1173.6 cGy), 1043.6 cGy (502.3 cGy if the highest dose is eliminated with a range of 53.4 to 4291.3 cGy) for patients with a partial response, and 279.4 cGy (range 100.6 to 451.4 cGy) for three out of five patients with stable disease that imaged well enough to calculate estimated tumor doses. It is important to point out that the value of these data is limited by the limited data per patient (usually one tumor site dose estimate) in patients that often had multiple sites of disease. In the two patients shown in Table 5 with two tumor dose estimates, individual tumor sites varied considerably in estimated doses (2.7 and 5.0 cGy/mCi in patient 3 and 21.5 and 365.1 cGy/mCi in patient 6). Tumor sites for dosimetric calculations were selected on the basis of size and surrounding contrast, both of which had to be sufficient for dose estimations, and did not necessarily represent disease sites with the most uptake. Furthermore, the validity of these estimates is also limited by a number of other factors including the inherent difficulty in accurately measuring activity in small, irregularly shaped tumor masses or regions of interest using gamma camera imaging (51), and by the inability to visualize all known sites of disease in all patients (52).

III. DOSIMETRY METHODS

Dosimetric studies are routinely performed prior to RIT in order to study radiolabeled MAb biodistribution and to identify patients who are most likely to benefit from therapy or to experience unacceptable toxicity. This information is used to determine which patients meet the criteria required to proceed to therapy. These studies utilize sequential gamma camera imaging and are frequently complemented by serial measurements of plasma and urine activity, as well as occasional tumor and bone marrow biopsies. In most cases there is considerable patient-to-patient variation, which demonstrates the importance of performing dosimetry studies in individual patients. Estimates of therapy doses in RIT are limited by the difficulty in imaging Bremsstrahlung radiation from ^{90}Y and the high activity levels of ^{131}I (53). Dose can be calculated from radioactivity quantitation, the equilibrium constant and the specific absorbed fraction for the target. The Medical Internal Radiation Dose (MIRD) Committee of the Society of Nuclear Medicine provides guidance for methods to calculate radiation absorbed dose estimates for the whole body and organs (54,55). This methodology has been adapted for

Table 3 Tumor and Normal Organ Dosimetry After IV or IA Administration: Range or Mean $\pm$ SD as cGy/mCi

Antibody conjugate (reference)	Tumor origin (route)	Dose/infusion (mCi) tumor uptake	Tumor	Whole body	Marrow	Liver	Spleen
[111]In-BrE-3 ^{90}Y-BrE-3 (127)	Breast (IV)	0.004–0.28% ID/g	5.2 ± 5.9	2.03 ± 1.6	2.10 ± 0.97	9.21 ± 3.67	—
[90]Y-BrE-3 (128)	Breast (IV) 9 pt.	15–20/m²	35–56 cGy/ mCi	1.6	1–6	6–27	9–59
[90]Y-chT84.66 (129)	Colorectal (IV) 3 pt.	5/m² 7.5–9.9	—	15–17 cGy total	38–67 cGy total	234–471 cGy total	197–258 cGy total
[131]I-chL6 (130)	Breast, 3 pt. (IV) × 3 q 8 wk	150/m²	112 Gy total	—	61–141 cGy/ infusion	—	—
[131]I-anti-CD45 (50)	AML	—	—	—	Grp 1: 3500–3675 Grp 2: 5250–5500	≤350 ≤525	—
[131]I-anti-ferritin (131,132)	Hepatoma (IV)	93–157	15–22 Gy total	1.1–2.2 Gy total	—	4–10 total	—
[90]Y-anti-ferritin (98)	Hepatoma (IV) 13 pt.	20–30 1st cycle	5.12–21.53 Gy total median 18.33	—	—	—	—
[90]Y-anti-ferritin (98)	Hodgkin's Disease (IV)	20 or 30	1 pt. 27 Gy tumor dose	—	—	—	—
99mTc-U36 (133)	Head & Neck	20.4 ± 12.4% ID/g/kg at 44 h	—	—	—	—	—
[186]Re-NR-LU-10 (134)	Metastatic epithelial carcinoma (IV) >25 pt.	25–120/m²	0.35–17.7 cGy/mCi mean 6.3 ± 4.8	0.6 ± 0.2	0.6 ± 0.2	2.9 ± 0.5	—
[186]Re-NR-CO-01 F(ab')₂ (134)	(IV) 5 pt. (IA)	25–200/m² 60–129/m²	4.0 ± 3.8 cGy/mCi	0.4 ± 0.1	0.4 ± 0.1	1.7 ± 0.3	—
^{131}I-PK4S (135)	Colorectal (IV)			$\bar{x}$ = 0.4 ± 0.2 range 0.2–0.7		$\bar{x}$ = 1.8 ± 1.0 range 1.2–3.6	—
^{131}I-PK4S (135)		38–60		$\bar{x}$ = 0.3 ± 0.1 range 0.1–0.5		$\bar{x}$ = 1.5 ± 0.3 range 1.2–1.9	—
[131]I-chB72.3 (136)	Colon 5 pt.	34–54	—	1.2–1.6	—	3–7	5–8
[131]I-ch 17-1A (136,137)	Colon	5 tracer	2.05	0.77–1.03	—	2–4	3–4

Kidneys	Lungs	Heart, other	Small intestine	Large intestine	Disease effect	Comments
6.47 ± 6.46	8.42 ± 5.93	—	—	—	—	Dose is ^{90}Y equivalent, using ^{111}In imaging
5–26	10–40	5–21	—	—	PR in 4 of 8 with measurable disease	Have not reached MTD using stem cell rescue
—	—	—	—	—	Progression at 6–10 wk	DTPA chelator and EDTA × 3 days
—	31 Gy total	—	—	—	↓ tumor markers ↓ symptoms	Stem cell rescue used
—	161.7	—	—	—	14/15 disease free 1–30 mo.	Targets marrow to eliminate residual leukemia
—	3.4	—	—	—	≥1/3 objective responses	Multimodality therapy
—	—	—	—	—	Partial responses with multi-modality Rx	Tumor dose rate 4.3–22.8 cGy/h median 14.5 cGy/h
—	—	—	—	—	2 CR, 1 PR	—
—	—	—	—	—	—	Mean tumor/marrow uptake 6.4 ± 3.5 Mean tumor/mucosa uptake 2.3 ± 1.5
5.7 ± 3.0	1.4 ± 0.0	Thyroid, 2.5 ± 1.7	0.2 ± 0.0	Upper = 0.5 ± 0.2 Lower = 1.4 ± 0.5	1.4 ± 0.5	^{99m}Tc-tracer preceded Rx; dose-limiting marrow toxicity at 120 mCi/m²
3.5 ± 1.5	0.9 ± 0.3	—	0.1 ± 0.0	Upper = 0.5 ± 0.2 Lower = 1.2 ± 0.4	1.2 ± 0.4	Mild non-marrow toxicity; dose-limiting marrow toxicity at 150 mCi/m²; 86% developed HAMA; similar serum clearance for IV vs IA
—	$\bar{x}$ = 1.1 ± 0.3 range 0.9–1.4	—	—	—	—	Results from initial antibody infusion
—	$\bar{x}$ = 0.9 ± 0.3 range 0.7–1.3	—	—	—	—	Results when a 2nd antibody against PK4S is given at 24 h at 50 mCi level
—	—	—	—	—	1 minor response	—
—	—	Thyroid 12–66	—	—	Tracer study	5 pts were same as received ^{131}I-ch B72.3

Table 3 Continued

Antibody conjugate (reference)	Tumor origin (route)	Dose/infusion (mCi) tumor uptake	Tumor	Whole body	Marrow	Liver	Spleen
[131]I-Mov18 (44)	Ovarian	5–75 mg MOV18 0.05–0.2 pre-op	4.2 ± 1.0% ID/kg	—	Blood act at 6 d = 6.7 ± 1.9% ID/L	—	—
[131]I-cG250 (138)	Renal cell CA 16 pt.	6; 5 protein doses: 2–50 mg	48	—	20–23 cGy	—	—
^{131}I-NP-4 (139)	57 pt. CEA expressing colorectal, lung, pancreas, breast, thyroid	8 = Tracer ≤2 wk before 44–268	2–218	31–344 cGy	45–706 cGy	—	—
^{90}Y-CYT-356 (140)	Prostate 12 pt	3.4–28.9	16.2 ± 21.9	2.1 ± 0.6	—	29.7 ± 58.9	7.4 ± 6.2
^{90}Y-KC4 (141)	Prostate	6–9/m² 11.5–20 total	—	—	—	—	—
^{131}I-CC49 (93)	Prostate	75/m² 126–193 total	1.4–7.9; total 1.8–10 Gy	—	—	—	—
^{131}I-CC49 (93)	Prostate	100/m² 211–230 + Cy and TBI	15.7	0.58–0.68 total 134–143 cGy	—	—	—
^{131}I-UJ13A (142)	Neuroblastoma	35–55	mean 13–21 Gy	—	—	—	—
[131]I-A6H (143)	Renal cell carcinoma 4 pt	50	0.53–13	—	—	—	—
^{131}I-CC49 (89)	Colon	100–300/m²	6.3–33	—	—	—	—
^{131}I-CC49 (144)	Colon	75/m²	16–33 Gy	—	—	—	—
^{111}In-CYT-356 (145)	Prostate 21 pt. 3 institutions	10–20 tracer	—	0.5	—	3.7	3.3
[131]NP-4F(ab′)₂ (146)	Colorectal, lung, pancreas, thyroid ≤3 cm	70–296	—	—	150–450 cGy	—	—

Kidneys	Lungs	Heart, other	Small intestine	Large intestine	Disease effect	Comments
—	—	—	—	—	—	Measured by Bx no HAMA normal tissue 1.8 ± 0.5% ID/kg, ratio same as previous studies with 3 mg IV
—	—	—	—	—	Imaging/ dosimetry study 13/16 imaged	Heterogeneous tumor uptake, normal tissue uptake low except liver at lowest protein dose
—	—	—	—	—	Anti-tumor effects 12/35 (1 PR, 4 minor/ mixed, 7 stable)	Pharmacokinetics varied with tumor origin
—	—	—	—	—	3/12 transient subjective improvement	Only 1/12 developed HAMA by 4 wk
—	—	—	—	—	3/9 symptom improvement	1/5 Gr 4 marrow suppression at 9 mCi/m^2
—	—	—	—	—	6/10 bone pain relief	13/15 imaged known lesion, 100% HAMA
—	—	—	—	—	2/3 objective response	Rx followed by stem cell reinfusion
—	—	—	—	—	1/5 CR	—
—	—	—	—	—	1/4 CLR bone marrow dose <25 cGy	Tumor doses for bone metastasis + 3 soft tissue masses
—	—	—	—	—	0/12	Stem cell rescue
—	—	—	—	—	0/10	—
0–2.5	—	Testes 0.5—2.0	—	—	—	Excretion thru GI tract was modeled & 10.8% of act was assigned to MIRDOSE 3 excretory path. This ↑ effective dose by 18%
—	—	—	—	—	6/13 stable	Marrow dose is higher than others report due to assumption in their calculation methods. Targeting to all tumors

Table 4 Tumor Dosimetry and Results of Selected Clinical RIT Trials in NHL

Antibody conjugate	No. Pts Tx	Dose/infusion	Tumor dose (cGy/mCi; mean ± SD)	Tumor dose (cGy)	Response rate	Ref.
90Y-anti-CD20	18	13.5–53.4 mCi	Mean: 26.9 ± 46.3 Range: 3.9–193.3	Mean: 740.4 Range: 53.4–4291.3	72.2%	108
131I-anti-B1	28	Variable (N/A)[a] to deliver 25–85 cGy to WB[b]	N/A	Mean: 734 for men 1197 for women (normalized to a WB dose of 75 cGy)	78.6%	109, 110
131I-anti-B1	21	127650–29045 GB to deliver 25–31 Gy to the normal organ receiving the highest dose	N/A	Max tumor dose— 925 ± 150 (mean ± SE) (range 141–2584)	85.7%	111
131I-MB-1, IF5 and B1	19	234–777 mCi to deliver 10–30.75 Gy to the normal organ receiving the highest dose	N/A	1010–9150	94.7%	13
131I-Lym-1	45	30–100 mCi/m² (includes fractionated Tx)	Median: 3.8[c] Range: 0.3–12.7	Median: 241 Range: 16–1485	54.5%	112[d]
131I-LL2	7	8–46.4 mCi	Mean: 5.2 Range: 2.9–9.3	Mean: 118 Range: 53.6–263.2	28.6%	112[e]

[a] N/A: Not available.
[b] WB: Whole body.
[c] Excluding tumors with a diameter <2 cm.
[d] Ref. 112; only 28% of patients had low-grade histologies.
[e] Ref. 38; only 2/7 patients had low-grade histologies.

Table 5 Tumor Dosimetry for Patients Treated with ^{90}Y-Anti-CD20 MAb[a]

Pt.	Administered dose (mCi/infusion)	Tumor dose (cGy/mCi)	Tumor dose (cGy)	Clinical response
1	13.6	7.4	100.6	SD[b]
2	13.5	11.1	149.9	CR[c]
3	13.7	3.9 (2.7, 5.0)[d]	53.4	PR[e]
4	21.6	20.9	451.4	SD
5	20.0	—[f]	—[f]	SD
6	22.2	193.3 (21.5, 365.1)[d]	4291.3	PR
7	21.3	55.1	1173.6	CR
8	31.1	36.9	1147.6	CR
9	31.4	10.1	317.1	PR
10	32.6	7.8	254.3	PR
11	41.6	14.3	594.9	CR
12	41.6	12.0	499.2	PR
13	43.5	16.2	704.7	PR
14	42.0	6.0	252.0	CR
15	51.7	—[f]	—[f]	SD
16	53.0	5.4	286.2	SD
17	53.4	7.2	384.5	CR
18	52.9	22.4	1185.0	PR

[a] Patients 1–4 were imaged and treated using B1 (Coulter Immunology, Hialeah FL) and patients 5–18 were imaged using IDEC-IN238 and treated with IDEC-Y2B8 (IDEC Pharmaceuticals Corp., San Diego, CA; Ref. 108).
[b] SD: stable disease.
[c] CR: complete response.
[d] Average of two tumor doses shown.
[e] PR: partial response.
[f] Tumor was imaged too poorly to compute an estimated dose.

radiolabeled antibody therapy and takes into account the time dependent accumulation/clearance of activity (56). The equations give the mean absorbed dose to a volume of tissue. This is the sum of absorbed doses from all source regions. For instance, dose to the liver from ^{131}I-labeled antibody includes the self dose from radiolabeled antibody localized to the liver and a smaller contribution from radioactivity in all other organs. The mean dose per unit of cumulated activity is a constant for a given radionuclide and each source-target combination. This has been designated as the S value by the MIRD committee. S values have been tabulated for the standard 70-kg reference man (55) as well as for humans ranging from the standard reference 55-kg adult female to infants (57). Computer programs have become available for implementing the MIRD system (56). With the advent of programs such as MIRDOSE 3, one may expect more dosimetry estimates for various organs. In previous reports, radiation doses have been reported only to a few large organs that may have adequate radiolabeled antibody concentration to be detected in Anger camera images such as the liver and spleen. Other organs that may be more sensitive to radiation, such as lungs and kidneys, are not reported. In many instances, the bladder may receive a higher dose than many other organs since it is a major path of excretion of unbound radioactivity. However, bladder doses are often not reported as toxicity has generally not been observed that has been attributed to bladder radiation. Normal organ doses from RIT have generally ranged from 0.7 to 8.2 cGy/mCi (0.2 to 2.2 mGy/MBq) with considerable interpatient variation in most studies despite differences in MAb and dosimetric techniques (51).

Since the MIRD tables are restricted to normal organs and do not contain S values for tumors, many investigators have used the MIRD tables for tumor dosimetry by assuming a tumor mass to be similar in configuration and location to a normal body organ. Other computer programs have also been developed with adaptation for RIT. This includes the MABDOS program by Johnson and Vessella. They used a Monte Carlo simulation similar to the original MIRD codes for estimating penetrating radiation contributions (58,59). Their program allows data entry for five tumor masses that act as sources and targets for radiation in the Standard Man Model. Other dosimetric methodologies have also been utilized for RIT and are discussed elsewhere (51,60).

Nearly all tumor doses reported from RIT studies have been obtained from whole body counting and gamma camera imaging methods. Organ and tumor volumes needed for dose calculation have been obtained from CT scans, MRI, or other special methods such as a ^{99m}Tc-sulfur colloid images for liver volumetrics (61). The study of Erdi and colleagues of resected specimens showed good correlation of imaging based dosimetry with biopsy quantitation (62). Such studies of distribution using conjugate view planar scintillation camera images have previously been limited by failure to account for overlapping structures (63). Published values of organs of interest from the MIRD committee have been extensively used and SPECT (single-photon emission computed tomography) is widely used for volume determination and to normalize time-activity data from planar imaging (64), which may improve the accuracy of the planar data, although the value of quantitative SPECT is unclear. More recently, regions of interest (organ and tumor volumetrics) have been defined by image fusion with CT (65) or MRI (65), or by projected shadows of an organ or structure (63). Image fusion combines the use of radiolabeled MAb imaging with conventional imaging modalities utilized for the localization of normal organs and/or tumor (64,65). This method may allow for improved determination of the activity concentration and ultimately for more accurate estimation of absorbed dose to regions of interest

(65). Nevertheless, none of the currently available dosimetry methods address microdosimetry, which is a more valid description of the energy deposited by beta particles but at this time is of unknown clinical significance (51).

Since bone marrow suppression remains the dose-limiting toxicity in most nonmyeloablative RIT applications, special attention has been given to bone marrow dosimetry (52,66,67). A standard technique currently used is based on the assumption that marrow activity is proportional to the blood activity and that the activity in the blood is uniformly distributed. From serial blood activity measurements, the area under the curve and S values from MIRD tables can be used to calculate marrow doses. This method assumes that the blood in the marrow is the major source organ contributing to marrow dose and that there is no specific marrow uptake, as could be the case with tumor infiltration of marrow or retention due to cross reactivity of antibody with normal marrow elements. Some investigators include an additional dose contribution from total body activity separate from the blood activity and sum the two for the total dose to the red marrow. Using ^{131}I-Lym-1, DeNardo et al. (66) reported that nonpenetrating radiation from the blood contributed 0.18 cGy/mCi and penetrating radiation from the total body contributed 0.18 cGy/mCi to the bone marrow. The mean total dose was 0.36 ± 0.14 cGy/mCi, and clearances and marrow doses were remarkably constant among different patients and among different therapy doses for the same patient. Wilder et al. have applied the linear-quadratic model (68) to RIT and bone marrow dosimetry in an effort to further improve the accuracy of these estimations (69).

IV. WHAT FACTORS INFLUENCE DOSE CALCULATION AND CORRELATION WITH EFFECTS

A wide range of tumor and normal organ radiation absorbed doses have been reported. Some of the variance is probably a true representation of a divergent range of doses delivered as evidenced by the fact that a fourfold range within multiple lesions in the same patient has been reported (70). However, a substantial portion of the variance may also reflect differences in dosimetry methods and assumptions used as well as inaccuracies inherent in the current stage of the development of individualized dosimetry. This situation may contribute to the lack of a correlation between dose and response in most clinical trials to date. However, higher doses are generally associated with more toxicity and a greater likelihood of tumor response in several studies. In addition, other factors such as toxicity related compromise from prior therapies or enhancement of efficacy with concurrent therapies may affect the dose/response relationship.

Differences in absorbed radiation dose for patients with similar hematologic toxicity may at least partially be accounted for by variance in assumptions of dosimetry calculations and the influence of outside factors such as prior chemotherapy (71). Much progress has been made for absorbed dose/toxicity comparison as investigators adopt similar methodology proposed from the AAPM Task Group (67,72) including ratios of marrow specific activity of 0.2 to 0.4 that of the whole blood. Most reports note marrow toxicity resulting from an absorbed dose of 100 to 200 cGy whereas Behr et al. (71) reported no significant bone marrow toxicity until 600 cGy based on utilization of a 1:1 ratio for marrow-specific and blood activity. This finding also applies to patients who have not had chemotherapy in the recent past. Variations are noted even among different tumor masses in the same patient (70). Although there are varying reports about factors that are expected to affect bone marrow toxicity from RIT or are found to have an influence on toxicity by retrospective analyses, there remains considerable uncertainty about the prediction of bone marrow toxicity.

Much work remains to be done regarding the correlation of toxicity with treatment/patient parameters. However, studies to date demonstrate modest correlation of toxicity with dose parameters and the existence of modifying factors. Several analyses of dose escalating studies have shown that toxicity increased with administered dose, but there were only a few patients treated at each dose level. In a dose escalation study, a University of Michigan analysis has shown that dosing based on lean body mass rather than actual mass provided a superior correlation between dose and hematologic toxicity with r values of .523 for the lean body mass versus .430 for actual total mass (73). Breitz et al. (74) found that expressing radioactivity administered relative to body size improved the correlation with marrow toxicity, but that a prior therapy index was needed to further improve the predictions for toxicity, such as noted by the Immunomedics group for prior chemotherapy.

Although individualized tracer dosimetry has been used in many studies in an effort to determine how much dose would be delivered to tumor and normal organs with a therapy dose of RIT, this methodology is not as practical for widespread community practice as a simple method of administration (e.g., based on per unit of body mass). Thus, there have been attempts to analyze data obtained from RIT studies to identify predictors of toxicity that can be utilized for determining individualized doses for patients based on factors such as body habitus and past chemotherapy-radiotherapy history. Analysis of data from three Phase II trials from the University of Alabama at Birmingham using ^{131}I-CC49 have shown modest correlation between variables related to marrow radiation dose, including the area under the curve (AUC), but not with clinical variables such as age and gender. These studies show that it is feasible to administer a dose considered to be the maximum tolerated dose (per body mass or surface area based on dose escalation trials) to diverse groups of patients with an acceptable and predictable toxicity range. Despite a relationship between toxicity and various predictors, this correlation would not be sufficient to dose escalate without the option of hematologic rescue.

Although often desirable when feasible, individualized tracer studies vary in their correspondence to subsequent therapeutic doses of the same agent (75). Therefore, tracer studies cannot always predict the dose limiting toxicity. This is illustrated by Macey et al. when adjunct treatment with interferon was felt to enhance marrow toxicity (76). In this case, current, rather than previous, therapy had an impact on toxicity that decreased the predictive capability of the tracer study. The DeNardo group also noted that marrow radiation from marrow and skeletal targeting (often from marrow disease involvement) affected toxicity (77). Tracer studies may be most feasible and helpful when immunogenicity is not problematic. Biodistribution can be markedly altered by tumor burden and possibly be a predictor of second organ toxicity when hematologic rescue is planned.

Another factor that may be critical to bone marrow and other organ toxicity (but not predicted or analyzed in the illustrations presented) is that of dose rate. For instance, Goddu and colleagues found a correlation between survival of GM-CFC with initial dose rate but a poor correlation with total absorbed dose (78). A dose rate effect is one of the factors for consideration in the comparison of continuous infusion versus multiple bolus administrations of RIT as studied by Roberson and Buchsbaum. They found in a murine model that three bolus injections resulted in a more uniform dose rate over a longer period of time and a 50% improvement in efficacy of the delivered dose (79,80).

In addition to dose rate, other factors may be equally if not more influential but are not reflected in dosimetry calculations. For instance, DeNardo and colleagues suggest that a major therapeutic effect of RIT may result from the activation of molecular pathways that trigger apoptosis. Their studies have included several RIT enhancement strategies that potentially synergize with RIT in the activation of apoptosis. They found the parameters of sequence, time, and dose to be critical for the optimization of combined therapy with agents such as the antimicrotubular agent Taxol and antibody c225 which is directed against the epidermal growth factor receptor (81), and in some cases suboptimal timing of agents resulted in increased toxicity but no increase in anti-tumor effects.

V. DOSE RESPONSE RELATIONSHIP AND RADIOSENSITIVITY TO RADIOIMMUNOTHERAPY

It is more difficult to establish a dose response relationship for clinical RIT than external beam radiation since the dose calculations are subject to more uncertainty, the dose delivered is usually much more heterogeneous and the probability for cure depends on the regions receiving the least dose which may be under-dosed, and there are several influential factors such as oxygenation status and proliferation rate that are not reflected in the number calculated to be the total dose delivered (82). Tumor doses have ranged from approximately 18.5 to 200 cGy/mCi (0.5 to 5.4 mGy/MBq) in patients with NHL with variable relationship between tumor response and estimated tumor dose (51). Nevertheless, there are some suggestions of a dose/response relationship as described above for patients with NHL treated with RIT as shown in Tables 4 and 5.

The lymphomas have shown the best overall response rate thus far (16), as is discussed in another chapter of this book. The extended survival of some lymphoma patients treated with low-dose RIT or high-dose RIT and stem cell transplantation after failing conventional therapies is encouraging (83). The greater success in treating lymphomas than other solid tumors to date is probably due to a variety of biological factors, including their greater radiosensitivity and possibly to immune mechanisms in some situations, which may also explain in part the relatively high response rate at relatively low tumor doses that has been observed (Table 4). As shown in Table 5, complete responses have occurred at estimated tumor doses as low as 150 cGy. Some of these estimated tumor doses at which clinical responses occurred were considerably lower than doses usually required to achieve similar responses using conventional fractionated high dose rate external beam radiation therapy. The surprising efficacy of low dose RIT in lymphoma is probably due to properties of both the low dose rate radiation associated with RIT and the particular antibody used in some situations.

Both MAbs (84) and low-dose rate radiation (85–87) have been reported to induce apoptosis in human lymphoma cell lines and recently apoptosis was found to be a predominant mechanism of cell killing following low-dose rate irradiation (87). Other studies suggest that the binding of some anti-CD20 antibodies is additive in the induction of apoptosis in lymphoma cell lines (88). These factors may be important determinants of RIT-mediated tumor cell killing, with the relative contribution of apoptosis to overall cell killing dependent upon the particular tumor or cell line, antibody, and radiation dose rate studied.

With nonlymphoma malignancies, there is generally a better response rate when higher RIT doses are given or when RIT is given in conjunction with potentially enhancing agents such as chemotherapy. However, high-dose RIT for patients with gastrointestinal tumors has resulted in significantly fewer objective responses than achieved in lymphomas and no complete remissions (89).

Local-regional rather than systemic routes of administration allow higher radiation doses to be delivered with RIT without excess toxicity. CNS malignancies that are often relatively resistant to external beam radiation show responses to RIT, but the doses delivered for these responses are generally severalfold higher than that tolerated with external beam therapy. Leukemias treated by intrathecal RIT may respond well because of their inherent radiosensitivity and the higher dose of radiation that can be delivered with compartmental administration.

The results of IP RIT for ovarian cancer suggest both a tumor size and radionuclide dose dependence. For instance, all patients receiving less than 50 mCi ^{131}I-2G3 antibody progressed whereas 75% of those given $\geq$50 mCi experienced palliation of ascites (90). Several studies suggest that the smaller the size of tumor masses, the greater the chance of control with IP RIT. This has been a general trend but not an unwavering observation among several groups studying this form of therapy. The initial trend of increasing control with decreasing tumor volume was reported by the London group (91,92), who noted no objective responses among patients with tumors $\geq$2 cm whereas 9/16 patients with smaller measurable nodules and 50% of patients with microscopic disease responded to therapy. It is also notable that failure to control ascites in one patient in their investigation was associated with a population of cells that did not react with the antibody used.

Ovarian cancer may be more radiosensitive than some other solid-tumor adenocarcinomas since a dose of 30 Gy or less to the whole abdomen shows some effectiveness against microscopic disease whereas doses of 45 Gy or higher appear to be needed for microscopic gastrointestinal adenocarcinomas. With this in mind, it is not surprising that delivering <30 Gy with RIT to solid tumors such as colorectal cancer often do not result in objective responses whereas higher doses delivered by IP administration for ovarian cancer can result in responses and prolonged survival. This is supported by the experience in which the same CC49 antibody labeled with ^{177}Lu and given IP resulted in higher doses and greater efficacy for ovarian cancer than when labeled with ^{131}I or ^{90}Y and given systemically for prostate, lung, breast and GI malignancies where the radiation dose achieved was lower (93–95). The greater radiosensitivity of ovarian cancer compared with other adenocarcinomas is also suggested by limited RIT studies where even lower absorbed doses of radiation were achieved with IV ^{131}I-MN-14 therapy and resulted in objective responses in ovarian cancer patients, but not in patients with CEA-reactive tumors of other origin (43,96).

Some of the most positive results with RIT of nonlymphoma solid tumors have been with hepatomas when external beam radiation therapy and RIT have been used together either alone or combined with nonradiation therapeutic modalities. A synergistic effect is possible and sometimes predicted from preclinical studies, but this has not been well studied in clinical trials (97). In nude mice bearing human colon cancer liver metastasis xenografts, an increased therapeutic effect was noted with the combination of RIT with external beam radiotherapy, and the best outcome was observed with simultaneous rather than sequential treatment (97). In clinical trials RIT appeared to contribute to the successful treatment of hepatomas when used in conjunction with other treatment modalities (98). This suggests that hepatomas may be relatively sensitive to RIT and/or that there was synergism between the treatment modalities utilized. However, the impact of the RIT component is difficult to discern from that of the other modalities used. Other factors such as blood supply to the tumors may be an important factor in treatment success compared to treatment of similar-size liver metastases which are poorly vascularized (99). Animal model studies of RIT combined with chemotherapy have also shown additive or synergistic antitumor effects (100).

RIT may be particularly useful as an adjuvant therapy for residual microscopic disease which cannot be detected by standard imaging. To further evaluate this, Dunn and colleagues have performed phantom studies using ^{131}I antibody adsorbed onto 0.004-cc beads. The radioactivity on the bead was equivalent to a maximum tumor uptake of 0.3% ID/g when a nonmyeloablative dose of 100 mCi was given. SPECT imaging was used in the dosimetry procedures which resulted in a calculated absorbed dose of 5400 cGy and an average dose rate of 78 cGy/hr. This dose would be expected to have therapeutic efficacy against micrometastases of most adenocarcinomas (101).

VI. FUTURE DIRECTIONS

There are a number of approaches being developed in preclinical animal model RIT studies and in Phase I clinical trials which may result in increased tumor uptake of radiolabeled MAb, reduced uptake in normal organs, and therefore an increased therapeutic ratio. These approaches involve three general strategies as detailed elsewhere (102): modifying antibodies including the production of dimeric and trimeric sFv or minibodies consisting of a sFv fused to a human IgG C_H3 domain, C_H2 domain deletions, or the use of new radiolabeling techniques and radionuclides; increasing blood and normal tissue clearance of radiolabeled MAb and/or the use of pretargeting; and modifying tumor delivery by local/regional administration, increasing tumor antigen expression with cytokines or gene transfer, or increasing tumor vascular permeability or blood flow with external beam irradiation, hyperthermia, and vasoactive agents or conjugates. The goal of ongoing clinical studies is to further investigate some of the more promising approaches to determine whether they increase the therapeutic efficacy of RIT. Preclinical studies are also evaluating the effects of the heterogeneity of radiolabeled antibody distribution on tumor dosimetry, tumor growth inhibition, and tumor control (82). The efficacy of RIT may be further enhanced by combining this form of therapy with other therapeutic modalities. A variety of such approaches are being investigated in preclinical studies (103–107). It is anticipated that the most promising of these approaches will be tested in clinical studies shortly.

ACKNOWLEDGMENTS

We gratefully acknowledge the critical reviews and suggestions from Dr. Daniel Macey and Dr. Barry Wessels, and Sally Lagan for the preparation of the manuscript. Supported in part by NIH grants CA44173, CA67828, CM-87215, and DOE grants DE-FG02-96ER62181 and DE-FG05-93ER61654.

REFERENCES

1. Goldenberg DM. Future role of radiolabeled monoclonal antibodies in oncological diagnosis and therapy. Semin Nucl Med 1989; 19:332–339.
2. Goldenberg DM. New developments in monoclonal antibodies for cancer detection and therapy. Cancer J Clin 1994; 44:43–64.
3. Meredith RF, Buchsbaum DJ. Radioimmunotherapy of solid tumors. In: Henkin RE, Boles MA, Dillehay GL, Halama JR, Karesh SM, Wagner RH, Zimmer AM, eds. Nuclear Medicine. St. Louis, MO: Mosby–Year Book, 1996:601–608.
4. Larson SM, Divgi CR, Scott A, Sgouros G, Graham MC, Kostakoglu L, Scheinberg D, Cheung NKV, Schlom J, Finn RD. Current status of radioimmunotherapy. Nucl Med Biol 1994; 21:785–792.
5. Sands H, Jones PL. Physiology of monoclonal antibody accretion by tumors. In: Goldenberg DM, ed. Cancer Imaging with Radiolabeled Antibodies. Boston: Kluwer Publishers, 1990:97–122.
6. Schlom J, Horan Hand P, Greiner JW, Colcher D, Shrivastav S, Carrasquillo JA, Reynolds JC, Larson SM, Raubitschek A. Innovations that influence the pharmacology of monoclonal antibody guided tumor targeting. Cancer Res 1990; 50(suppl): 820s–827s.
7. Jain RK, Baxter LT. Mechanisms of heterogeneous distribution of monoclonal antibodies and other macromolecules in tumors: significance of elevated interstitial pressure. Cancer Res 1988; 48:7022–7032.
8. Baxter LT, Yuan F, Jain RK. Pharmacokinetic analysis of the perivascular distribution of bifunctional antibodies and haptens: comparison with experimental data. Cancer Res 1992; 52:5838–5844.
9. Neuwelt EA, Barnett PA, Hellstrom KE, Hellstrom I, McCormick CI, Ramsey FL. Effect of blood-brain barrier disruption on intact and fragmented monoclonal antibody localization in intracerebral lung carcinoma xenografts. J Nucl Med 1994; 35:1831–1841.
10. van Osdol W, Fujimori K, Weinstein JN. An analysis of monoclonal antibody distribution in microscopic tumor nodules: consequences of a "binding site barrier." Cancer Res 1991; 51:4776–4784.
11. Press OW, Eary JF, Appelbaum FR, Bernstein ID. Radiolabeled antibody therapy of lymphomas. In: DeVita VT, Hellman S Rosenberg SA, eds. Biologic Therapy of Cancer. Philadelphia: Lippincott Healthcare Publications, 1994:1–13.
12. Press OW, Eary JF, Appelbaum FR, Bernstein ID. Treatment of relapsed B cell lymphomas with high-dose radioimmunotherapy and bone marrow transplantation. In: Goldenberg DM, ed. Cancer Therapy with Radiolabeled Antibodies. Boca Raton, FL: CRC Press, 1995:229–237.
13. Press OW, Eary JF, Appelbaum FR, Martin PJ, Badger CC, Nelp WB, Glenn S, Butchko G, Fisher D, Porter B, Matthews DC, Fisher LD, Bernstein ID. Radiola

beled-antibody therapy of B-cell lymphoma with autologous bone marrow support. N Engl J Med 1993; 329:1219–1224.

14. Bunn PA Jr, Carrasquillo JA, Keenan AM, Schroff RW, Foon KA, Hsu SM, Gazdar AF, Reynolds JC, Perentesis P, Larson SM. Imaging of T-cell lymphoma by radiolabelled monoclonal antibody. Lancet 1984; 2:1219–1221.

15. Shen S, DeNardo GL, O'Donnell RT, Yuan A, DeNardo DA, DeNardo SJ. Impact of splenomegaly on I-131-Lym-1 dosimetry and response for radioimmunotherapy in patients with B-lymphocytic malignancies. Tumor Targeting 1996; 2:175.

16. Kaminski MS, Zasadny KR, Frances IR, Milik AW, Ross CW, Moon SD, Crawford SM, Burgess JM, Petry NA, Butchko GM, Glenn SD, Wahl RL. Radioimmunotherapy of B-cell lymphoma with [^{131}I]anti-B1 (anti-CD20) antibody. N Engl J Med 1993; 329:459–465.

17. Knox SJ, Goris ML, Trisler K, Negrin R, Davis T, Liles TM, Grillo-Lopéz A, Chinn P, Varns C, Ning SC, Fowler S, Deb N, Becker M, Marquez C, Levy R. ^{90}Y-labeled anti-CD20 monoclonal antibody therapy of recurrent B cell lymphoma. Clin Cancer Res 1996; 2:457–470.

18. Buchsbaum DJ. Experimental radioimmunotherapy and methods to increase therapeutic efficacy. In: Goldenberg DM, ed. Cancer Therapy with Radiolabeled Antibodies. Boca Raton, FL: CRC Press, 1995:115–140.

19. Knox SJ. Overview of studies on experimental radioimmunotherapy. Cancer Res 1995; 55(suppl):5832s–5836s.

20. Paganelli G, Magnani P, Siccardi AG, Fazio F. Clinical application of the avidin-biotin system for tumor targeting. In: Goldenberg D, ed. Cancer Therapy with Radiolabeled Antibodies. Boca Raton, FL: CRC Press, 1995:239–254.

21. Kuhn JA, Beatty BG, Wong JYC, Esteban JM, Wanek PM, Wall F, Buras RR, Williams LE, Beatty JD. Interferon enhancement of radioimmunotherapy for colon carcinoma. Cancer Res 1991; 51:2335–2339.

22. Greiner JW, Ullmann CD, Nieroda C, Qi C-F, Eggensperger D, Shimada S, Steinberg SM, Schlom J. Improved radioimmunotherapeutic efficacy of an anticarcinoma monoclonal antibody (^{131}I-CC49) when given in combination with γ-interferon. Cancer Res 1993; 53:600–608.

23. Roselli M, Guadagni F, Buonomo O, Belardi A, Vittorini V, Mariani-Costantini R, Greiner JW, Casciani CU, Schlom J. Systemic administration of recombinant interferon alfa in carcinoma patients upregulates the expression of the carcinoma-associated antigens tumor-associated glycoprotein-72 and carcinoembryonic antigen. J Clin Oncol 1996; 14:2031–2042.

24. Murray JL, Macey DJ, Grant EJ, Rosenblum MG, Kasi LP, Zhang HZ, Katz RL, Riger PT, LeBherz D, Bhadkamkar V, Greiner JW, Schlom J, Podoloff DA. Enhanced TAG-72 expression and tumor uptake of radiolabeled monoclonal antibody CC49 in metastatic breast cancer patients following α-interferon treatment. Cancer Res 1995; 55(suppl):5925s–5928s.

25. Meredith R, Alvarez R, Partridge E, Khazaeli MB, Grizzle W. Enhanced intraperitoneal radioimmunotherapy with adjuvant interferon and Taxol. Int J Radiat Oncol Biol Phys 1997; 39(suppl 2):303.

26. Blumenthal RD, Sharkey RM, Goldenberg DM. Dose escalation of radioantibody in a mouse model with the use of recombinant human interleukin-1 and granulocyte-

macrophage colony-stimulating factor intervention to reduce myelosuppression. J Natl Cancer Inst 1992; 84:399–407.

27. Wheeler RH, Meredith RF, Saleh MN, Khazaeli MB, Murray JL, LoBuglio AF. A phase II trial of IL-1 + radioimmunotherapy (RIT) in patients (Pts) with metastatic colon cancer. Proc ASCO 1994; 13:295.

28. Leichner PK, Akabani G, Colcher D, Harrison KA, Hawkins WG, Eckblade M, Baranowska-Kortylewica J, Augustine SC, Wisecarver J, Tempero MA. Patient-specific dosimetry of indium-111 and yttrium-90-labeled monoclonal antibody CC49. J Nucl Med 1997; 38:512–516.

29. Vriesendorp HM, Shao Y, Blum JE, Quadri SM, Williams JR. Fractionated intravenous administration of ^{90}Y-labeled B72.3 GYK-DTPA immunoconjugate in beagle dogs. Nucl Med Biol 1993; 20:571–578.

30. Vriesendorp HM, Quadri SM, Stinson RL, Onyekwere OC, Shao Y, Klein JL, Leichner PK, Williams JR. Selection of reagents for human radioimmunotherapy. Int J Radiat Oncol Biol Phys 1991; 22:37–45.

31. Humm JL. Dosimetric aspects of radiolabeled antibodies for tumor therapy. J Nucl Med 1986; 27:1490–1497.

32. Wessels BW, Buchsbaum DJ. Dosimetry of radiolabeled antibodies. In: Smith AR, ed. Radiation Therapy Physics. New York: Springer-Verlag, 1995:365–384.

33. Volkert WA, Goeckeler WF, Ehrhardt GJ, Ketring AR. Therapeutic radionuclides: production and decay property considerations. J Nucl Med 1991; 32:174–185.

34. Mausner LF, Srivastava SC. Selection of radionuclides for radioimmunotherapy. Med Phys 1993; 20:503–509.

35. Muthuswamy M, Roberson PL, Ten Haken RK, Buchsbaum DJ. A quantitative study of radionuclide characteristics for radioimmunotherapy from 3D reconstructions using serial autoradiography. Int J Radiat Oncol Biol Phys 1996; 35:165–172.

36. DeNardo DA, DeNardo GL, Yuan A, Shen S, DeNardo SJ, Macey DJ, Lamborn KR, Mahe M, Groch MW, Erwin WD. Prediction of radiation doses from therapy using tracer studies with iodine-131 labeled antibodies. J Nucl Med 1996; 37:1970–1975.

37. Press OW, Eary JF, Appelbaum FR, Badger CC, Bernstein ID. Radiolabeled antibody therapy of lymphoma. In: Dana B, ed. Malignant Lymphomas, Including Hodgkin's Disease: Diagnosis, Management and Special Problems. Boston: Kluwer Academic Publishers, 1993:127–145.

38. Goldenberg DM, Horowitz JA, Sharkey RM, Hall TC, Murthy S, Goldenberg H, Lee RE, Stein R, Siegel JA, Izon DO. Targeting, dosimetry, and radioimmunotherapy of B-cell lymphomas with iodine-131-labeled LL2 monoclonal antibody. J Clin Oncol 1991; 9:548–564.

39. Miyamoto C, Brady LW, Rackover M, et al. Utilization of ^{125}I monoclonal antibody in the management of primary glioblastoma multiforme. Radiat Oncol Invest 1995; 3:126–132.

40. Brady LW, Miyamoto C, Woo DV, Rackover M, Emrich J, Bender H, Dadparvar S, Steplewski Z, Koprowski H, Black P, Lazzaro B, Nair S, McCormack T, Nieves J, Morabito M, Eshleman J. Malignant astrocytomas treated with iodine-125 labeled monoclonal antibody 425 against epidermal growth factor receptor: a phase II trial. Int J Radiat Oncol Biol Phys 1991; 22:225–230.

41. Brown MT, Coleman RE, Friedman AH, Friedman HS, McLendon RE, Reiman R, Felsberg GJ, Tien RD, Bigner SH, Zalutsky MR, Zhao XG, Wikstrand CJ, Pegram CN, Herndon JE II, Vick NA, Paleologos N, Fredericks RK, Schold SC Jr, Bigner DD. Intrathecal ^{131}I-labeled antitenascin monoclonal antibody 81C6 treatment of patients with leptomeningeal neoplasms or primary brain tumor resection cavities with subarachnoid communication: phase I trial results. Clin Cancer Res 1996; 2:963–972.

42. Richardson RB, Kemshead JT, Davies AG, Staddon GE, Jackson PC, Coakham HB, Lashford LS. Dosimetry of intrathecal iodine[131] monoclonal antibody in cases of neoplastic meningitis. Eur J Nucl Med 1990; 17:42–48.

43. Juweid M, Sharkey RM, Swayne LC, Dunn R, Rubin A, Herskovic T, Hanley D, Goldenberg DM. Phase I dose-escalation trial of ^{131}I-labeled MN-14 anti-carcinoembryonic antigen (CEA) monoclonal antibody in patients with epithelial ovarian cancer. Tumor Targeting 1996; 2:189.

44. Molthoff C, Prinssen W, van Hof A, Kenemans P, den Hollander W, Verheijen R. Chimeric monoclonal antibody MOv18 IgG in ovarian cancer patients: Influence of escalating doses of c-MOv18 protein. Tumor Targeting 1996; 2:190–191.

45. Larson SM, Carrasquillo JA, Colcher DC, Yokoyama K, Reynolds JC, Bacharach SA, Raubitchek A, Pace L, Finn RD, Rotman M, et al. Estimates of radiation absorbed dose for intraperitoneally administered iodine-131 radiolabeled B72.3 monoclonal antibody in patients with peritoneal carcinomatoses. J Nucl Med 1991; 32:1661–1667.

46. Stewart JSW, Hird V, Snook D, Sullivan M, Myers MJ, Epenetos AA. Intraperitoneal [131]I- and ^{90}Y-labeled monoclonal antibodies for ovarian cancer: pharmacokinetics and normal tissue dosimetry. Int J Cancer 1988; 3(suppl):71–76.

47. Williams LE, Duda RB, Proffitt RT, Beatty BG, Beatty JD, Wong JYC, Shively JE, Paxton RJ. Tumor uptake as a function of tumor mass: a mathematic model. J Nucl Med 1988; 29:103–109.

48. O'Donoghue JA, Bardies M, Wheldon TE. Relationships between tumor size and curability for uniformly targeted therapy with beta-emitting radionuclides. J Nucl Med 1995; 36:1902–1909.

49. Mayer R, Dillehay LE, Shao Y, Zhang Y-G, Song S, Bartholomew RM, Mackenson DG, Williams JR. Direct measurement of intratumor dose-rate distributions in experimental xenografts treated with ^{90}Y-labeled radioimmunotherapy. Int J Radiat Oncol Biol Phys 1995; 32:147–157.

50. Matthews DC, Appelbaum FR, Eary JF, Fisher DR, Durack LD, Bush SA, Hui TE, Martin PJ, Mitchell D, Press OW, et al. Development of marrow transplant regimen for acute leukemia using targeting hematopoietic irradiation delivered by ^{131}I-labeled anti-CD45 antibody, combined with cyclophosphamide and total body irradiation. Blood 1995; 85:1122–1131.

51. Siegel JA, Goldenberg DM, Badger CC. Radioimmunotherapy dose estimation in patients with B-cell lymphoma. Med Phys 1993; 20:579–582.

52. Eary JF, Press OW, Badger CC, Durack LD, Richter KY, Addison SJ, Krohn KA, Fisher DR, Porter BA, Williams DL, Martin PJ, Appelbaum FR, Levy R, Brown SL, Miller RA, Nelp WB, Bernstein ID. Imaging and treatment of B-cell lymphoma. J Nucl Med 1990; 31:1257–1268.

53. Pollard KR, Bice AN, Eary JF, Durack LD, Lewellen TK. A method for imaging therapeutic doses of iodine-131 with a clinical gamma camera. J Nucl Med 1992; 33:771–776.
54. Dillman LT, Van der Lage FC. Radionuclide decay schemes and nuclear parameters for use in radiation-dose estimation. Soc Nuc Med MIRD pamphlet #10, 1975.
55. Snyder WS, Ford MR, Warner GG, Warner GG, Watson SB. "S" absorbed dose per unit cumulated activity for selected radionuclides and organs. Soc Nuc Med MIRD pamphlet #11, 1975.
56. Watson EE, Stabin MG, Siegel JA. MIRD formulation. Med Phys 1993; 20:511–514.
57. Cristy M, Eckerman EF. Specific absorbed fractions of energy at various ages from internal photon source. ORNL/TM 1987; 1–7:8381.
58. Johnson TK. MABDOS: A generalized program for internal radionuclide dosimetry. Comput Meth Prog Biomed 1988; 27:159–176.
59. Johnson TK, Vessella RL. A generalized dosimetry schema for preferential uptake of monoclonal antibodies in radionuclide immunotherapy. J Nucl Med 1987; 28(suppl):680.
60. Strand SE, Jonsson BA, Ljungberg M, Tennvall J. Radioimmunotherapy dosimetry—a review. Acta Oncol 1993; 32:807–817.
61. Yang N-C, Leichner PK, Fishman EK, Siegelman SS, Frenkel TL, Wallace JR, Loudenslager DM. CT volumetrics of primary liver cancers. J Comput Assist Tomogr 1986; 10:621–628.
62. Erdi AK, Wessels BW, DeJager R, Erdi YE, Atkins FB, Yorke ED, Smith L, Huang E, Smiddy M, Murray J, et al. Tumor activity confirmation and isodose curve display for patients receiving iodine-131-labeled 16.88 human monoclonal antibody. Cancer 1994; 73:932–944.
63. Goris ML, Knox SA, Nielsen KR, Bouillant O. Organ modeling in the quantitation of planar images for distribution studies. Cancer 1994; 73:919–922.
64. Koral KF, Zasadny KR, Swailem FM, Buchbinder SF, Francis IR, Kaminski MS, Wahl RL. Importance of intra-therapy single-photon emission tomographic imaging in calculating tumour dosimetry for a lymphoma patient. Eur J Nucl Med 1991; 18:432–435.
65. Larson SM, Macapinlac HA, Scott AM, Divgi CR. Recent achievements in the development of radiolabeled monoclonal antibodies for diagnosis, therapy and biologic characterization of human tumors. Acta Oncol 1993; 32:709–715.
66. DeNardo GL, Mahe MA, DeNardo SJ, Macey DJ, Mirick GR, Erwin WD, Groch MW. Body and blood clearance and marrow radiation dose of ^{131}I-Lym-1 in patients with B-cell malignancies. Nucl Med Commun 1993; 14:587–595.
67. Siegel JA, Wessels BW, Watson EE, Stabin MG, Vriesendorp HM, Bradley EW, Badger CC, Brill AB, Kwok CS, Stickney DR, Eckerman KF, Fischer DR, Buchsbaum DJ, Order SE. Bone marrow dosimetry and toxicity for radioimmunotherapy. Antib Immunoconjug Radiopharm 1990; 3:213–233.
68. Fowler JF. The linear-quadratic formula and progress in fractionated radiotherapy. Br J Radiol 1989; 62:679–694.
69. Wilder RB, DeNardo GL, Sheri S, Fowler JF, Wessels BW, DeNardo SJ. Application of the linear-quadratic model to myelotoxicity associated with radioimmunotherapy. Eur J Nucl Med 1996; 23:953–957.

70. Meredith RF, Johnson TK, Plott G, Macey DJ, Vessella RL, Wilson LA, Breitz HB, Williams LE. Dosimetry of solid tumors. Med Phys 1993; 20:583–592.
71. Behr TM, Sharkey RM, Juweid MI, Dunn RM, Ying Z, Zhang C-H, Siegel JA, Gold DV, Goldenberg DM. Factors influencing the pharmacokinetics, dosimetry, and diagnostic accuracy of radioimmunodetection and radioimmunotherapy of carcinoembryonic antigen-expressing tumors. Cancer Res 1996; 56:1805–1816.
72. Sgouros G. Bone marrow dosimetry for radioimmunotherapy: theoretical considerations. J Nucl Med 1993; 34:689–694.
73. Zasadny KR, Gates VL, Fisher SJ, Kaminski MS, Wahl RL. Correlation of dosimetric parameters with hematological toxicity after radioimmunotherapy of non-Hodgkin's lymphoma with I-131 anti-B1. Utility of a new parameter: "total body dose-lean." J Nucl Med 1995; 36:214P.
74. Breitz HB, Fisher DR, Wessels B. Correlation of bone marrow absorbed dose estimates with marrow toxicity. Tumor Targeting 1996; 2:173.
75. Meredith R, Khazaeli MB, Plott G, Wheeler R, Russell C, Shochat D, Norvitch M, Saletan S, LoBuglio A. Comparison of diagnostic and therapeutic doses of ^{131}I-LYM-1 in patients with non-Hodgkin's lymphoma. Antibody Immunoconj Radiopharm 1993; 6:1–11.
76. Macey DJ, Murray JL, Grant EJ, Podoloff DA. Failure of the tracer principle for predicting red marrow doses in radioimmunotherapy patients challenged with interferon. Tumor Targeting 1996; 2:175–176.
77. DeNardo DA, Lim S, DeNardo GL, Shen S, O'Donnell RT, Yuan A, DeNardo SJ. Validity of marrow radiation dose estimation and semi-quantitative marrow indices for improved prediction of myelotoxicity. Tumor Targeting 1996; 2:178–179.
78. Goddu SM, Howell RW, Rao DV. Biologic dosimetry of bone marrow: implications for radionuclide therapy. Tumor Targeting 1996; 2:146.
79. Buchsbaum DJ, Khazaeli MB, Mayo MS, Roberson PL. Comparison of multiple bolus and continuous injections of ^{131}I-labeled CC49 for therapy in a colon cancer xenograft model. Clin Can Res 1999; 5(suppl):3153s–3159s.
80. Roberson PL, Dudek S, Buchsbaum DJ. Dosimetric comparison of bolus and continuous injections of CC49 monoclonal antibody in a colon cancer xenograft model. Cancer 1997; 80:2567–2575.
81. DeNardo SJ, Lamborn KR, Kroger LA, Miers LA, Kukis DL, Salako Q, Meares CF, DeNardo GL. The importance of time dose relationships in enhancement strategies for RIT of breast cancer. Tumor Targeting 1996; 2:148–149.
82. Roberson PL, Buchsbaum DJ. Reconciliation of tumor dose response to external beam radiotherapy versus radioimmunotherapy with [131]iodine-labeled antibody for a colon cancer model. Cancer Res 1995; 55(suppl):5811s–5816s.
83. Press OW, Eary JF, Badger CC, Martin PJ, Appelbaum FR, Levy R, Miller R, Brown S, Nelp WB, Krohn KA, Fisher D, DeSantes D, Porter B, Kidd P, Thomas ED, Bernstein ID. Treatment of refractory non-Hodgkin's lymphoma with radiolabeled MB-1 (anti-CD37) antibody. J Clin Oncol 1989; 7:1027–1038.
84. Valentine MA, Licciardi KA. Rescue from anti-IgM-induced programmed cell death by the B cell surface proteins CD20 and CD40. Eur J Immunol 1992; 22:3141–3148.

85. Macklis RM, Beresford BA, Palayoor S, Sweeney S, Humm JL. Cell cycle alterations, apoptosis, and response to low-dose-rate radioimmunotherapy in lymphoma cells. Int J Radiat Oncol Biol Phys 1993; 27:643–650.

86. Macklis RM, Beresford BA, Humm JL. Radiobiologic studies of low-dose-rate ^{90}Y-lymphoma therapy. Cancer Res 1994; 73(suppl):966–973.

87. Murtha A, Rupnow B, Knox S. Low dose rate radiation favors apoptosis as a mechanism of cell death. Int J Radiat Oncol Biol Phys 1997; 39(suppl):242.

88. Illidge T, Cragg M, Glennie M. Cell cycle alterations, apoptosis and response to radioimmunotherapy in lymphoma cells. Proc ASCO 1997; 16:545a.

89. Tempero M, Colcher D, Dalrymple G, Harrison K, Augustine S, Schlom J, Linder J, Leichner P. High dose therapy with ^{131}I conjugated monoclonal antibody CC49: a phase I trial. Antib Immunoconj Radiopharm 1993; 6:90.

90. Buckman R, De Angelis C, Shaw P, Covens A, Osborne R, Kerr I, Reed R, Michaels H, Woo M, Reilly R, Law J, Baumal R, Groves E, Marks A. Intraperitoneal therapy of malignant ascites associated with carcinoma of ovary and breast using radioiodinated monoclonal antibody 2G3. Gynecol Oncol 1992; 47:102–109.

91. Epenetos AA, Munro AJ, Stewart S, Rampling R, Lambert HE, McKenzie CG, Soutter P, Rahemtulla A, Hooker G, Sivolapenko GB, Snook D, Courtenay-Luck N, Dhokia B, Krausz T, Taylor-Papadimitrou J, Durbin H, Bodmer WF. Antibody-guided irradiation of advanced ovarian cancer with intraperitoneally administered radiolabeled monoclonal antibodies. J Clin Oncol 1987; 5:1890–1899.

92. Stewart JSW, Hird V, Snook D, Sullivan M, Hooker G, Courtenay-Luck N, Sivolapenko G, Griffiths M, Myers MJ, Lambert HE, Munro AJ, Epenetos AA. Intraperitoneal radioimmunotherapy for ovarian cancer: pharmacokinetics, toxicity, and efficacy of I-131 labeled monoclonal antibodies. Int J Radiat Oncol Biol Phys 1989; 16:405–413.

93. Meredith RF, Khazaeli MB, Carabasi MH, LoBuglio AF. Radioimmunotherapy of prostate cancer. In: Riva P, ed. Therapy of Malignancies with Radioconjugate Monoclonal Antibodies: Present Possibilities and Future Perspectives. Langhorne, PA: Harwood Academic Publishers, 1999:321–331.

94. Murray JL. Radioimmunotherapy of colorectal cancer. In: Goldenberg DM, ed. Cancer Therapy with Radiolabeled Antibodies. Boca Raton, FL: CRC Press, 1995: 173–188.

95. Tempero M, Leichner P, Dalrymple G, Harrison K, Augustine S, Schlom J, Anderson J, Wisecarver J, Colcher D. High-dose therapy with iodine-131-labeled monoclonal antibody CC49 in patients with gastrointestinal cancers: a phase I trial. J Clin Oncol 1997; 15:1518–1528.

96. Juweid M, Sharkey RM, Alavi A, Swayne LC, Herskovic T, Hanley D, Rubin AD, Pereira M, Goldenberg DM. Regression of advanced refractory ovarian cancer treated with iodine-131-labeled anti-CEA monoclonal antibody. J Nucl Med 1997; 38:257–260.

97. Sun L-Q, Vogel C-A, Mirimanoff R-O, Coucke P, Donath A, Slosman DO, Mach J-P, Buchegger F. Increased therapeutic effect of concurrent radioimmunotherapy and radiotherapy of a human colon carcinoma in nude mice. Tumor Targeting 1996; 2:179.

98. Order SE, Vriesendorp HM, Klein JL, Leichner PK. A phase I study of ^{90}Yttrium

antiferritin: dose escalation and tumor dose. Antib Immunoconj Radiopharm 1988; 1:163–168.

99. Order SE, Klein JL, Leichner PK, Frincke J, Lollo C, Carlo DJ. ^{90}Yttrium antiferritin—a new therapeutic radiolabeled antibody. Int J Radiat Oncol Biol Phys 1986; 12:277–281.

100. Tschmelitsch J, Welt S, Barendswaard E, Yao T, Cohen A, Old L. Enhanced antitumor activity of combination radiotherapy (^{131}I-monoclonal antibody A33) with chemotherapy (fluorouracil). Proc Am Assoc Cancer Res 1996; 37:469.

101. Dunn RM, Juweid M, Behr TM, Siegel JA, Sharkey RM, Goldenberg DM. Therapeutic potential in patients with minimal residual disease using ^{131}I-labeled antibodies for radioimmunotherapy (RAIT). Tumor Targeting 1996; 2:145–146.

102. Buchsbaum DJ. Experimental tumor targeting with radiolabeled ligands. Cancer 1997; 80:2371–2377.

103. Scheinberg DA. Current applications of monoclonal antibodies for the therapy of hematopoietic cancers. Curr Opin Immunol 1991; 3:679–684.

104. Chatal J-F, Peltier P, Bardies M, Chetanneau A, Thedrez P, Faivre-Chauvet A, Gestin JF. Does immunoscintigraphy serve clinical needs effectively? Is there a future for radioimmunotherapy? Eur J Nucl Med 1992; 19:205–213.

105. Goldenberg DM. Monoclonal antibodies in cancer detection and therapy. Am J Med 1993; 94:297–312.

106. Goldenberg DM, Blumenthal RD, Sharkey RM. Biological and clinical perspectives of cancer imaging and therapy with radiolabeled antibodies. Semin Cancer Biol 1990; 1:217–225.

107. Sharkey RM, Blumenthal RD, Goldenberg DM. Development of cancer radioimmunotherapy and its potential use as an adjuvant treatment. In: Goldenberg DM, ed. Cancer Therapy with Radiolabeled Antibodies. Boca Raton, FL: CRC Press, 1995:101–114.

108. Knox SJ, Goris ML, Trisler K, Negrin R, Davis T, Liles T-M, Grillo-Lopez A, Chinn P, Varns C, Ning S-C, Fowler S, Deb N, Becker M, Marquez C, Levy R. Yttrium-90-labeled anti-CD20 monoclonal antibody therapy of recurrent B-cell lymphoma. Clin Cancer Res 1996; 2:457–470.

109. Kaminski MS, Zasadny KR, Francis IR, Fenner MC, Ross CW, Milik AW, Estes J, Tuck M, Regan D, Fisher S, Glenn SD, Wahl RL. Iodine-131-anti-B1 radioimmunotherapy for B-cell lymphoma. J Clin Oncol 1996; 14:1974–1981.

110. Zasadny KR, Gates VL, Francis I, Fisher S, Kaminski MS, Wahl RL. Normal organ and tumor dosimetry of I-131-anti-B1 (anti-CD20) radioimmunotherapy at non-marrow ablative doses. J Nucl Med 1997; 38(suppl):230.

111. Press OW, Eary JF, Appelbaum FR, Martin PJ, Nelp WB, Glenn S, Fisher DR, Porter B, Matthews DC, Gooley T, Bernstein ID. Phase II trial of ^{131}I-B1 (anti-CD20) antibody therapy with autologous stem cell transplantation for relapsed B cell lymphomas. Lancet 1995; 346:336–340.

112. Lamborn KR, DeNardo GL, DeNardo SJ, Goldstein DS, Shen S, Larkin EC, Kroger LA. Treatment-related parameters predicting efficacy of Lym-1 radioimmunotherapy in patients with B-lymphocytic malignancies. Clin Cancer Res 1997; 3:1253–1260.

113. Kalofonos HP, Pawlikowska TR, Hemingway A, Courtenay-Luck N, Dhokia B,

Snook D, Sivolapenko GB, Hooker GR, McKenzie CG, Lavender PJ, Thomas DGT, Epenetos AA. Antibody guided diagnosis and therapy of brain gliomas using radiolabeled monoclonal antibodies against epidermal growth factor receptor and placental alkaline phosphatase. J Nucl Med 1989; 30:1636–1645.
114. Riva P, Arista A, Tison V, Sturiale C, Franceschi G, Spinelli A, Riva N, Casi M, Moscatelli G, Frattarelli M. Intralesional radioimmunotherapy of malignant gliomas. An effective treatment in recurrent tumors. Cancer 1994; 73:1076–1082.
115. Riva P, Marangolo M, Tison V, Armaroli L, Moscatelli G, Franceschi G, Spinelli A, Vecchietti G, Morigi P, Tassini R, et al. Treatment of metastatic colorectal cancer by means of specific monoclonal antibodies conjugated with iodine-131: A phase II study. Nucl Med Biol 1991; 18:109–119.
116. Westlin J-E, Snook D, Nilsson S, Husin S, Enblad P, Stavrou S, Epenetos AA, Bergh J. Intravenous and intratumoural therapy of patients with malignant gliomas with ⁹⁰yttrium-labelled monoclonal antibody MUC 2-63. In: Epenetos A, ed. Monoclonal Antibodies 2: Applications in Clinical Oncology. London: Chapman & Hall Medical, 1993:17–25.
117. Riva P, Arista A, Sturiale C, Moscatelli G, Tison V, Mariani M, Seccamani E, Lazzari S, Fagioli L, Franceschi G, Sarti G, Riva N, Natali PG, Zardi L, Scassellati GA. Treatment of intracranial human glioblastoma by direct intratumoral administration of ¹³¹I-labeled anti-tenascin monoclonal antibody BC-2. Int J Cancer 1992; 51:7–13.
118. Franceschi G, Arista A, Casi M, Cremonini AM, Riva N, Vergoni M, Riva P. Intralesional radioimmunotherapy of high grade glioma: clinical experiences in 59 patients. Tumor Targeting 1996; 2:164.
119. Hird V, Stewart JS, Snook D, Dhokia B, Coulter C, Lambert HE, Mason WP, Soutter WP, Epenetos AA. Intraperitoneally administered ⁹⁰Y-labelled monoclonal antibodies as a third line of treatment in ovarian cancer. A phase 1-2 trial: problems encountered and possible solutions. Br J Cancer 1990; 10(suppl):48–51.
120. Hnatowich DJ, Mardirossian G, Rose PG, Kinders B, Rusckowski M, Stevens S, Hunter R, Griffin T, Brill AB. Intraperitoneal therapy of ovarian cancer with yttrium-90-labeled monoclonal antibodies, preliminary observations. Antib Immunoconj Radiopharm 1991; 4(3):359–371.
121. Jacobs AJ, Fer M, Su FM, Breitz H, Thompson J, Goodgold H, Cain J, Heaps J, Weiden P. A phase I trial of a rhenium 186-labeled monoclonal antibody administered intraperitoneally in ovarian carcinoma: toxicity and clinical response. Obstet Gynecol 1993; 82:586–593.
122. Breitz HB, Durham JS, Fisher DR, Weiden PL. Radiation-absorbed dose estimates to normal organs following intraperitoneal ¹⁸⁶Re-labeled monoclonal antibody: methods and results. Cancer Res 1995; 55(suppl):5817s–5822s.
123. Breitz HB, Durham JS, Fisher DR, Weiden PL, DeNardo GL, Goodgold HM, Nelp WB. Pharmacokinetics and normal organ dosimetry following intraperitoneal rhenium-186-labeled monoclonal antibody. J Nucl Med 1995; 36:754–761.
124. Meredith RF, Partridge EE, Alvarez RD, Khazaeli MB, Plott G, Russell CD, Wheeler RH, Liu T, Grizzle WE, Schlom J, LoBuglio AF. Intraperitoneal radioimmunotherapy of ovarian cancer with lutetium-177-CC49. J Nucl Med 1996; 37: 1491–1496.

125. Meredith RF, Macey DJ, Plott WE, Brezovich IA, Khazaeli MB, Alvarez R, Partridge E, Russell CD, Wheeler RH, Liu T, Elliott G, Schlom J, LoBuglio AF. Radiation dose estimates from intraperitoneal radioimmunotherapy with ^{177}Lu-CC49. Proc 6th Int Radiopharm Dosimetry Symp 1999; 1:158–171.

126. Alvarez RD, Partridge EE, Khazaeli MB, Plott G, Austin M, Kilgore L, Russell CD, Liu T, Grizzle WE, Schlom J, LoBuglio AF, Meredith RF. Intraperitoneal radioimmunotherapy of ovarian cancer with ^{177}Lu-CC49: a phase I/II study. Gynecol Oncol 1997; 65:94–101.

127. Kramer EL, DeNardo SJ, Liebes L, Kroger LA, Noz ME, Mizrachi H, Salako QA, Furmanski P, Glenn SD, DeNardo GL, et al. Radioimmunolocalization of metastatic breast carcinoma using indium-111-methyl benzyl DTPA BrE-3 monoclonal antibody: phase I study. J Nucl Med 1993; 34:1067–1074.

128. Schrier DM, Stemmer SM, Johnson T, Kasliwal R, Lear J, Matthes S, Taffs S, Dufton C, Glenn SD, Butchko G, Ceriani RL, Rovira D, Bunn P, Shpall EJ, Bearman SI, Purdy M, Cagnini P, Jones RB. High-dose [90]Y Mx-diethylenetriaminepentaacetic acid (DTPA)-BrE-3 and autologous hematopoietic stem cell support (AHSCS) for the treatment of advanced breast cancer: a phase I trial. Cancer Res 1995; 55(suppl):5921s–5924s.

129. Wong JYC, Williams LE, Yamauchi DM, Odom-Maryon T, Esteban JM, Neumaier M, Wu AM, Johnson DK, Primus FJ, Shively JE, Raubitschek AA. Initial experience evaluating [90]yttrium-radiolabeled anti-carcinoembryonic antigen chimeric T84.66 in a phase I radioimmunotherapy trial. Cancer Res 1995; 55(suppl):5929s–5934s.

130. Richman CM, DeNardo SJ, O'Grady LF, DeNardo GL. Radioimmunotherapy for breast cancer using escalating fractionated doses of ^{131}I-labeled chimeric L6 antibody with peripheral blood progenitor cell transfusions. Cancer Res 1995; 55(suppl):5916s–5920s.

131. Leichner PK, Klein JL, Garrison JB, Jenkins RE, Nickoloff EL, Ettinger DS, Order SE. Dosimetry of ^{131}I-labeled anti-ferritin in hepatoma: a model for radioimmunoglobulin dosimetry. Int J Radiat Oncol Biol Phys 1981; 7:323–333.

132. Order SE, Stillwagon GB, Klein JL, Leichner PK, Siegelman SS, Fishman EK, Ettinger DS, Haulk T, Kopher K, Finney K, et al. Iodine-131-antiferritin, a new treatment modality in hepatoma: a radiation therapy oncology group study. J Clin Oncol 1985; 3:1573–1582.

133. de Bree R, Roos JC, Quak JJ, den Hollander W, Snow GB, van Dongen GAMS. Radioimmunoscintigraphy and biodistribution of technetium-99m-labeled monoclonal antibody U36 in patients with head and neck cancer. Clin Cancer Res 1995; 1:591–598.

134. Breitz HB, Weiden PL, Vanderheyden J-L, Appelbaum JW, Bjorn MJ, Fer MF, Wolf SB, Ratliff BA, Seiler CA, Foisie DC, Fisher DR, Schroff RW, Fritzberg AR, Abrams PG. Clinical experience with rhenium-186-labeled monoclonal antibodies for radioimmunotherapy: results of phase I trials. J Nucl Med 1992; 33:1099–1112.

135. Begent RHJ, Ledermann JA, Green AJ, Bagshawe KD, Riggs SJ, Searle F, Keep PA, Adam T, Dale RG, Glaser MG. Antibody distribution and dosimetry in patients receiving radiolabeled antibody therapy for colorectal cancer. Br J Cancer 1989; 60:406–412.

136. Meredith RF, Khazaeli MB, Plott WE, Brezovich IA, Russell CD, Wheeler RH, Spencer SA, LoBuglio AF. Comparison of two mouse/human chimeric antibodies in patients with metastatic colon cancer. Antib Immunoconj Radiopharm 1992; 5: 75–80.

137. Meredith RF, LoBuglio AF, Plott WE, Orr RA, Brezovich IA, Russell CD, Harvey EB, Yester MV, Wagner AJ, Spencer SA, Wheeler RH, Saleh MN, Rogers KJ, Polansky A, Salter MM, Khazaeli MB. Pharmacokinetics, immune response, and biodistribution of iodine-131-labeled chimeric mouse/human IgGI, 17-1A monoclonal antibody. J Nucl Med 1991; 32:1162–1168.

138. Steffens MG, Boerman OC, Oosterhof GON, Koenders E, Oosterwijk-Wakka JC, Witjes JA, Cebruyne FMJ, Corstens FHM, Oosterwijk E. Targeting and therapeutic potential of ^{131}I-labeled chimeric monoclonal antibody G250 in renal cell carcinoma patients. Tumor Targeting 1996; 2:164.

139. Behr TM, Sharkey RM, Juweid ME, Dunn RM, Vagg RC, Swayne LC, Ying Z, Siegel JA, Goldenberg DM. Radioimmunotherapy of CEA-expressing cancers: results of a phase I/II trial with ^{131}I-labeled murine anti-CEA NP-4 IgG_1. Tumor Targeting 1996; 2:162.

140. Deb N, Goris M, Trisler K, Fowler S, Saal J, Ning S, Becker M, Marquez C, Knox S. Treatment of hormone-refractory prostate cancer with ^{90}Y-CYT-356 monoclonal antibody. Clin Cancer Res 1996; 2:1289–1297.

141. Abdel-Nabi HH, Spaulding M, Farrell E, Derby L, Lamonica D. Treatment of refractory prostate carcinoma with Y-90 KC4. J Nucl Med 1995; 36(suppl):213P.

142. Lashford L, Jones D, Pritchard J, Gordon I, Breatnach F, Kemshead JT. Therapeutic application of radiolabeled monoclonal antibody UJ13A in children with disseminated neuroblastoma. NCI Monogr 1987; 3:53–57.

143. Vessella RL. Radioimmunoconjugates in renal cell carcinoma. In: Debruyne FMJ, Bukowski RM, Pontes JE, et al., eds. Immunotherapy of Renal Cell Carcinoma. Heidelberg: Springer-Verlag, 1991:38–46.

144. Murray JL, Macey DJ, Kasi LP, Rieger P, Cunningham J, Bhadkamkar V, Zhang HZ, Schlom J, Rosenblum MG, Podoloff DA. Phase II radioimmunotherapy trial with ^{131}I-CC49 in colorectal cancer. Cancer 1994; 73(suppl):1057–1066.

145. Mardirossian G, Brill AB, Dwyer KM, Kahn D, Nelp W. Radiation absorbed dose from indium-111-CYT-356. J Nucl Med 1996; 37:1583–1588.

146. Juweid ME, Sharkey RM, Behr T, Swayne LC, Dunn R, Siegel J, Goldenberg DM. Radioimmunotherapy of patients with small-volume tumors using iodine-131-labeled anti-CEA monoclonal antibody NP-4 F(ab')$_2$. J Nucl Med 1996; 37:1504–1510.

3
Metallic Radionuclides for Radioimmunotherapy

Alan R. Fritzberg
NeoRx Corporation, Seattle, Washington

Claude F. Meares
University of California, Davis, California

I. INTRODUCTION

Many elements have radioisotopes of radiotherapeutic potential. Based on considerations of type of emission, energy, half-life, production capability, and cost, a significant number have been evaluated for application to radioimmunotherapy. A listing of various of these radionuclides is provided in Table 1, adapted from Fritzberg and Wessels (1). As can be easily seen, the majority of the radionuclides that have been of interest are metals and a great deal of work has been carried out to stably attach them to antibody proteins in ways that do not interfere with the tumor targeting of the antibody. This chapter will describe the various approaches used for the attachment of metals to antibodies, evaluations in vitro and in vivo, and a perspective on current status of metallic radionuclides in radiotherapy. As space and time limitations preclude an exhaustive review of all studies of therapeutic radionuclides, the chapter will focus on those that are representative and have had significant developmental effort applied to them. Several reviews are available that describe properties and production of therapeutic radionuclides, and they are recommended for more details (2–4).

Metal chemistry is organized by groups as related to their properties of oxidation levels, bonding characteristics, and size. The review will describe radionuclides as groups that are chemically related. Thus, yttrium-90 will be discussed in a section with other related radionuclides including lutetium-177, and imaging

Table 1 Physical Properties of Selected Radiotherapy Radionuclides

Radionuclide	Half-life (hr)	E_{max} beta (Mev)	Mean range (mm)	Imaging gamma energy in keV (% abundance)
^{32}P	342	1.71	1.85	—
^{64}Cu	12.8	0.57 (β^-)	0.40	511 (positron), 38%
		0.66 (β^+)		
^{67}Cu	62	0.57	0.27	92 (11%)
				185 (49%)
^{90}Y	64	2.27	2.76	—
^{131}I	193	0.61	0.40	364 (81%)
^{153}Sm	47	0.80	0.53	103 (28%)
^{177}Lu	162	0.50	0.28	113 (6.4%)
				208 (11%)
^{186}Re	89	1.07	0.92	137 (9%)
^{188}Re	17	2.12	2.43	155 (15%)
^{211}At$^+$	7.2	5.9 (α, 42%)	0.06[a]	670 (0.3%)
		7.5 (ec, 58%)[b]	0.08[a]	
^{212}Bi	1.0	1.36 (β, 64%)[c]	0.09[a]	727 (7%)
		6.1 (α, 36%)	0.06[a]	
^{213}Bi	0.78	5.8	0.06[a]	440
		8.4[d]	0.08[a]	

[a] Maximum alpha particle range.
[b] Product ^{211}Po decays to ^{207}Pb with 0.52-sec half-life.
[c] Product ^{212}Po decays with 0.3-μsec half-life via 8.8 MeV α.
[d] Alpha particle energy via product ^{213}Po pathway.

radionuclides gallium-67 and indium-111. Other sections will discuss copper-64 and -67, rhenium-186 and -188, and related imaging radionuclide technetium-99m, and alpha-emitting bismuths, ^{212}Bi and ^{213}Bi with the generator precursor, lead (^{212}Pb).

II. GROUP IIIa/b AND LANTHANIDE RADIONUCLIDES

A. Indium (^{111}In)

1. Nuclear Properties and Production

Indium-111 is the radioisotope of interest in radioimmunotherapy. It is cyclotron produced and is routinely used in nuclear medicine. It has a half-life of 2.8 days and decays by electron capture with abundant gamma rays at 184 and 296 keV energies. Its half-life is well matched to whole antibody IgG of 150 kD with slow pharmacokinetics.

2. Indium Chemistry: Useful Chelates and Methodology

Indium is a group III metal and not a transition metal, but many of its uses are related to its similarity with iron. In acidic solutions In(III) is preferably in the form of a hexacoordinated $[In(H_2O)_6]^{3+}$. Above pH 3 to 4 indium tends to precipitate as the hydroxide $In(OH)_3$. If a metal complexing buffer like citrate, acetate, or tartrate is added, the pH at which precipitation begins can be considerably increased. The In-DTPA complex can be formed at low pH using a citrate buffer; the pH may then be raised to neutral, without precipitation of the indium hydroxide. In contrast, if indium is added directly to a solution of DTPA at the elevated pH, indium hydroxide precipitates. The chelate can either be labeled before or after the conjugation to the antibody. Labeling of the antibody conjugate is simpler than prelabeling of the free chelate. The use of a buffer to optimize the chelation yield is of particular importance (5).

C-functionalized EDTA and DTPA (6–10) ligands are used successfully for labeling with ^{111}In. In-DTPA has a slightly higher thermodynamic stability at physiological pH than In-EDTA, whereas the macrocyclic In-DOTA is much less stable thermodynamically. However, dissociation kinetics are of more practical importance; surprisingly, C-functionalized EDTA indium complexes dissociate more slowly in serum than C-functionalized DTPA complexes (11), and macrocyclic complexes such as In-DOTA decompose at even slower rates (12). Therefore macrocycles are preferred for use in vivo. The structures of the various chelating agents for indium and other +3 metals are shown in Figure 1.

B. Gallium (^{67}Ga, ^{68}Ga)

1. Nuclear Properties and Production

Gallium-67 and -68 are the gallium radioisotopes of interest in nuclear medicine. ^{67}Ga is readily available from a cyclotron. A physical half-life of 3.26 d and various δ radiations from electron capture (EC) decay allow its use for diagnostic purposes. ^{68}Ga is one of the few useful positron-emitting radionuclides that can be obtained from a generator, the long-lived germanium-68 (^{68}Ge) isotope ($T_{1/2} =$ 275 d).

2. Chemical Properties

In aqueous chemistry, only the oxidation state Ga(III) is important. The coordination chemistry of Ga(III) is very similar to that of Fe(III). The hexaqua ion $[Ga(H_2O)_6]^{3+}$ is formed only under acidic conditions. As the pH is raised, hydrol-

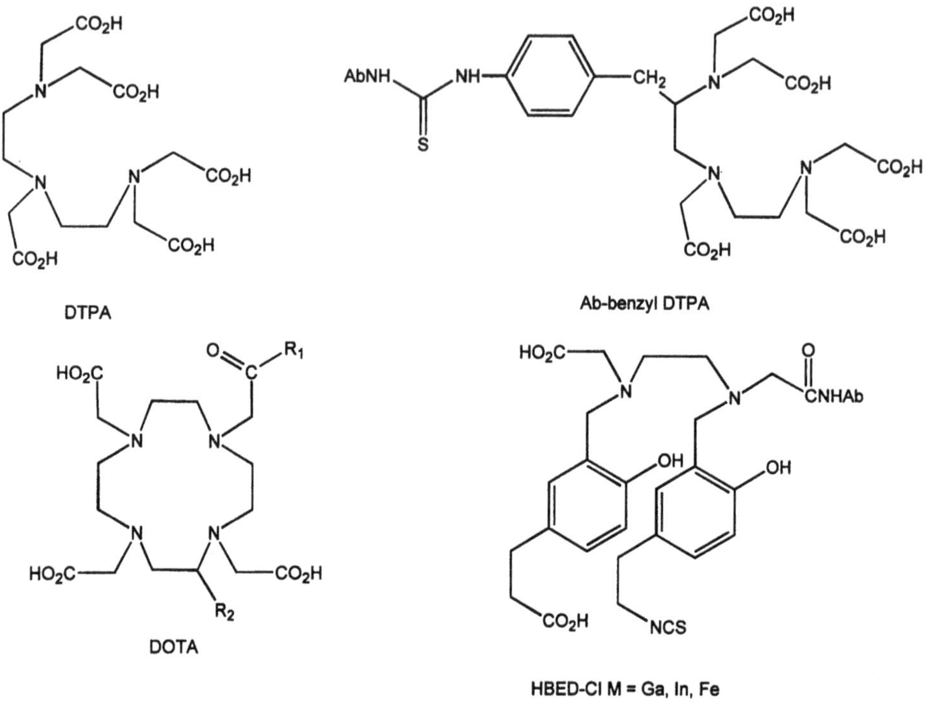

Figure 1 Structures of various chelating agents used for the lanthanides and other metals of similar +3 metal chemistry. 2-Benzyl-DOTA: R_2 = Benzyl-linker; R_1 = OH. DOTA-peptide: R_2 = H$_1$; R_1 = NH-linker.

ysis is observed leading to the formation of the insoluble gallium trihydroxide, Ga(OH)$_3$(s). Addition of a buffer like citrate (13,14) or acetate (15) is widely used. In the case of citrate, it is possible to keep gallium in solution up to pH 8. Due to its high charge and small ionic radius (0.62 Å), Ga(III) is considered as a "hard acid" (16). Therefore it prefers hard bases such as oxygen and nitrogen for coordination, with oxygen favored over nitrogen.

3. Useful Chelates and Methodology

Several chelates have been developed for the use of ^{67}Ga and ^{68}Ga in radioimaging (13–15,17–21). In general, the different properties of these ligands (structure, charge, lipophilicity) affect the biological pathway of their gallium complexes in vivo. Therefore imaging of different organs can be accomplished by the choice of the chelate. The introduction of bifunctional chelates which allow conjugation to an antibody seems to be not as important as for other radionuclides. There are only a few examples for gallium where this technique has been used (22–24).

Some of the chelates are derivatives of EDTA where two of the carboxymethyl groups are replaced by phenolic functions (PLED; HBED) (15). Other ligands are based on tricatecholamide functions, which are enterobactin analogs (TriP-MECAM(S);3,4-DiP-LICAM(S) (13), or on salicylaldimine (H$_3$[(5-MeOsal)$_3$TAME]) (19). The latter is one of only a few radiopharmaceuticals where an x-ray structure of the gallium complex is reported. Besides the traditional open-chain ligands EDTA and DTPA, the macrocyclic polyaminopolycarboxylate DOTA (21) and NOTA (20) seem to be useful chelates.

In serum, the gallium complexes of these ligands are in competition with the protein transferrin. This property has been used by injecting a gallium complex with a weak chelator like citrate (17). Within a short amount of time, transchelation of the gallium to transferrin occurs (25) followed by transport to the tumor. This method has limited selectivity toward imaging of particular organs, mainly liver and marrow. It is of interest to avoid such transchelation in order to achieve more specificity and to reduce background activity. In fact the kinetics of gallium loss from the strong chelators above seem to be slow enough to permit their use in radioimaging.

C. Yttrium (^{90}Y)

1. Nuclear Properties and Preparation

The radioisotope yttrium-90 has a pure beta emission which is useful in radiotherapy. In comparison to ^{131}I, which has a maximum beta energy of 600 keV, ^{90}Y has a maximum of 2300 keV. The higher energy results in greater tissue penetration with superior potential for treating larger tumors (see O'Donoghue, Chapter 1). The absence of any gamma radiation makes this radioisotope a particularly attractive therapeutic agent. Yttrium-90 is prepared from strontium-90 via a generator system (26,27). Thus, it is available in high specific activity.

2. Yttrium Chemistry: Useful Chelates and Methodology

Yttrium, which lies in the periodic table over lanthanum, has atomic and ionic radii close to those for terbium and dysprosium. Its chemistry is similar to the lanthanides. Like indium, only the trivalent ion has thermodynamic stability in solution. Y(III) is a hard Lewis acid, like the 3+ charged lanthanides. The ionic radius is 15% larger than indium and this results in yttrium binding relatively larger numbers of water molecules or other ligands, the most common coordination numbers being 8 and 9.

Yttrium hydrolyzes below pH 7, so that in seeking a suitable ligand for yttrium, similar criteria to those for indium are imposed. The ligand must bind yttrium quickly and at low ligand concentration, and must form a kinetically inert complex with respect to protein-promoted dissociation. Yttrium prefers octadentate coordination. Compared to the indium complexes with EDTA, the analogous Y-complexes exchange rapidly.

Significant amounts of ^{90}Y can be incorporated into bone when ^{90}Y is injected as the DTPA chelate in vivo (28). Recent studies of benzyl-DTPA based bifunctional chelating agents showed that the loss of Y(III) in vitro in human serum was much slower than with unsubstituted DTPA (29) and that Y(III) loss in vivo from these chelates may be decreased by the addition of methyl groups on the DTPA backbone (30). The low stability of Y-EDTA complexes may be a result of the availability of only six binding sites; backbone-substituted DTPA has eight coordinating sites.

Ligands having a macrocyclic cavity that can accommodate the large metal ion are preferred. From comparisons of many yttrium chelates for stability it is clear that macrocyclic ligands based on DOTA have excellent properties. Early work from Desreux et al. (31) with lanthanides demonstrated the high thermodynamic stability of complexes of DOTA. A bifunctional chelating agent, a C-functionalized DOTA ligand (p-nitrobenzyl-DOTA), was prepared by Moi et al. (29). This ligand binds yttrium and also other metals including copper, cobalt, and indium. Serum stability studies of the Y(III) chelate of this ligand showed no detectable loss of yttrium to serum proteins after 18 days under physiological conditions (32).

Because there were earlier reports of potential immunogenicity of DOTA conjugates (33–35) and slow kinetics of chelation, efforts have continued to find improved polyamino acid derivatives. As backbone substitution of DTPA improves stability, derivatives based on vicinal cyclohexane substitution for further rigidity were synthesized and studied (36,37). Depending on the stereochemistry of the cyclohexyl substitution, diastereomers result, designated CHX-A and CHX-B (36). These were compared to DOTA with ^{88}Y and the results indicated that CHX-A was lower in bone accumulation than CHX-B, but still not as low as DOTA. Further work on resolving enantiomers of the CHX-A and CHX-B (37) indicated that both forms of CHX-A were quite low in bone (4.0% vs. 4.6% ID/g at 168 h, while the CHX-B enantiomers differed significantly and were higher at 12% and 22% ID/g in bone at 168 h postinjection. For comparison, Y-DOTA in bone was about 0.5% ID/g at 168 h (36).

With recent improvements in the purity of radiopharmaceutical quality ^{90}Y, the kinetics of chelation with DOTA have improved so that antibody DOTA conjugates can be radiolabeled under practical conditions (38). Further, the development of DOTA-peptide reagents has preserved the kinetic properties of the C-substituted DOTA reagents while (so far) giving no problems with immunogenicity (39,40).

III. COPPER RADIOISOTOPES (^{62}Cu, ^{64}Cu, ^{67}Cu)

A. Physical Properties and Radiochemistry of Copper

Besides copper-67 (41), copper-62 (42) and copper-64 (43) have been developed as medical radionuclides. Due to its short half-life of 9.8 min, ^{62}Cu is not useful for radiotherapy. Copper-64 has a half-life of 12.4 hours and has been studied in radioimmunotherapy (44). It can be made in large amounts by accelerator production. Copper-67 has excellent physical and biological properties for radioimmunotherapy. Its physical half-life of 2.58 d is similar to the residence time of a typical antibody on the tumor. Copper-67 releases moderate energy beta particles which can penetrate to a few millimeters (4). It also emits gamma radiation (184 keV), which allows it to be traced in the body for imaging and dosimetry.

B. Radionuclide Production

Copper-64 is produced by a number of approaches. Low specific activity results from neutron irradiation of copper. High-energy neutron (n,p) irradiation of zinc results in high-specific-activity ^{64}Cu (45). Use of the latter approach at the University of Missouri Research Reactor has resulted in specific activities over 100 mCi/μg Cu. More recently, production of ^{64}Cu via cyclotron resulting from proton irradiation of ^{64}Ni in a cyclotron has been optimized (46). In addition to providing very high specific activity ^{64}Cu, availability is not limited by the weekly access to the fast neutron flux trap of the reactor.

Copper-67 has been made via irradiation of natural zinc targets with high-energy protons from accelerators at Los Alamos and Brookhaven (47,48). The spallation reaction produced several radioactive byproducts with the ^{67}Cu isolated by an electrolytic method. While the theoretical specific activity is high by this approach, contamination from stable copper resulted in variable levels of specific activity.

C. Copper Chemistry: Useful Chelates and Methodology

The most important oxidation state of copper is Cu(II). In general Cu(II) salts dissolve well in water to form the aqua ion $[Cu(H_2O)_6]^{2+}$. Many of its complexes have four short equatorial Cu-L bonds and two longer axial Cu-L bonds (where L represents a ligand atom such as N or O). Cu(II) is flexible in the number of ligands coordinated, but six ligands are present in most stable complexes for medical use. Most of the complexes form easily at neutral or acidic pH. In general Cu(II) favors nitrogen over oxygen donor atoms.

There are several ligands which form thermodynamically stable complexes with Cu(II). Some are based on macrocyclic polyamines (e.g., cyclam) which form $+2$ charged complexes with Cu(II). Others are based on macrocyclic (TETA, DOTA, NOTA) polyaminopolycarboxylates and form anionic complexes at neutral pH.

In the case of TETA, the thermodynamic stability constant K_s for the formation of the complex between Cu^{2+} ions and $TETA_4^-$ ions at 298°K is given by:

$$K_s = f([CuTETA_2^-]/[TETA_4^-] [Cu_2^+]) = 1021.6$$

Though thermodynamic stability constants provide useful information about the potential of these chelates, they do not refer to practical conditions in serum. All the chelates mentioned above contain highly basic groups and therefore will bind H^+ avidly. This competition between metal ion and H^+ leads to a decrease in thermodynamic stability (49). For TETA the thermodynamic proton binding constants are given as $\log K_1 = 10.68$, $\log K_2 = 10.14$, $\log K_3 = 4.09$ and $\log K_4 = 3.35$ (note that, e.g., $\log K_1 = f([HTETA_3^-]/[TETA_4^-] [H^+])$). Furthermore, association of OH^- to the metal ion can play an important role at higher pH. The equilibrium constants for binding of OH^- are $\log bCuOH = 6.1$, $\log bCu(OH)_2 = 12.8$, $\log bCu(OH)_3 = 14.5$, and $\log bCu(OH)_4 = 16$ (note that, e.g., $\log bCu(OH)_4 = f([Cu(OH)_4^{2-}]/[Cu^{2+}] [OH^-]_4)$). The result is that the conditional stability constant $\log K_{scond} = 15.4$ at pH 7.5. In human serum Cu(II) binds predominantly to albumin (50). The stability constant for the binding of copper to human serum albumin (HSA) at physiologic pH 7.5 is $\log K_{HSA} = 16.2$ (51). The concentration of albumin in human serum is approximately 5×10^{-4} M (51). In a realistic clinical experiment the concentration of the antibody bound chelate will be less than 10^{-7} M, so at equilibrium all the copper will be bound to albumin. The challenge to the synthetic chemist is to design and synthesize molecules such as TETA (41) that lose copper extremely slowly.

The chelates of interest in radioimmunotherapy are bifunctional. They need a functional side chain that allows conjugation to an antibody. This is achieved either by attachment of the sidechain to the carbon backbone of the chelate (8,9,41) or by a substitution at one nitrogen atom (52–54). Substitution at the carbon backbone can decrease the rates of dissociation of metal complexes (8). C-substituted macrocyclic derivatives of TETA (41,55,56), and cyclam (57) bind copper with practical stability in vivo. For the TETA derivative, in vitro serum studies show only a loss of about 1% copper per day whereas the open chain derivatives of EDTA and DTPA lose their copper rapidly to serum albumin (50,58). This indicates that the loss of the metal ion is controlled by kinetic factors that depend on the structure of the chelate (Fig. 2).

The complexation of copper is usually complete within a few minutes. The excess free or nonspecifically bound copper is removed from the antibody by chelation with EDTA or DTPA followed by gel filtration.

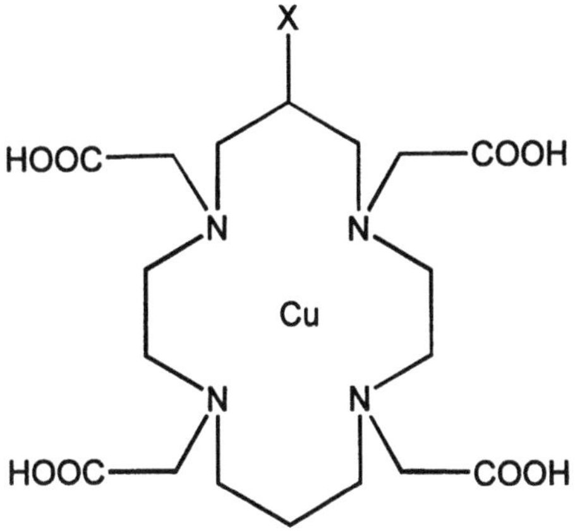

17 TETA, Cu; X = linker

Figure 2 Structure of the macrocyclic TETA bifunctional chelating agent.

IV. RHENIUM RADIOISOTOPES (^{186}Re, ^{188}Re)

A. Physical Properties and Radiochemistry of Rhenium Radioisotopes

Rhenium has two radioisotopes with favorable physical properties for use in targeted radiotherapy (Table 1). Rhenium-186 with its half-life of 3.71 days, 1.07 MeV maximum beta energy, and a primary gamma emission of 137 keV (9%) is favorably matched with slower tumor targeting and normal organ loss of radioactivity forms such as whole IgG antibody (150 kD) and F(ab')$_2$ (100 kD) antibody fragments. Rhenium-188 has a half-life of 17.0 hours, maximum beta energy of 2.12 MeV, and gamma emissions of 155 keV (15%). Its shorter half-life is more limited to applications with rapid target uptake, shorter tumor retention, and rapid normal organ loss of radioactivity. The beta particle energies of ^{186}Re are moderate and average tissue penetration is 0.9 mm, about 40 cell diameters, while ^{188}Re with its high-energy beta particles (2.12 MeV$_{max}$) has an average penetration of 2.4 mm. The greater penetration may have some advantage in larger lesions (59), but controlled in vivo studies demonstrating more effective therapy remain to be done. Both rhenium radioisotopes have favorable energies for imaging and the low fractional abundances of their gamma radiation that result in minimal contribution to non-specific irradiation of normal organs. When the radiation delivery potential is considered, which is a combination of equilibrium dose constant and the average lifetime, ^{186}Re provides about 2.5 times more rads/mCi than ^{188}Re assuming tissue retention until decay. For further comparison, ^{90}Y results in about 4.5 times more rads/mCi than ^{188}Re, again assuming rapid uptake and tissue retention for the physical decay lifetime of the radionuclide.

B. Radionuclide Production of $^{186/188}$Re

Rhenium-186 has been produced by reactor neutron irradiation of enriched ^{185}Re. Production at the University of Missouri Research Reactor with a neutron flux of 2×10^{14} neutrons/cm^2-sec has resulted in specific-activity levels on the order of 3 Ci/mg (60). At this level of specific activity, sufficient carrier protein must be used in order to avoid the impact of derivatization or loading on the antigen binding and biological targeting properties of the antibody. Studies addressing this concern will be described later. The target form of ^{185}Re typically used has been Re metal. While pure metal results in minimal byproduct radioactivity, the chemical conversion of the ^{186}Re in metal form into the useful $+7$ perrhenate oxidation level requires oxidation. This has been done by treatment with either HCl/HNO$_3$ or H$_2$O$_2$. In the case of the HCl/HNO$_3$ reagents, significant effort was required to remove residual nitrate which interfered with radiolabeling chemistry or, in the latter case, residual peroxide would consume the reducing agent necessary to reduce the $+7$ perrhenate to lower oxidation level rhenium required for chelation. An improved Al(ReO$_4$)$_3$ target was developed that only required simple dissolution with water to produce a solution of ^{186}Re perrhenate (61).

Rhenium-188 has been prepared either from enriched ^{187}Re via neutron irradiation or from the radioactive decay of tungsten-188. The reactor production is simple, but with the short half-life of ^{188}Re, the process is inconvenient and carrier ^{187}Re is present in the ^{188}Re. As ^{188}W decays to ^{188}Re with a 69.4-day half-life, ^{188}W/^{188}Re generators have been developed that allow production of ^{188}Re over a several-month lifetime. These generators have been based on either gel (62) or alumina (63) separation technologies. Tungsten-188 requires neutron irradiation of ^{186}W to achieve a capture of two neutrons. The low probability of a double neutron capture has limited production of generators that provide therapeutically useful amounts of ^{188}Re to the Oak Ridge high-flux reactor (63). Curie level generators of ^{188}Re are currently being produced there for research studies. A significant advantage of the generator production of ^{188}Re is the resultant ''carrier-free'' high specific activity.

C. Protein ^{188}Re/^{188}Re Radiolabeling Chemistry

The similarities of rhenium and technetium structural chemistry have provided a basis for approaches to the attachment of rhenium radionuclides to proteins. In early work on the radiopharmaceutical chemistry of ^{99m}Tc (64,65), stable rhenium contributed to the characterization of ^{99m}Tc radiopharmaceutical chemistry, particularly in providing structural information without requiring use of radioactive materials. Thus, the relationships between Tc and Re of group VII (Mn group) were well appreciated as interest developed in the application of radiolabeled antibodies for radioimmunotherapy. Initial interest was in ^{99m}Tc antibodies for imaging and the studies with ^{99m}Tc and antibody proteins lead the way for application with antibody labeling with rhenium radioisotopes.

Early success in imaging tumors with whole and fragment forms of monoclonal antibodies using iodine-131 and subsequently Indium-111 suggested further improvement by using ^{99m}Tc with its superior imaging properties. As discussed above, success with ^{99m}Tc would then provide a basis for application of ^{186}Re or ^{188}Re with the similarities in chelate chemistry. Proteins contain the donor atoms typically found in chelating agents used in ^{99m}Tc radiopharmaceuticals including carboxylate oxygen, thiol, amine, and amide nitrogen. Thus, early work with ^{99m}Tc protein radiolabeling leads to approaches using direct radiolabeling via endogenous donor atom groups as well as indirect radiolabeling via bifunctional chelating agents.

1. Direct Radiolabeling of Proteins with Rhenium Radioisotopes

The basis for direct attachment of ^{99m}Tc to proteins using endogenous donor atoms has relied on the strong binding interaction of these metals with sulfhydryl group(s). With the sulfhydryl group mediating attachment, other nearby donor atoms in proteins, chiefly amide nitrogens, become involved to give chelates similar to the N,S amide thiolate series. Representative structures of N,S amide thiolate chelates and derived chelates in peptide/protein amino acid sequences mediated by cysteine moiety point of attachment are shown in Figure 3. Based on model chelate studies, the ability of the N,S donor atoms to form a spatially ideal tetradentate donor set may be limited when protein tertiary structural interactions restrict donor atom availability (66,67). Thus, stability of endogenous metal complexes is likely to be of variable stability.

Immunoglobulin proteins have a number of interchain and intrachain disulfide bonds and cleavage of these disulfides can form the desired sulfhydryl groups for metal Tc/Re binding. Various disulfide reducing reagents have been used to provide metal binding sulfhydryl groups with subsequent exchange of the stannous reduced radiometal to the protein. Optimization of ratios of reducing reagent to antibody protein and exchange chelates such as gluconate, tartrate, or citrate resulted in high yields of radio-Re-immunoglobulin. Biodistribution studies in tumor xenograft models generally have resulted in reduced tumor uptake at 24 hours or later post injection as well as reduced levels of radioactivity remaining in the blood when compared to control radioiodinated antibodies that were simultaneously injected. Thus, the tumor to blood and normal organs ratios were favor-

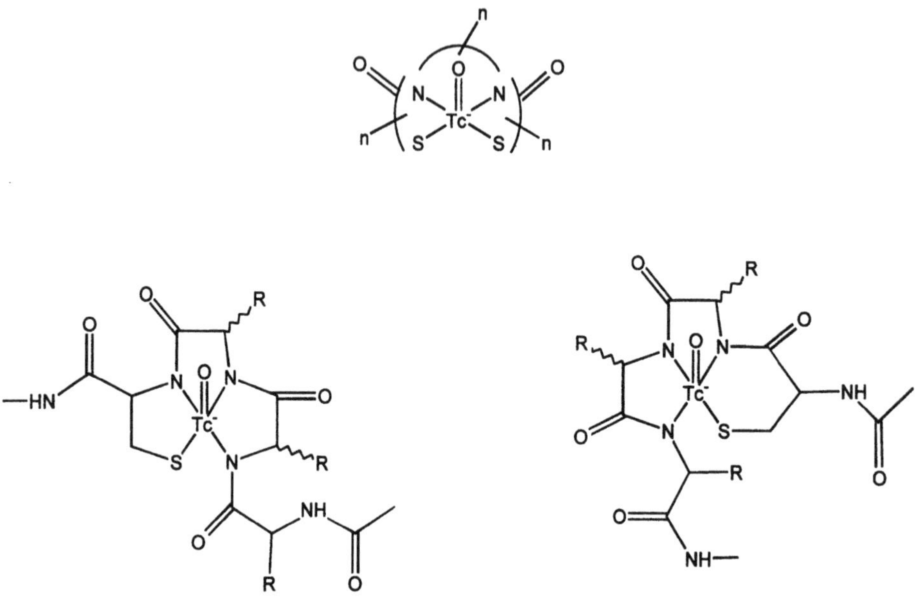

5,5,5   5,5,6

Figure 3 N,S-amide thiolate chelating agents showing basis for chelate ring size (n) and examples of such endogenous N,S-amide thiolate chelation in cysteine containing peptides and proteins.

able, but the efficiency of rhenium radioisotope was compromised on a tumor delivery basis (68–70). For the shorter half-lived ^{188}Re, the lower retention at tumor at later times are of lower impact on radiation delivered and the more favorable tumor to blood ratio provides an advantage.

The direct radiolabeling method is inherently very simple and thus attractive. As the reduction of perrhenate is more difficult than with technetium and the kinetics of exchange are slower, the conditions for direct labeling have required considerably larger amounts of stannous ion for the perrhenate reduction step and extended the time required for the exchange of rhenium to protein.

2. Indirect Radiolabeling of Proteins with Rhenium Radioisotopes

The indirect attachment of ^{186}Re/^{188}Re to antibody proteins involves use of a bifunctional chelating group designed to stably hold the rhenium and also modified to be covalently linked to a protein functional group such as lysine amine via active ester conjugation or cysteine sulfhydryl via maleimide addition. Because of the slow exchange kinetics of rhenium, most work has centered on formation of a rhenium complex and subsequent conjugation reaction of the preformed chelate with the protein. This approach has the advantage of allowing low pH and high temperatures, relatively harsh conditions, to be used to form the metal chelate in high yield and then mild conditions to be used for the protein conjugation step. This avoids the extreme conditions that would damage the protein. While, this approach leads to additional steps and time in the radiolabeling, the metal chelation is controlled and covalent and stable attachment to protein results by using reagent functional groups such as active esters that have a large body of experience in protein modification chemistry.

Early efforts with DTPA as a bifunctional chelating agent lead to inefficient incorporation of ^{186}Re and low levels of immunoreactivity (71). The N,S amide thiolate chelate series provided an attractive starting point for improved attachment of rhenium radioisotopes to antibody proteins. These tetradentate chelates provide stable complexes with rhenium and allow chemistry to be carried out independently on functional groups attached to chelate backbone carbons. The lack of carboxylate group interaction with the metal oxo center in the tetradentate amide thiolate system was indicated by earlier work in the HPLC behavior of chelate ring substituent diastereomers (72) and confirmed by the determination of crystal structures of Tc and Re N_2S_2-carboxylate complexes (67). Thus, a carboxylate group can be converted to an active ester after chelation or a chelate can be formed in the presence of reactive groups such as active esters.

The results of Re protein labeling applications with N_2S_2 (73) and N_3S (74,75) amide thiolate bifunctional chelating agents have been described. Preliminary evaluation of active esters indicated tetrafluorophenyl to have a superior balance of protein lysine amine acylation versus the undesired hydrolysis pathway. The sulfur donor atom of the N,S chelating group must be protected to avoid oxidation during storage or prevent reaction with the active ester. The hemithioacetal group has been found to effectively protect the sulfur and give high yields of N,S chelate at low pH and with heating over a several minute period. A typical sequence for radiolabeling is shown in Figure 4 for the MAG_2GABA, an N_3S bifunctional chelating agent. This chemistry has allowed attachment of nearly 600 mCi of ^{186}Re on 100 mg of protein and patient administration of 560 mCi in a single dose (75). The approach using in situ esterification of the similar N_3S chelating agent, ^{186}Re-MAG$_3$, has been optimized to good yields and applied in animal studies (76). A peptide as a base for a modified N_3S chelate has also been synthesized and evaluated (77). Tumor targeting was shown, although very low yields of ^{186}Re protein were reported.

Loading studies on antibody forms with ^{186}Re-MAG$_2$-GABA have been carried out on whole IgG and F(ab')$_2$ (78). Ratios of 4:1 ^{186}Re-MAG$_2$-

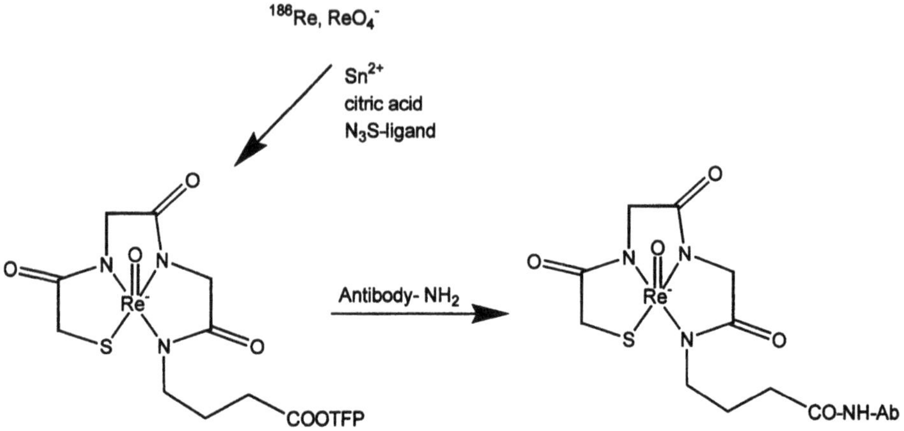

Figure 4 Preformed chelate labeling of proteins with rhenium radioisotopes using the MAG₂-GABA tetrafluorophenyl (TFP) bifunctional chelating agent.

GABA:F(ab')₂ did not alter immunoreactivity or tumor targeting and normal organ biodistribution while on whole IgG with antibody NR-LU-10, ratios of up to 10 metal chelates to antibody did not alter immunoreactivity, but tumor uptake was reduced at that level while five metal chelates to antibody resulted in no change in tumor uptake or normal organ biodistribution.

The radioactivity excreted in urine and bile for the ^{186}Re N,S chelates was shown to be composed of the starting radiometal chelate with lysine attached (79). This supported conjugation via the lysine groups as expected. However, the abnormal amide linkage formed by acylation of the e-amino group was not degraded by the lysosomes. Thus, the product of protein catabolism following liver or kidney uptake was readily excreted and resulted in relatively low normal organ radiation doses. However, the product lysine-Re chelate had a much greater propensity to be excreted in the intestines. A number of modifications to the amide thiolate chelates were made including additional carboxylate groups for increased hydrophilicity (80) and ester linkage for release of parent chelate (81). The derivatives with increased charge decreased intestinal excretion, but increased kidney retention. In the case of an ester linkage via mercaptoacetyl-glycyl-glycyl-seryl-succinate, decreased intestinal radioactivity as well as increased urinary excretion of radioactivity while maintaining tumor uptake and retention was observed.

D. Radiotherapy with ^{186}Re in Animal Model Systems

A number of animal tumor model studies have been reported demonstrating therapeutic effect using ^{186}Re antibodies. These include xenografts of small-cell lung cancer (82), colon cancer and lymphoma (83), and squamous head and neck cancer (84). The studies indicated that single doses as large as 600 μCi of ^{186}Re antibodies could be given to mice and that small, established solid tumors (ca. 20 mm^3) could be cured with a single dose of 200 μCi. Higher doses were required to effectively treat larger tumors (100–250 mm^3). In this case, a single 400-μCi dose resulted in regression with about 50% cured and the remainder regrowing.

V. METAL ALPHA-EMITTING RADIONUCLIDES

A. Nuclear Properties of Alpha-Emitters

Alpha particles are helium atoms and are about 8000 times larger than beta particles (electrons). When emitted from radionuclides that decay via an alpha pathway, they release enormous amounts of energy over a distance of several cell diameters. Thus, they have high LET (linear energy transfer). Properties of high LET are low numbers of particle emissions required to kill a cell, lack of repair potential and lack of oxygen effects on cytotoxicity (85,86). Thus, few atoms are needed to kill a cell. Killing is effective in hypoxic tumor areas and such therapy should be effective for micrometastases and isolated cells which may escape lethality from beta emitters in which insufficient crossfire for cytotoxicity is developed (see discussion by O'Donoghue in Chapter 1 regarding tumor size and therapeutic efficiency) (59).

There are several metals that decay by alpha emission and others that are generators of alpha emitters which are of interest for targeted radiotherapy. Bismuth radioisotopes ^{212}Bi (60.6 min $t_{1/2}$) and ^{213}Bi (47 min $t_{1/2}$) are short-lived alpha emitters that may be useful in applications of rapid targeting such as leukemias (87) or local applications such as intraperitoneal treatment of ovarian cancers (88) or brain tumors (89). However, for systemic targeting of tumors, tumor uptake and disappearance from normal tissues (i.e., generation of a favorable therapeutic index) before major loss of potency is unlikely from these short-lived emitters. Lead (^{212}Pb) with a 10.6-hr half-life offers the potential of targeting and generating the ^{212}Bi alpha emitter in vivo. The longer-lived alpha emitter, ^{225}Ac, with a 10-day half-life and several alpha events per decay chain ending in ^{213}Bi, is also under consideration (90). The discussion following will focus on the lead and bismuth radionuclides as significant effort has taken place and progress toward demonstration of potential via antibody mediated targeting has been gained. Importantly, ^{213}Bi is in Phase I clinical studies for anti-CD33 targeting of leukemia (91).

B. Radionuclide Production

Bismuth (^{213}Bi) is derived from long-lived thorium (^{229}Th) with a 7340-year $t_{1/2}$, which comes from uranium (^{233}U). The ^{229}Th decays to ^{225}Ra with a 12-day half-life subsequently decaying to [225]Ac. As mentioned above, it can be used directly or as a generator of [213]Bi. A generator has been developed to supply the preclinical and clinical amounts needed for [213]Bi (92,93). Bismuth ([212]Bi) is produced by decay of [212]Pb. The [212]Pb is supplied by a generator based on [224]Ra which decays with a 3.6 day $t_{1/2}$ to [212]Pb via [220]Rn with a 55-sec $t_{1/2}$ (94). By varying conditions, the [212]Bi can be eluted by itself or in equilibrium with the [212]Pb.

C. Antibody Radiolabeling Chemistry

A significant amount of effort has gone into developing the chemistry for attachment of [212]Pb and [212]Bi to antibodies for radioimmunotherapy. The macrocyclic chelating agent DOTA was shown to form kinetically inert complexes with both lead and bismuth (95). A linker form of DOTA, p-SCN-benzyl-DOTA, was conjugated to antibody B72.3 for evaluation of radioisotopic Pb antibody radiolabeling (96). Essentially identical biodistribution and tumor targeting results were obtained in LS-174T xenografts in mice based on [203]Pb as a model for [212]Pb. However, things were not so simple with [212]Pb. When [212]Pb-DOTA was characterized with respect to chemical form of radionuclide daughter [212]Bi, it was found that about a third of the [212]Bi was not chelated by the DOTA (97). Free bismuth localizes in the kidneys and thus the [212]Bi that escapes may result in increased kidney radiation dose. A study of [212]Pb attached to antibody AE1 reactive against the HER2/neu oncoprotein was recently reported (98). Therapy model studies were reported that indicated efficacy against minimal tumor (treated 3 days post tumor cell injection) and small tumors (15 mm³) and no effect on larger tumors (150 mm³). Marrow toxicity was seen at 25 μCi limiting the amount of dose that could be given. Unfortunately, no analysis was reported of the actual [212]Pb and [212]Bi localization.

VI. DEVELOPMENT OF METAL RADIONUCLIDES FOR RADIOIMMUNOTHERAPY

Although there are a significant number of metal radionuclides that emit particles with energies and half-lives suitable for consideration for radioimmunotherapy applications, the number of radionuclides for whom substantial development has taken place is small. This is a result of the combination of physical properties and practical considerations. Most of the current effort involves ^{90}Y, which has several key advantages: availability, high specific activity, favorable half-life, high energy, and lack of normal tissue-exposing gamma radiation. Its high energy is most suitable for larger tumors, which translates to potential for treating tumors that can be monitored for response by CT or MRI modalities. The major limitation of ^{90}Y, instability of antibody protein attachment, seems to have been solved by the use of DOTA. The moderate energy ^{186}Re has very favorable physical properties and can be conveniently produced in large amounts, but as it is produced in a reactor, its lower specific activity has been a limitation, especially for use in antibody pretargeting (Chapters 7 and 8).

While lower energy beta emitters such as lutetium (^{177}Lu) and ^{67}Cu may have advantages for small tumors, determining responses may require observation for time to tumor progression. This is also a concern for alpha emitters with their short path lengths that makes them theoretically advantageous for micrometastases and indicated for adjuvant treatment. These properties offer great promise for cancer control or cure through adjuvant treatment, but longer-term clinical studies will be required for efficacy demonstration.

REFERENCES

1. Fritzberg AR, Wessels BW. Therapeutic radionuclides. In: Wagner HN, Szabo Z, Buchanan J, eds. Principles of Nuclear Medicine, 2nd ed. Philadelphia: W.B. Saunders Company, 1995:229–234.
2. Volkert WA, Goeckeler WF, Ehrhardt GJ, Ketring AR. Therapeutic radionuclides: production and decay property considerations. J Nucl Med 1991; 32:174–185.
3. Mausner LF, Srivastava SC. Selection of radionuclides for radioimmunotherapy. Med Phys 1993; 19:503–509.
4. Wessels BW, Rogus RD. Radionuclide selection and model absorbed dose calculations for radiolabeled tumor associated antibodies. Med Phys 1984; 11:638–645.
5. Meares CF, Goodwin DA, Leung CS, Girgis AY, Silvester DJ, Nunn AD, Lavender PL. Covalent attachment of metal chelates to proteins: the stability in vivo and in vitro of the conjugate of albumin with a chelate of 111-indium. Proc Natl Acad Sci USA 1976; 73:3803–3806.
6. Meares CF, McCall MJ, Reardan DT, Goodwin DA, Diamanti CI, McTigue M. Conjugation of antibodies with bifunctional chelating agents: isothiocyanate and bromoacetamide reagents, methods of analysis, and subsequent addition of metal ions. Anal Biochem 1984; 142:68–78.
7. Brechbiel MW, Gansow OA, Atcher RW. Synthesis of 1-(p-isothiocynatobenzyl)-derivatives of DTPA and EDTA. Antibody labeling and tumor imaging studies. Inorg Chem 1986; 25:2772–2778.
8. Yeh SM, Sherman DG, Meares CF. A new route to "bifunctional" chelating agents: conversion of amino acids to analogs of ethylenedinitroilotetraacetic acid. Anal Biochem 1979; 100:152–159.
9. Sundberg MW, Meares CF, Goodwin DA, Diamanti CI. Selective binding of metal ions to macromolecules using bifunctional analogs of EDTA. J Med Chem 1974; 17:1304–1307.
10. Roselli M, Schlom J, Gansow OA, Raubitschek A, Mirzadeh S, Brechbiel MW, Colcher D. Comparative biodistributions of yttrium and indium-labeled monoclonal

antibody B72.3 in athymic nude mice bearing human colon carcinoma xenografts. J Nucl Med 1989; 30:672–682.

11. Deshpande SV, Subramanian R, McCall MJ, DeNardo SJ, DeNardo GL, Meares CF. Metabolism of indium chelates attached to monoclonal antibody: minimal transchelation of indium from Benzyl-EDTA chelate in vivo. J Nucl Med 1990; 31:218–224.

12. Meares CF, Moi MK, Diril H, Kukis DL, McCall MJ, Deshpande SV, DeNardo SJ, Snook D, Epenetos AA. Macrocyclic chelates of radiometals for diagnosis and therapy. Br J Cancer 1990; 62(suppl):21–26.

13. Moerlein SM, Welch MJ, Raymond KN, Weitl FL. Tricatecholamide analogs of enterobactin as gallium- and indium-binding radiopharmaceuticals. J Nucl Med 1981; 22:710–719.

14. Hunt FC. Potential radiopharmaceuticals for the diagnosis of biliary atresia and neonatal hepatitis: EHPG and HBED chelates of ^{67}Ga and [111]In. Nucl Med Biol 1988; 15:659–664.

15. Mathias CJ, Sun Y, Welch MJ, Green MA, Thomas JA, Wade KR, Martell AE. Targeting radiopharmaceuticals: comparative biodistribution studies of gallium and indium complexes of multidentate ligands. Nucl Med Biol 1988; 15:69–81.

16. Pearson RG. Hard and soft acids and bases. J Am Chem Soc 1963; 85:3533–3539.

17. Hayes RL, Carlton JE, Byrd BL. Bone scanning with gallium-68: a carrier effect. J Nucl Med 1965; 6:605–610.

18. Weiner RE, Thakur ML, Goodman M, Hoffer PB. Relative stability of In-111 and Ga-67 desferrioxamine and human transferrin complexes. In: Radiopharmaceuticals II. New York: Society of Nuclear Medicine, 1979:331–340.

19. Green MA, Welch MJ, Mathias CJ, Fox KAA, Knabb RM, Huffman JC. Gallium-68 1,1,1-tris(5-methoxysalicylaldiminomethyl)ethane: a potential tracer for evaluation of regional myocardial blood flow. J Nucl Med 1985; 26:170–180.

20. Broan CJ, Cox JPL, Craig AS, Kataky R, Parker D, Harrison A, Randall AM, Ferguson G. Structure and solution stability of indium and gallium complexes of 1,4,7-triazacyclononanetriacetate and of yttrium complexes of 1,4,7,10-tetraazacyclododecanetetraacetate and related ligands: kinetically stable complexes for use in imaging and radioimmunotherapy. X-ray molecular structure of the indium and gallium complexes of 1,4,7-triazacyclononane-1,4,7-triacetic acid. J Chem Soc Perkin Trans 1991; 2:87–91.

21. Clarke ET, Martell AE. Stabilities of trivalent metal ion complexes of the tetraacetate derivatives of 12-, 13- and 14-membered tetraazamacrocycles. Inorg Chim Acta 1991; 190:37–46.

22. Wagner SJ, Welch MJ. Gallium-68 labeling of albumin and albumin microspheres. J Nucl Med 1979; 20:428–433.

23. Yokohama A, Ohmomo Y, Horiuchi K, Saji R, Tanaka H, Yamamoto K, Ishii Y, Torizuka K. Desferrioxamine, a promising bifunctional chelating agent for labeling proteins with gallium: Ga-67 DF-HSA. J Nucl Med 1982; 23:909–914.

24. Janoki AG, Harwig JF, Wolf W. Studies on high specific activity labeling of proteins using bifunctional chelates. Nucl Med Biol 1982; 1:689–692.

25. Larson SM, Allen DR, Ramsey JS, Grunbaum Z. Kinetics of binding of carrier-free Ga-67 to human transferrin. J Nucl Med 1978; 19:1245–1249.

26. Wike JS, Guyer CE, Ramey DW, Phillips BP. Chemistry for commercial scale production of yttrium-90 for medical research. Appl Radiat Isot 1990; 41:861.
27. Dietz ML, Horwitz EP. Improved chemistry for the production of yttrium-90 for medical applications. Appl Radiat Isot 1992; 43:1093–1101.
28. Rowlinson G, Snook D, Stewart S, Epenetos AA. Intravenous EDTA to reduce bone uptake of Y-90 following Y-90 labeled antibody administration. Br J Cancer 1989; 59:322–328.
29. Moi MK, Meares CF, DeNardo SJ. The peptide way to macrocyclic bifunctional chelating agents: Synthesis of 2-(p-nitrobenzyl)-1,4,7,10-tetraazacyclododecane-N-N′,N″,N‴-tetraacetic acid and study of its yttrium (III) complex. J Am Chem Soc 1988; 110:6266–6267.
30. Kozak RW, Raubitschek A, Mirzadeh S, Brechbiel MW, Junghaus R, Gansow OA, Waldmann TA. Nature of the bifunctional chelating agent used for radioimmunotherapy with yttrium-90 monoclonal antibodies: critical factors in determining in vivo survival and organ toxicity. Cancer Res 1989; 49:2639–2644.
31. Loncin E, Desreux MF, Merciny JF. Coordination of lanthanides by two polyamino polycarboxylic macrocycles: formation of highly stable lanthanide complexes. Inorg Chem 1986; 25:2646–2648.
32. Deshpande SY, DeNardo SJ, Kukis DL, McCall ML, DeNardo GL, Meares CF. Yttrium-90 labeled monoclonal antibody for therapy: labeling by a new macrocyclic bifunctional chelating agent. J Nucl Med 1990; 31:473–479.
33. Watanabe N, Goodwin DA, Meares CF, et al. Immunogenicity in rabbits and mice of an antibody-chelate conjugate: comparison of (s) and (R) macrocyclic enantiomers and an acyclic chelating agent. Cancer Res 1994; 54:1049–1054.
34. Kosmas C, Snook D, Gooden CS, et al. Development of humoral immune responses against a macrocyclic chelating agent (DOTA) in cancer patients receiving radioimmunoconjugates for imaging and therapy. Cancer Res 1992; 52:904–911.
35. Kosmas C, Maraveyas A, Gooden CS, Snook D, Epenetos AA. Anti-chelate antibodies after intraperitoneal yttrium-90-labeled monoclonal antibody immunoconjugates for ovarian cancer therapy. J Nucl Med 1995; 36:746–753.
36. Camera L, Kinuya S, Garmestani K, Wu C, Brechbiel MW, Pai LH, McMurry TJ, Ganson OA, Pastan I, Paik CH, Carrasquillo JA. Evaluation of the serum stability and in vivo biodistribution of CHX-DTPA and other ligands for yttrium labeling of monoclonal antibodies. J Nucl Med 1994; 35:882–889.
37. Kobayashi H, WU C, Yoo TM, Sun B-F, Drumm D, Pastan I, Paik CH, Gansow OA, Carrasquillo JA, Brechbiel MW. Evaluation of the in vivo biodistribution of yttrium-labeled isomers of CHX-DTPA-conjugated monoclonal antibodies. J Nucl Med 1998; 39:829–836.
38. DeNardo SJ, Kukis DL, Miers LA, Winthrop MD, Kroger LA, Salako Q, Shen S, Lamborn KR, Gumerlock PH, Meares CF, DeNardo GL. Yttrium-90-DOTA-peptide chimeric L6 radioimmunoconjugate: efficacy and toxicity in mice bearing p53 mutant human breast cancer xenografts. J Nucl Med 1998; 39:842–849.
39. Li M, Meares CF. Synthesis, metal chelate stability studies, and enzyme digestion of A peptide-linked DOTA derivative and its corresponding radiolabeled immunoconjugates. Bioconj Chem 1993; 4:275–283.
40. DeNardo SJ, Kukis DL, Kroger LA, O'Donnell RT, Lamborn KR, Miers LA, De-

Nardo DG, Meares CF, DeNardo GL. Synergy of taxol and radioimmunotherapy with yttrium-90-labeled chimeric L6 antibody: efficacy and toxicity in breast cancer xenografts. Proc Natl Acad Sci USA 1997; 94:4000–4004.

41. Moi MK, Meares CF, McCall MJ, Cole WC, DeNardo SJ. Copper chelates as probes of biological systems: stable copper complexes with a macrocyclic bifunctional chelating agent. Anal Biochem 1985; 148:249–253.

42. Green MA, Mathias CJ, Welch MJ, McGuire AH, Perry D, Fernandez-Rubio F, Perlmutter JS, Raichle ME, Bergman SR. Copper-62-labeled pyruvaldehyde bis(N-4-methylthiosemicarbazonato)copper(II): synthesis and evaluation as a positron emission tomography tracer for cerebral and myocardial perfusion. J Nucl Med 1990; 31:1989–1996.

43. Anderson CJ, Connett JM, Schwarz SW, Rocque PA, Guo LW, Philpott GW, Zinn KR, Meares CF, Welch MJ. Copper-64-labeled antibodies for PET imaging. J Nucl Med 1992; 33:1685–1691.

44. Connett JM, Anderson CJ, Guo L-W, Schwarz SW, Zinn KR, Rogers BE, Siegel BA, Philpott GW, Welch MJ. Radioimmunotherapy with a ^{64}Cu-labeled monoclonal antibody: a comparison with ^{67}Cu. Proc Natl Acad Sci USA 1996; 93:6814–6818.

45. Zinn KR, Chaudhuri TR, Cheng TP, Meyer WA, Morris JS. Production of no-carrier added ^{64}Cu from zinc metal irradiated under boron shielding. Cancer 1994; 73:774–778.

46. McCarthy DW, Shefer RE, Klinkowstein RE, Bass LA, Margeneau WH, Cutler CS, Anderson CJ, Welch MJ. Efficient production of high specific activity ^{64}Cu using a biomedical cyclotron. Nucl Med Biol 1997; 24:35–43.

47. Mirzadeh S, Mausner LF, Srivastava SC. Production of no-carrier added ^{67}Cu. Appl Radiat Isot 1986; 37:29.

48. Troutner DE. Chemical and physical properties of radionuclides. Int J Radiat Appl Instrum Part B 1987; 14:171–176.

49. Ringborn A. Complexation in Analytical Chemistry. New York: Interscience, 1963.

50. Lau SJ, Sarkar B. Ternary coordination complex between human serum albumin, copper (II), and L-histidine. J Biol Chem 1971; 246:5938–5943.

51. White A, Handler P, Smith EL. Principles of Biochemistry 4th ed. New York: McGraw-Hill, 1968:711.

52. Studer M, Kaden TA, Maecke HR. Reactivity studies of the pendant carboxylic group in a macrocyclic Cu^{2+} complex towards amide formation and its use as a protein-labeling agent. Helv Chim Acta 1990; 73:149–153.

53. Franz J, Freeman GM, Barefield EK, Volkert WA, Ehrhardt GJ, Holmes RA. Labeling of antibodies with ^{64}Cu using a conjugate containing a macrocyclic amine chelating agent. Nucl Med Biol 1987; 14:479–484.

54. Deshpande SV, DeNardo SJ, Meares CF, McCall MJ, Adams GP, Moi K, DeNardo GL. Copper-67-labeled monoclonal antibody Lym-1, a potential radiopharmaceutical for cancer therapy: labeling and biodistribution in RAJI tumored mice. J Nucl Med 1988; 29:217–225.

55. DeNardo GL, DeNardo SJ, Meares CF, Kukis D, Moody DC, Deshpande SV. Pharmacokinetics of copper-67 conjugated Lym-1, a potential therapeutic radioimmunoconjugate, in mice and in patients with lymphoma. Antibody Immunoconj Radiopharm 1991; 4:777–785.

56. Morphy JR, Parker D, Kataky R, Eaton MAW, Millican AT, Alexander R, Harrison A, Walker C. Towards tumour targeting with copper-radiolabeled macrocycle-antibody conjugates: synthesis, antibody linkage, and complexation behaviour. J Chem Soc Perkin Trans 1990; 2:573–585.

57. Cole WC, DeNardo SJ, Meares CF, McCall MJ, DeNardo GL, Epstein AL, O'Brien HA, Moi MK. Comparative serum stability of radiochelates for antibody radiopharmaceuticals. J Nucl Med 1987; 28:83–90.

58. Kukis DL, Diril H, Greiner DP, DeNardo SJ, DeNardo GL, Salako QA, Meares CF. A comparative study of copper-67 radiolabeling and kinetic stabilities of antibody-macrocyclic chelate conjugates. Cancer 1994; 73(suppl):779–786.

59. O'Donoghue JA, Bardies M, Wheldon TE. Relationships between tumor size and curability for uniformly targeted therapy with b-emitting radionuclides. J Nucl Med 1995; 36:1902–1909.

60. Jia W, Ehrhardt GJ. Progress toward enhanced specific activity Re-186 using inorganic Szilard-Chalmers methods. In: Nicolini M, Bandoli G, Mazzi U, eds. Technetium and Rhenium in Chemistry and Nuclear Medicine 4. Padova, Italy: SGE Editoriali, 1995:379–381.

61. Blumer M, Ehrhardt GJ, Su F-M. Experience with aluminum perrhenate targets for production of Re-186 and Re-188. J Nucl Med 1994; 35:242. Abstract.

62. Ehrhardt GJ, Ketring AR, Liang Q, Miller RA, Holmes RA, Wolfangel RG. Refinement of the peroxide process for making W-188/Re/188 and Mo-99/Tc-99m gel radioisotope generators for nuclear medicine. In: Nicolini M, Bandoli G, Mazzi U, eds. Technetium and Rhenium in Chemistry and Nuclear Medicine 4. Padova, Italy: SGE Editoriali, 1995:313–317.

63. Knapp FF Jr, Mirzadeh S, Beets AL, Sharket R, Griffiths G, Juweid M, Goldenberg DM. Curie-scale tungsten-188/rhenium-188 generators for routine clinical applications. In: Nicolini M, Bandoli G, Mazzi U, eds. Technetium and Rhenium in Chemistry and Nuclear Medicine 4. Padova, Italy: SGE Editoriali, 1995:319–323.

64. Deutsch EA, Libson K, Vanderheyden J-L, Ketring AR, Maxon HR. The chemistry of rhenium and technetium as related to the use of isotopes of these elements in therapeutic and diagnostic nuclear medicine. Nucl Med Biol 1986; 13:465–477.

65. Jones AG, Davison A. The relevance of basic technetium chemistry to nuclear medicine. J Nucl Med 1982; 23:1041–1043.

66. Davison A, Jones A, Orvig C, Sohn MG. A new class of oxotechnetium(5^+)chelate complexes containing a $TcON_2S_2$ core. Inorg Chem 1981; 20:1629–1632.

67. Rao TN, Adhikesavalu D, Camerman A, Fritzberg AR. Technetium(V) and rhenium(V) complexes of 2,3-bis(mercaptoacetamido)-propanoate. Chelate ring stereochemistry and influence on chemical and biological properties. J Am Chem Soc 1990; 112:5798–5804.

68. Griffiths GL, Goldenberg DM, Diril H, Hansen HJ. Technetium-99m, rhenium-186, and rhenium-188 direct-labeled antibodies. Cancer 1994; 73:761–768.

69. John E, Thakur ML, DeFulvio J, McDevitt MR, Damjanov I. Rhenium-186-labeled monoclonal antibodies for radioimmunotherapy: preparation and evaluation. J Nucl Med 1992; 34:260–267.

70. Griffiths GL, Goldenberg DM, Jones AL, Hansen HJ. Radiolabeling of monoclonal

antibodies and fragments with technetium and rhenium. Bioconj Chem 1992; 3:91–99.

71. Quadri SM, Wessels BW. Radiolabeled biomolecules with [186]Re: potential for radio-immunotherapy. Nucl Med Biol 1986; 13:447–451.

72. Fritzberg AR, Nunn AD. Radio HPLC application to organics and metal chelate chemistry. In: Wieland D, Tobes M, Manger T, eds. Analytical and Chromatographic Techniques in Radiopharmaceutical Chemistry. Los Angeles: Springer-Verlag, 1985:183–212.

73. Fritzberg AR, Abrams PG, Beaumier PL, Kasina S, Morgan AC, Rao TN, Reno JM, Sanderson JA, Srinivasan A, Wilbur DS, Vanderheyden, J-L. Specific and stable labeling of antibodies with technetium-99m using a diamide dimercaptide (N_2S_2) chelating agent. Proc Natl Acad Sci USA 1988; 85:4025–4029.

74. Fritzberg AR, Vanderheyden J-L, Morgan AC, Schroff RW, Abrams PG. Rhenium-186/-188 labeled antibodies for radioimmunotherapy. In: Nicolini M, Bandoli G, Mazzi U, eds. Technetium and Rhenium in Chemistry and Nuclear Medicine 3. Verona, Italy: Cortina International, 1990:615–622.

75. Su F-M, Lyen L, Breitz HB, Weiden PL, Fritzberg AR. [186]Rhenium Mag_2GABA antibody radiolabeling. In: Nicolini M, Bandoli G, Mazzi U, eds. Technetium and Rhenium in Chemistry and Nuclear Medicine 4. Padova, Italy: SGE Editoriali, 1995: 511–517.

76. Visser GWM, Gerretsen M, Herscheid JDM, Snow GB, van Dongen G. Labeling of monoclonal antibodies with rhenium-186 using the MAG_3 chelate for radioimmunotherapy of cancer: a technical protocol. J Nucl Med 1993; 34:1953–1963.

77. Ram S, Buchsbaum DJ. A peptide-based bifunctional chelating agent for [99m]Tc- and [186]Re-labeling of monoclonal antibodies. Cancer 1994; 73:769–773.

78. Vanderheyden J-L, Su F-M, Venkatesan P, Beaumier P, Bugaj J, Fritzberg A. The chemistry of rhenium-186 labeled antibodies and F(ab′)$_2$ fragments for RIT in animals and man. J Nucl Med 1990; 31:823. Abstract.

79. Su F-M, Axworthy D, Galster J, Weiden P, Vanderheyden J-L, Fritzberg AR. Characterization of patients urinary catabolites from Re-186 radiolabeled monoclonal antibodies and fragments. J Nucl Med 1990; 31:823. Abstract.

80. Srinivasan A, Kasina S, Fitzner JN, Gustavson LG, Reno JM, Rao TN, Sanderson JA, Gray MA, Axworthy D, Fritzberg AR. Modified bifunctional amide thiolate ligands: enhanced utility of Tc-99m Fab for radioimmunodetection. J Nucl Med 1990; 31:747. Abstract.

81. Su F-M, Axworthy DB, Vanderheyden J-L, Srinivasan A, Fitzner J, Galster J, Kasina S, Reno J, Beaumier P, Fritzberg AR. Evaluation of a cleavable N_3S-hydroxyl ester ligand for improved targeting of rhenium-186 antibodies. J Nucl Med 1991; 32: 1020. Abstract.

82. Beaumier P, Venkatesan P, Vanderheyden J-L, Burgua WD, Kunz LL, Fritzberg AR, Abrams PG, Morgan AC Jr. [186]Re radioimmunotherapy of small cell lung carcinoma xenografts in nude mice. Cancer Res 1991; 51:676–681.

83. Najafi A, Alauddin MM, Sosa A, Ma GQ, Chen DCP, Epstein AL, Siegel ME. The evaluation of [186]Re-labeled antibodies using N_2S_4 chelate in vitro and in vivo using tumor-bearing nude mice. Nucl Med Biol 1992; 19:205–212.

84. Gerretsen M, Visser GWM, van Walsum M, Meijer CJLM, Snow GB, van Dongen

GAMS. [186]Re-labeled monoclonal antibody E48 immunoglobulin G-mediated therapy of human head and neck squamous cell carcinoma xenografts. Cancer Res 1993; 53:3524–3529.

85. Zalutsky MR, Bigner DD. Radioimmunotherapy with a-particle emitting radioimmunoconjugates. Acta Oncol 1996; 35:373–379.

86. Zalutsky MR, Schuster JM, Garg PK, Archer GE Jr., Dewhirst MW, Bigner DD. Two approaches for enhancing radioimmunotherapy: α emitters and hyperthermia. Recent Results Cancer Res 1996; 141:101–122.

87. Huneke RB, Pippin CG, Squire RA, Brechbiel MW, Gansow OA, Strand M. Effective a-particle-mediated radioimmunotherapy of murine leukemia. Cancer Res 1992; 52:5818–5821.

88. Rotmensch J, Whitlock JL, Schwartz JL, Hines JJ, Reba RC, Harper PV. In vitro and in vivo studies on the development of the a-emitting radionuclide bismuth 212 for intraperitoneal use against microscopic ovarian carcinoma. Am J Obstet Gynecol 1997; 176:833–841.

89. Zalutsky MR, McLendon RE, Garg PK, Archer GE, Schuster JM, Bigner DD. Radioimmunotherapy of neoplastic meningitis in rats using an a-particle-emitting immunoconjugate. Cancer Res 1994; 54:4719–4725.

90. Beyer GJ, Offord RE, Kunz G, Jones RMI, Ravn U, Aleksandrova Y, Werlen RC, Macke H, Lindroos M, Jahn S, Tengblad D. Biokinetics of monoclonal antibodies labeled with radio-lanthanides and 225-Ac in xenografted nude mice. Proc. 12th Int Symp Radiopharm Chem, Uppsala, Sweden, 1997:529–530.

91. Scheinberg DA. Presentation of Phase I clinical study in leukemia patients. AAAS, 163rd Meeting, Seattle WA, 1997.

92. Wu C, Brechbiel MW, Gansow OA. An improved generator for the production of [213]Bi from [225]Ac. Radiochim Acta 1997; 79:141–144.

93. Boll RA, Mirzadeh S, Kennel SJ. Optimizations of radiolabeling of immunoproteins with [213]Bi. Radiochim Acta 1997; 79:145–149.

94. Atcher RW, Friedman AM, Hines JJ. An improved generator for the production of [212]Pb and [212]Bi from [224]Ra. Appl Radiat Isot 1988; 39:283–286.

95. Kumar K, Magerstädt M, Gansow OA. Lead (II) and bismuth (III) complexes of the polyazacycloalkane-N-acetic acids nota, dota, and teta. Chem Comm 1989; 145–146.

96. Pippin CG, McMurry TJ, Brechbiel MW, McDonald M, Lambrecht R, Milenic D, Roselli M, Colcher D, Gansow OA. Lead (II) complexes of 1,4,7,10-tetraazacyclododecane-N,N′,N″,N‴-tetraacetate: solution chemistry and application to tumor localization with [203]Pb labeled monoclonal antibodies. Inorg Chim Acta 1995; 239: 43–51.

97. Mirzadeh S, Kumar K, Gansow OA. The chemical fate of [212]Bi-DOTA produced by β-decay of [212]Pb(DOTA)$^{2-}$. Radiochim Acta 1993; 60:1–10.

98. Horak E, Hartmann F, Garmestani G, Wu C, Brechbiel M, Gansow OA, Landolfi NF, Waldmann TA. Radioimmunotherapy targeting of HER2/neu oncoprotein on ovarian tumor using lead-212-DOTA-AE1. J Nucl Med 1987; 38:1944–1950.

4

Radiohalogens for Radioimmunotherapy

Michael R. Zalutsky
Duke University Medical Center, Durham, North Carolina

I. INTRODUCTION

The selective delivery of cytotoxic radionuclides to malignant cell populations is the central objective of radioimmunotherapy. The impact of radioimmunotherapy on the clinical management of cancer has generally been limited, particularly for the treatment of solid tumors. Nonetheless, labeled monoclonal antibody (mAb) therapy remains an attractive approach for cancer treatment with the caveat that its success will depend on improving mAb specificity, delivery, and radiolabeling. In preclinical settings, promising advances have been achieved in these three areas and they will be investigated soon in clinical trials. First, molecular biological techniques have demonstrated that malignant transformation can lead to gene rearrangement, yielding truly tumor-specific targets. For example, an epidermal growth factor receptor deletion mutant has been identified which is present on several tumor cell populations but not on normal tissues, and mAbs specific for this receptor have been developed (1). Second, efforts to improve mAb tumor delivery not only have involved the generation of novel molecular constructs (2,3) but also have been directed at augmenting mAb tumor uptake through modification of tumor hemodynamics (4). And third, a considerable effort has been directed at improving mAb radiolabeling. In that regard, the current status of mAb radiohalogenation approaches will be summarized in this review.

II. SELECTION OF THE RADIONUCLIDE

The selection of a nuclide with characteristics that are well matched to those of the intended tumor target is an important consideration for radioimmunotherapy. A key element of this process is the identification of radionuclides that emit radiation with a range in tissue that is compatible with the size, location, and geometry of a particular tumor. Clearly, different types of radiation would be expected to be more effective for use with large, solid tumors than would be preferred for treating metastasis consisting of only a few hundred cells. The degree of homogeneity of mAb localization in tumor is an additional factor pertinent to radiation range which must be considered. By utilizing radiation with a relatively long range, heterogeneities of antibody deposition in tumor can be overcome through the crossfire irradiation of cancer cells that do not accumulate the labeled mAb.

Other factors are relevant to the decision whether to pursue a radiohalogen or radiometal. Although the number of metallic radionuclides far exceeds the number of halogen radionuclides, appropriate chemistries must be developed for each element to provide a labeled mAb with high immunoreactivity and in vivo stability. From a practical perspective, radionuclide availability is an important issue. For example, ^{67}Cu has excellent properties for mAb labeling including β emissions of similar energy as those of ^{131}I; however, ^{67}Cu is at best available only sporadically, and at a cost considerably higher than that of ^{131}I. In addition, the catabolites created during the degradation of the labeled mAb should clear rapidly from normal tissues. This is of particular concern for metallic radionuclides which localize in bone when released in ionic form, with the potential consequence of creating dose-limiting bone marrow toxicity. Finally, the physical half life of the radionuclide should be compatible with the pharmacokinetics of the labeled mAb or fragment.

Radiohalogen nuclides are available which emit radiation of multicellular to subcellular range (Table 1). Iodine-131 is a β-emitter with a range in tissue of several millimeters and the majority of clinical radioimmunotherapy trials have used ^{131}I (5,6). At the other extreme are radionuclides emitting radiation of subcellular range. The radiohalogens ^{77}Br, ^{125}I, and ^{123}I, by virtue of their Auger and Coster-Kronig electrons, fall within this category. These radionuclides have therapeutic potential when combined with mAbs that are internalized into the tumor cell after binding. These low-energy electrons act as high linear energy transfer (LET) radiation and are extremely cytotoxic when localized in close proximity to the cell nucleus. A potential advantage of low-energy electron emitters is the low toxicity to antigen-negative normal cells which lack the capacity for internalization of the labeled mAb. In other settings, it might be ideal to use radiation with a range of only a few cell diameters, particularly when the tumor is located in close proximity to highly radiation sensitive normal tissues such as bone mar-

Table 1 Radiohalogen Nuclides of Potential Utility for Radioimmunotherapy

Nuclide	Half-life	Decay mode	Energy (keV)	Yield (%)
^{77}Br	57.0 hours	Auger	1.3	113
		Auger	0.04–0.08	357
^{123}I	13.0 hours	Auger	<0.001	851
		Coster-Kronig	<0.001	531
^{125}I	60.1 days	Auger	<0.001	1418
		Coster-Kronig	<0.001	887
^{131}I	8.1 days	β	336	13
		β	606	86
^{211}At	7.2 hours	α	5866	42
		α	7450	58

row. Alpha particles such as those emitted by ^{211}At have a range in tissue of 55 to 80 μm and thus offer the possibility of matching the cellular specificity of mAb targeting with radiation of similar dimensions.

In the following sections, the current status and future prospects of radioimmunotherapy using radiohalogen nuclides will be discussed. Emphasis will be placed on radioiodination methodologies and the impact of mAb cellular processing on the nature of the radiolabeling approach. In addition, because it is anticipated that their evaluation in patients will soon commence, studies with ^{211}At-labeled mAbs will be highlighted.

III. IODINE RADIONUCLIDES

A. Rationale for Radioimmunotherapy

1. Iodine-131

Iodine-131 was the first radionuclide used for clinical radioimmunodiagnosis and radioimmunotherapy; however, its 364-keV γ-ray is not ideal for imaging and complicates its use for therapy. This motivated the development of methods for labeling mAbs with other β-emitting radionuclides including ^{67}Cu, ^{186}Re, and ^{90}Y; the current status of this work is discussed in the previous chapter. Nonetheless, ^{131}I remains the most frequently used radionuclide for radioimmunotherapy (5,6) and a strong rationale exists for continuing to label mAbs with ^{131}I and other iodine radionuclides. For example, paired-label experiments can be performed using ^{125}I- and ^{131}I-labeled mAbs to compare directly different mAbs, routes of injection, and labeling methods in the same animal or patient. In this way, variations in tumor size, antigen expression, and hemodynamics among different groups can be factored out.

The ability to image and treat with radionuclides of the same element greatly facilitates the use of quantitative mAb imaging to estimate dosimetry prior to therapy. In contrast, the lack of a suitable γ-emitting yttrium radionuclide necessitates the calculation of ^{90}Y-labeled mAb dosimetry on the basis of imaging studies performed with ^{111}In-labeled mAbs. This could result in an underestimation of dose to bone marrow (7); however, improved labeling methods should minimize this problem in the future. In contrast, radionuclides of the same element suitable for quantitative, tomographic imaging are available for use in tandem with ^{131}I-labeled mAb therapy. Single-photon emission tomography using ^{123}I-labeled mAbs have been used to estimate tumor and normal tissue dosimetry in patients with glioma (8), and dosimetric calculations based on positron emission tomographic images of ^{124}I-labeled mAb distributions also have been reported (9,10).

Yttrium-90 is perhaps the most extensively evaluated alternative radionuclide to ^{131}I for radioimmunotherapy. The higher β-particle energy of ^{90}Y may help compensate for heterogeneities in mAb uptake, particularly in large tumors, but the lower β-energy of ^{131}I might be advantageous for other applications. If radioimmunotherapy is ultimately to be utilized as an adjuvant for treating small metastasis, then shorter-range β-emitters would be preferable since they would deposit a greater fraction of their decay energy in the tumor (11,12). Iodine-131 also may be better for treating compartmental tumors such as neoplastic meningitis, which is characterized by free-floating tumor cells in the cerebrospinal fluid and tumor on the surface of the cavity. Dose ratios of cerebrospinal fluid to normal spinal cord absorbed for ^{131}I-labeled mAbs have been estimated to be six to nine times higher than for mAbs labeled with ^{90}Y (13). An additional advantage of ^{131}I for radioimmunotherapy is that the clearance of activity from normal tissue is generally more rapid than with metallic radionuclides. This may account for the fact that in preclinical studies comparing ^{131}I- and ^{90}Y-labeled mAbs at equitoxic doses, considerably higher radiation dose could be delivered to tumor using ^{131}I (14,15).

2. Iodine-125 and Iodine-123

Radionuclides which emit short-range Auger and Coster-Kronig electrons are exquisitely cytotoxic when localized in close proximity to the cell nucleus. The potential for utilizing low-energy electron emitters for radiotherapy has been demonstrated in extensive investigations with the thymidine analogue 5-iodo-2'-deoxyuridine (IUdR) which can be incorporated into cellular DNA (reviewed in Ref. 16). With IUdR as the carrier molecule, ^{125}I exhibits high-LET cytotoxic effects and ^{131}I does not; the mean activity required to reduce survival to 37% was 0.10 pCi per cell for ^{125}I compared with 1.16 pCi per cell for ^{131}I. The feasibility of combining ^{125}I with an internalizing mAb for radioimmunotherapy has been demonstrated by Bender et al. (17). When a mAb directed against the external domain of the epidermal growth factor receptor was radioiodinated, its cytotoxic effectiveness against human glioma cells both in vitro and in vivo was significantly higher with ^{125}I than with ^{131}I.

The 13.1-hour half-life radionuclide ^{123}I might be a more useful Auger emitter than ^{125}I despite the fact that the number of low-energy electrons emitted per decay is higher for ^{125}I (13.8 vs. 23.1) (18). The half-life of ^{123}I is more compatible with the pharmacokinetics of mAbs and mAb fragments. An additional consequence of the shorter half-life of ^{123}I is that fewer atoms must be localized per cell to accumulate a sufficient number of decays to achieve a given cytotoxic dose (19). Studies with [^{123}I]IUdR have demonstrated that ^{123}I can exert high-LET type cytotoxic effects when localized in proximity to the cell nucleus (20).

B. Radioiodination of mAbs by Direct Electrophilic Methods

To date, all clinical radioimmunotherapy trials with radioiodinated mAbs have involved mAbs labeled via electrophilic substitution of the radioiodine directly onto its constituent amino acids. Although under certain conditions, labeling of phenylalanine, cysteine, tryptophan, or histidine residues can occur, at neutral pH, iodination of tyrosine residues predominates (21). Various oxidants have been utilized to generate the electrophilic radioiodinating species; however, the vast majority of therapy-level radioiodinations have been performed using either chloramine-T (22) or Iodogen (23) because these methods are readily adaptable to remote or semiremote preparation.

Although they are convenient, a number of potential problems are associated with direct protein iodination methods. Because they involve exposure of the mAb to oxidizing agents, chemical damage to the protein can occur. Chloramine-T and N-chlorosuccinimide can oxidize methionine, tryptophan, and cysteine residues with the extent of the modification varying from protein to protein (24). These structural alterations may be sufficient to alter the immunoreactivity of the labeled mAb; in fact, some mAbs cannot be labeled successfully using direct methods. For example, incubation of the anti–breast carcinoma mAb DF-3 with as little as 1 μg of Iodogen even in the absence of radioiodine reduced mAb affinity for an antigen-positive tumor cell line to <25% (25).

The most significant disadvantage of mAbs labeled by direct methods for radioimmunotherapy is that they frequently undergo extensive dehalogenation in the in vivo environment. The observation of high activity levels in the stomach and thyroid of animals and patients injected with radioiodinated mAbs (26,27) is indicative of deiodination because these are the organs with the highest proclivity for free iodide. More recent analyses of the chemical form of species created during the catabolism of a mAb F(ab')$_2$ fragment radioiodinated by the Iodogen method have demonstrated that radioiodide is the principal low-molecular-weight catabolite (28). While normal tissue radiation dose can be minimized through the use of blocking agents, dehalogenation is still problematic because it decreases the activity associated with mAb and thus available for binding to tumor.

The increased rate of deiodination of proteins in vivo has generally been considered to be mediated by enzymes involved in the metabolism of thyroid hormones. The rationale for this belief is based on the structural similarity of the labeled template created on the mAb with iodotyrosines and iodothyronines, both of which are rapidly deiodinated in the presence of tissue. The thyroid, liver, kidney, and other normal tissues posses deiodinases of varying specificity for the phenolic and nonphenolic rings of iodothyronines and the phenolic ring of iodotyrosines (29–31). The role of deiodinases in tumor is less clear. Several tumors have been reported to possess deiodinases with a significantly lower K_m than those present in normal tissue (32–34), while other tumors appear to lack deiodinases (35).

C. Radioiodination Methods for Circumventing Deiodination

1. Introduction

If strategies could be devised for minimizing the dehalogenation of mAbs in vivo, then the advantages associated with the use of radioiodine nuclides noted in previous sections could be more fully exploited. Based on the expectation that deiodination could be minimized by decreasing the structural similarity of the iodination site to thyroid hormones, a number of groups including our own have developed protein iodination reagents that do not involve iodination *ortho* to a hydroxyl group on an aromatic ring. The prototypical method consists of two steps: synthesis of N-succinimidyl 3- or 4-[^{131}I]iodobenzoate (SIB) from the corresponding N-succinimidyl (tri-n-butylstannyl)benzoate precursor via iododestannylation followed by conjugation of SIB to lysine ε-amino groups on the mAb (36,37). Several structural modifications of SIB have been investigated including methoxy (38) and methyl (39) substituted SIB analogs as well as the use of vinyl (40) and pyridine (41,42) templates. For an excellent review of the chemistry of these and other radioiodination methods, the reader is referred to an excellent review by Wilbur (43). The following section will focus on results obtained with

SIB because the most promising results to date have been obtained with this reagent.

2. *N*-Succinimidyl Iodobenzoates (SIB)

Direct iodination methods as well as the commercially available Bolton-Hunter reagent (44) result in the substitution of the iodine *ortho* to a hydroxyl group on an aromatic ring. As noted above, this substitution pattern could increase dehalogenation due to the action of endogenous deiodinases. Moreover, the hydroxyl group activates the ring toward hydrolytic dehalogenation. Therefore, a radiohalogenation approach not requiring a hydroxyl group to activate the aromatic ring toward electrophilic iodination was sought. The target compound, SIB, is conceptually similar to the Bolton-Hunter agent with two important changes (Fig. 1). First, SIB lacks a hydroxyl group *ortho* to the iodination site. And second, the two-carbon spacer present in the Bolton-Hunter reagent between the aromatic ring and the active ester was omitted in an attempt to maximize mAb coupling efficiency by minimizing competitive hydrolysis. SIB was synthesized from *N*-succinimidyl 3-(tri-*n*-butylstannyl)benzoate via iododestannylation using *t*-butylhydroperoxide as the oxidant (36). Yields for this step of greater than 85% have been obtained and similar iodination efficiencies have been achieved with the *para* SIB isomer using *N*-chlorosuccinimide as the oxidant (37). Coupling of SIB to mAbs was found to be dependent on mAb concentration and pH; conjugation efficiencies of 70% or more are readily achievable at pH 8.5 and protein concentrations of at least 5 mg/mL. In a direct comparison study, conjugation efficiencies obtained with SIB were about twice those obtained with the Bolton-Hunter reagent (45), confirming the supposition that omitting the two-carbon spacer would increase mAb coupling yields.

Because normal tissue toxicity must be minimized in radioimmunotherapy, it is important to ascertain the normal tissue retention of potential labeled catabolites associated with a particular mAb labeling method. Because SIB labeling generates *m*-iodobenzoic acid-mAb conjugates, a paired-label tissue distribution experiment was performed with *m*-[^{125}I]iodobenzoic acid and [^{131}I]iodide, a likely catabolite from mAbs labeled by direct methods. Clearance of ^{125}I from normal tissues was considerably faster than that of ^{131}I such that by 1 hr, a sixfold difference in whole body activity was observed (46). The fact that this behavior was due in part to the in vivo formation of an iodobenzoic acid-glycine conjugate that is eliminated rapidly via the kidney was demonstrated in a subsequent study (47).

The potential utility of SIB for the radioiodination of intact mAbs has been investigated in studies with murine 81C6, an IgG$_{2b}$ mAb reactive with an epitope of tenascin, an extracellular matrix antigen present on gliomas as well as other tumors. Experiments were performed both in vitro and in athymic mice bearing

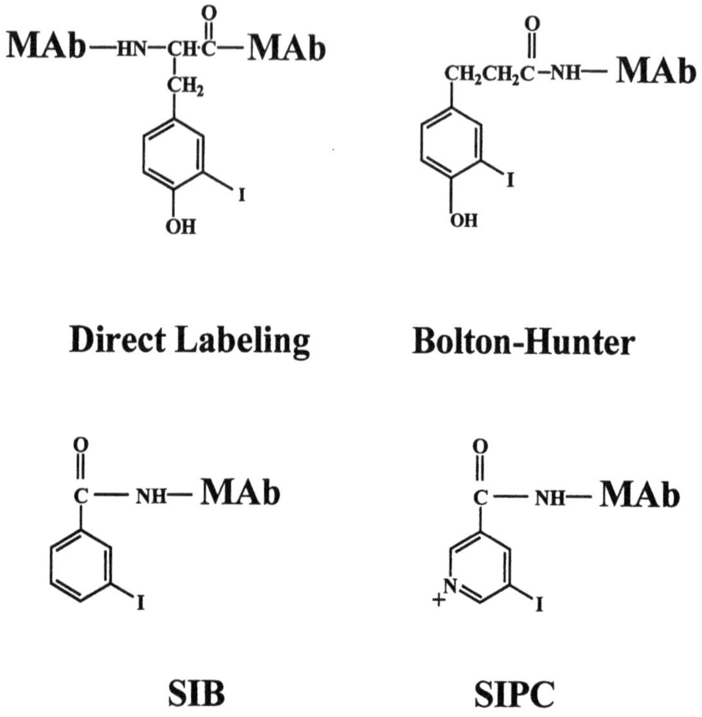

Figure 1 Structure of the iodination site created with various antibody radioiodination approaches. Direct labeling involves substitution of the iodine *ortho* to a hydroxyl group of a constituent tyrosine residue while the Bolton-Hunter, SIB (*N*-succinimidyl 3-iodobenzoate), and SIPC (*N*-succinimidyl 5-iodo-3-pyridinecarboxylate) reagents all react with ε-amino groups on lysine residues on the antibody.

subcutaneous D-54 MG human glioma xenografts to compare the properties of 81C6 labeled using SIB with those when Iodogen was used (48). The immunoreactivity and affinity of 81C6 labeled using SIB were slightly higher than those of the Iodogen preparations. Paired-label tissue distribution experiments demonstrated that labeling 81C6 using SIB decreased thyroid uptake by 40- to 100-fold, suggesting that an increased resistance to deiodination had been achieved. In addition, labeling 81C6 with SIB dramatically increased tumor uptake; the tumor delivery advantage for the SIB preparation increased from twofold to five-fold over 8 days. Finally, superior tumor-to-normal-tissue ratios for 81C6-labeled using SIB were observed consistently. Similar results have been obtained in studies performed with intracranial D-54 MG xenografts as well as in other tenascin-positive human glioma tumor models.

Radiation dose calculations based on these biodistribution data predicted that labeling the 81C6 mAb using SIB would deliver a threefold higher dose to subcutaneous D-54 MG xenografts (48). To determine whether the more favorable tumor accumulation and tumor-to-normal-tissue ratios observed at tracer levels resulted in improved therapeutic efficacy, the treatment potential of 81C6 labeled by the SIB and Iodogen methods were compared (49). SIB could be used for labeling 81C6 at high specific activity; at 24 to 26 µCi/µg, ^{131}I-labeled 81C6 had an affinity constant of 2 to 3 $\times$ 10^8 M^{-1}, a range about twofold higher than observed for mAb labeled at therapy levels using Iodogen. More importantly, treatment outcome was influenced by radioiodination method; with 500 µCi of ^{131}I-labeled 81C6, the tumor growth delay in the SIB group was significantly longer than that observed in the animals receiving mAb labeled using Iodogen. In addition, there were 3 of 10 long-term survivors in the SIB group with no long-term survivors from the Iodogen group. Whether a similar advantage can be obtained in clinical radioimmunotherapy with mAbs labeled using the SIB method remains to be ascertained.

D. Radioiodination Methods for Internalizing mAbs

1. Introduction

The ideal labeling method for a particular mAb is governed by a number of factors not the least of which is the processing of the mAb after binding to tumor cells. Internalizing antigens are some of the most attractive molecular targets for radioimmunotherapy. B-cell lymphoma (50), T-cell leukemia (51), and neuroblastoma (52) all possess antigens that internalize, and a number of clinical radioimmunotherapy trials with mAbs directed against these antigens are under way. In addition, mAbs directed at growth factor receptors, such as the p185 c-*erb*B-2 oncogene product found on breast and ovarian carcinomas (53), and the mutant epidermal growth factor receptor variant III (EGFRvIII) found on breast, lung, and ovarian carcinomas as well as glioma (1), internalize after binding. An additional advantage of using mAbs directed at internalizing antigens for radioimmunotherapy is that internalization can significantly increase the absorbed dose received by the cell nucleus. Even for radiation of multicellular range such as the β-particles of ^{131}I, decay sites located in cytoplasmic vesicles and the cell nucleus increased the dose to the nucleus by factors of about 2 and 10, respectively, compared with decays occurring on the cell membrane (54).

Unfortunately, internalization of conventionally radioiodinated mAbs creates problems from a radiolabeling perspective. Lysosomal degradation of the mAb occurs after internalization with the result that radioactivity from the tumor cell is released in the form of iodotyrosine (51,55). Labeling internalizing mAbs using the SIB method offers no advantages compared with direct labeling methods (56). Two approaches for residualizing radioactivity in tumor cells following mAb internalization will be described in the following sections.

2. Oligosaccharide Conjugates

A number of oligosaccharides are known to be resistant to degradation by lysosomal hydrolases. This property has been exploited for "residualizing" radioiodine in lysosomes by labeling proteins via oligosaccharide-tyramine conjugates (57). The most extensively utilized approach involves the coupling of radioiodinated tyramine-cellobiose (TCB) to the protein (58). In this procedure, TCB is synthesized by reductive amination, radioiodinated using chloramine-T, and the labeled conjugate is coupled to the protein using cyanuric chloride. Labeling mAbs using the TCB method can significantly increase the retention of radioiodine in target cells following internalization compared with mAbs labeled using a conventional method (59,60). In addition, proteins labeled using TCB have exhibited higher tumor retention in mouse (58,59) and rat (61) models.

Our results utilizing TCB for labeling the anti-EGFRvIII mAbs L8A4 and H10 are representative of the advantages that this method can offer for labeling internalizing mAbs (60). An in vitro internalization and cellular processing assay was performed with the HC2 20 d2 EGFRvIII-positive cell line to compare the properties of L8A4 labeled using TCB and Iodogen. Cell-associated activity (76%, TCB; 27%, Iodogen at 20 hr) and protein-associated activity in cell culture supernatants were considerably higher with TCB. Similar comparisons were made in athymic mice bearing subcutaneous HC2 20 d2 xenografts. Two days after injection, tumor retention of radioiodine was two to three times higher for both mAbs when labeled using TCB, and the tumor delivery advantage for TCB rose to 3.4 for L8A4 and 6.7 for H10 at 7 days.

Unfortunately, there also are several disadvantages associated with the TCB method that have been observed by other investigators (59) as well as ourselves (60). Although affinities of the anti-EGFRvIII mAbs labeled via the two methods were comparable, TCB labeling resulted in lower immunoreactivity than seen with Iodogen. In addition, about 10% to 20% of the activity in some TCB mAb preparations was present as aggregates. This probably reflects the potential for creating cross-links due to the three replaceable chlorines in cyanuric chloride. In vivo, significantly higher retention of radioiodine activity in both the spleen and the liver was observed with TCB. Finally, tumor localization indices for TCB-labeled mAbs (measured by paired-label comparison with isotype-matched control mAbs) reached maximum values of about 3, values considerably lower than those generally obtained with non-internalizing mAbs.

Another reagent that has been investigated for the radioiodination of internalizing mAbs is dilactitol-tyramine (DLT). DLT has been radioiodinated using Iodogen and the labeled conjugate coupled to mAbs via the generation of aldehydes with galactose oxidase, followed by reductive amination using sodium cya-noborohydride (57). Unfortunately, the labeling efficiency with this method is quite low, ranging from 3% to 6% (62). Labeling mAbs using DLT increased retention in Calu-3 xenografts by a factor of 6 compared with conventionally radioiodinated mAb; however, liver, spleen and kidney levels were about 50% to 100% higher with DLT. Recently, the therapeutic potential of a mAb labeled with ^{131}I using DLT has been investigated. Tumor regressions of up to 7 weeks' duration were observed in 73% of animals with Calu-3 adenomas of the lung with DLT compared with a 14% regression rate when the Iodogen method was used (63). However, the low specific activity of DLT mAb preparations necessi-tated the use of mAb protein doses in excess of those where optimal tumor tar-geting was achieved.

3. Positively Charged Templates

We have been pursuing an alternative strategy for labeling internalizing mAbs that involves the generation of a template on the mAb that is positively charged at lysosomal pH. Positively charged molecules such as neutral red and chlo-roquine are taken up by lysosomes to such a degree that they are used as markers of this organelle. We hypothesized that if positively charged catabolites were created during mAb proteolysis, then they should also be trapped in the lysosome. *N*-succinimidyl 5-iodo-3-pyridinecarboxylate (SIPC) was utilized to test this hy-pothesis because the positive charge on its pyridine ring (Fig. 1) should lead to labeled catabolites which are positively charged at lysosomal pH. SIPC may be particularly useful for this purpose because noninternalizing mAbs labeled using this reagent did not undergo dehalogenation in vivo and exhibited low retention in normal tissues including liver and spleen (41).

Anti-EGFRvIII mAb L8A4 was radioiodinated using Iodogen, SIPC and SIB, a reagent which renders mAbs inert to deiodination but unlike SIPC, is not positively charged. Internalization and cell retention assays with HC2 20 d2 cells demonstrated that SIPC labeling increased cellular retention of radioiodine by up to 65% compared with mAb labeled using either SIB or Iodogen (56). Analysis of lower-molecular-weight catabolites by HPLC indicated that the radioiodide activity was retained within the cell primarily as an iodonicotinic acid–lysine conjugate, a positively charged molecule.

The tissue distribution of L8A4 radioiodinated using SIPC and Iodogen was compared in athymic mice with HC2 20 d2 xenografts. The SIPC method provided significantly higher tumor uptake over the first 72 hr after injection and more favorable tumor:normal tissue ratios including in the liver (16:1 vs. 5:1 at 72 hr) and in the spleen (26:1 vs. 8:1 at 72 hr). A subsequent study was performed to determine the specificity of mAb uptake in tumor with SIPC label-ing (64). Tumor localization indices for L8A4 of up to 14.8 at 120 hr were observed, compared with a maximum of 3.1 ± 0.5 for TCB (56). This suggests that the specificity of mAb uptake in these xenografts was nearly five times higher with SIPC. A final paired-label experiment compared the tissue distribution of L8A4 labeled with ^{125}I using SIPC and with ^{131}I using TCB (64). The coupling efficiency for labeling mAb L8A4 with SIPC was 50% to 60% compared with 30% for the conjugation of TCB to this mAb at similar protein concentrations. Similar tumor levels of both radionuclides were observed; however, tumor-to-tissue ratios for kidneys, liver, and spleen, organs known to be involved in the catabolism of exogenous proteins, were three times higher for SIPC at later time points. In summary, SIPC appears to be a useful method for labeling internalizing mAbs and it is anticipated that clinical evaluation of the anti-EGFRvIII mAb L8A4 labeled by the SIPC method will soon be initiated.

IV. BROMINE RADIONUCLIDES

A. Rationale for Radioimmunotherapy

Most investigations of the therapeutic potential of Auger and Coster-Kronig electron emitters have utilized ^{125}I; however, there is a strong rationale for pursuing other radionuclides such as 56-h half-life ^{77}Br for therapeutic applications requiring radiation of subcellular range. The feasibility of using ^{77}Br for generating high-LET cell kill was demonstrated by Kassis et al. (65) using the thymidine analogue, 5-[^{77}Br]bromo-2'-deoxyuridine. A potential disadvantage of ^{77}Br is that fewer electrons are emitted per decay than by ^{125}I with a range of <100 nm (5.6 vs. 23.1) (18); nonetheless, ^{77}Br offers several potential advantages. First, the half-life of ^{77}Br is more compatible with the residence time of labeled mAbs on tumor cells. Thus, even though the number of electrons emitted per decay is higher for ^{125}I, as a consequence of its 60-day half-life, most of these decays would be expected to occur after the ^{125}I has become dissociated from the tumor cell. In addition, the carbon-halogen bond strength for bromine is higher than with iodine which should enhance in vivo stability. Finally, bromide, unlike iodide, does not localize in the thyroid, obviating the need for blocking regimes to minimize thyroid toxicity during radioimmunotherapy.

B. Radiobromination of mAbs

Methods for labeling proteins with bromine radionuclides are largely based on those previously developed for radioiodine; however, direct labeling of proteins with bromine may require harsher oxidizing conditions due to the lower oxidation potential of bromine. This may require compromising between obtaining a high labeling efficiency and maximizing the immunoreactivity of the radiobrominated mAb. The labeling of an anti-CEA mAb with ^{76}Br via the chloramine-T and bromoperoxidase methods has been reported (66). Use of chloramine-T resulted in low and irreproducible mAb labeling efficiencies and poor immunoreactivity. More favorable results were obtained with an optimized bromoperoxidase procedure which involved a 40-min reaction at 0°C and quenching the reaction with the addition of sodium metabisulfite. When this protocol was used, the immunoreactivity of ^{76}Br-labeled anti-CEA mAb 38S1 was 74 ± 7%. Separation of the labeled mAb from bromoperoxidase must be accomplished, particularly if the enzyme itself becomes labeled.

Conjugation methods have also been employed for labeling mAbs with ^{77}Br. N-succinimidyl 4-[^{77}Br]bromobenzoate was synthesized via the electrophilic bromodestannylation of N-succinimidyl 4-(tri-n-butylstannyl)benzoate in 44% yield and then coupled to the Fab fragment of anti-melanoma mAb NR-ML-05 (67). Even though several labeled impurities were present in the preparation, mAb conjugation efficiencies were good (60% to 70%). The ^{77}Br-labeled Fab fragment had an immunoreactivity of 80%, equivalent to that obtained with radioiodinated NR-ML-05 Fab.

A potential advantage of labeling mAbs with ^{77}Br (and ^{76}Br for PET imaging) instead of radioiodine nuclides is that they may exhibit more favorable in vivo behavior due to differences in stability and distribution of labeled catabolites. A recent study has compared the tissue distribution of anti-CEA mAb 38S1 labeled with ^{76}Br and ^{125}I labeled using bromoperoxidase and chloramine-T, respectively (68). Athymic rats bearing LS174T human colonic adenocarcinoma xenografts were used as the animal model. Uptake of ^{76}Br in tumor was slightly higher than that of ^{125}I; however, an even more pronounced increase in ^{76}Br uptake was seen in normal organs, resulting in less favorable tumor-to-normal tissue ratios for the ^{76}Br-labeled mAb. In an attempt to understand the reason for these differences, the nature of the labeled catabolites generated during the degradation of the ^{76}Br- and ^{125}I-labeled mAbs was analyzed. In both tumor and normal tissues, levels of radioactivity associated with intact mAb were quite similar for both radionuclides; however, the amount of [^{76}Br]bromide was significantly higher than [^{125}I]iodide. An additional experiment comparing the tissue distribution patterns of the two radiohalides demonstrated that the retention of [^{76}Br]bromide in tissues was much more prolonged than [^{125}I]iodide. Thus, although the dehalogenation rates for the two labeled mAbs were similar, normal tissue levels with ^{76}Br were higher due to the slower clearance of [^{76}Br]bromide from normal tissues.

Because the envisioned therapeutic applications of ^{77}Br would involve internalizing mAbs, it is important to consider the fact that intracellular processing or radiohalogenated mAbs primarily results in the generation of labeled amino acids, not halides (69). In addition, if ^{77}Br is utilized in this context, it would be anticipated that it would be beneficial to utilize a residualizing labeling approach analogous to those described above for iodine radionuclides.

V. ASTATINE RADIONUCLIDES

A. Properties of Astatine-211

For a number of reasons, [211]At has generally been considered to be the most promising α-emitting radionuclide for radioimmunotherapy. First, its 7.2-hr half-life is more compatible with the pharmacokinetics of mAbs and mAb fragments than the alternative α-emitters [212]Bi or [213]Bi, which have half-lives of 61 and 47 min, respectively. In addition, the decay of both bismuth radionuclides also involves the emission of abundant β particles and thus, these radionuclides emit a mixture of high- and low-LET radiations. A simplified version of the double-branched decay scheme of [211]At is presented in Figure 2 illustrating that each decay of [211]At results in the emission of an α-particle. One branch (42%) involves decay to [207]Bi via emission of 5.87-MeV α-particles and the other (58%) is by electron capture to 0.5-sec [211]Po which in turn de-excites by the emission of 7.45-MeV α-particles. The [211]At and [211]Po α-particles have mean ranges in tissue of about 55 and 80 μm, respectively, equivalent to only a few cell diameters. A fortuitous consequence of the [211]At electron capture decay branch is the emission of polonium K x-rays with an energy range of 77 to 92 keV. These x-rays are of sufficient energy to permit external imaging of [211]At distributions by planar methods as well as by single-photon emission computed tomography (70,71).

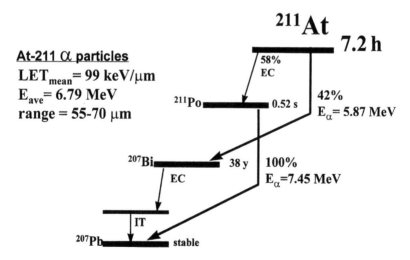

Figure 2   Simplified decay scheme of the 7.2-h half life α-emitter [211]At and properties of its α-particles relevant to radioimmunotherapeutic application.

A significant problem with ^{211}At is that only a few institutions have access to a medium-energy cyclotron equipped with an α particle beam, facilities which are needed for its production via the ^{207}Bi(α,2n)^{211}At reaction. However, advances in ^{211}At production methodologies have made it possible to routinely produce ^{211}At at activity levels sufficient for multiple clinical doses envisioned for ^{211}At-labeled mAbs. We have developed an internal target system which is capable of running at α-particle beam current of up to 85 µA with yields of about 40 Mbq/µAhr (72). Using this system, we have routinely produced in excess of 2 GBq (ca. 60mCi) of ^{211}At and target enhancements currently under evaluation should be able to further increase ^{211}At production.

B. Rationale for Radioimmunotherapy Using α-Emitters

Tumor size, geometrical configuration, and location relative to radiation-sensitive normal tissues are factors that must be considered in selecting the type of radionuclide for a particular radioimmunotherapeutic setting. A number of comparisons have been made between the absorbed dose that would be received from the α-particles of ^{211}At and the β-particles of ^{90}Y. For example, the absorbed fraction ratio for ^{211}At α-particles to ^{90}Y β-particles increases from 9 to 33 as tumor diameter decreases from 1 mm to 0.2 mm (73). Under single-cell conditions, the mean number of cell surface decays of ^{211}At required to achieve cell kill was predicted to be 1200 times lower than needed with ^{90}Y (74). This suggests that radioimmunotherapeutic application of ^{211}At might be well suited for treating lymphomas and other cancers in the circulation, micrometastatic disease, and compartmental cancers such as ovarian carcinoma and neoplastic meningitis. With regard to compartmental application, Roeske and Chen (75) have calculated that treatment of cystic brain tumors might be possible with ^{211}At cystic fluid concentrations as low as 6 µCi/mL compared with 60 µCi/mL for ^{90}Y. An advantage in surface dose per mCi administered for ^{211}At compared with ^{90}Y also was calculated for mAb delivered intraperitoneally for the treatment of ovarian carcinomas (76).

Alpha particles such as those emitted by ^{211}At also offer several advantages from a radiobiological perspective. As a consequence of their high energy and short range in tissue, the LET_{mean} of ^{211}At α-particles is 97 keV/µm, a value about 500 times higher than the LET for the β particles of ^{90}Y and close to that where the biological effectiveness of radiation is maximum (77). This is due to the fact that the distance between ionizing events at this LET is about the same as that between DNA strands resulting in a high probability of creating irreparable double DNA strand breaks, thereby enhancing cytotoxicity (78). Finally, high-LET radiation is attractive for radioimmunotherapy because its cytotoxic effectiveness is nearly independent of cell cycle position, dose rate, and oxygen concentration (77).

C. Astatine-211-Labeled mAbs

1. Labeling Chemistry

Although astatine is the element directly below iodine in the periodic table, their chemistries are sufficiently different that attempts to label proteins cannot be labeled with ^{211}At using direct electrophilic iodination techniques (79). A two-step procedure involving the synthesis of p-[^{211}At]astatobenzoic acid followed by its conjugation with the protein via a mixed anhydride reaction improved in vivo stability; however, radiochemical yields were low and specific activities were less than desirable for radioimmunotherapy (80).

To circumvent these limitations, we investigated the feasibility of labeling proteins using an analog of SIB, N-succinimidyl 3-[^{211}At]astatobenzoate (SAB) (81). Initially, SAB was synthesized by electrophilic astatodestannylation of N-succinimidyl 3-(tri-n-butylstannyl)benzoate using the same reaction conditions developed for the synthesis of SIB; however, radiochemical yields were some-what lower with ^{211}At. One factor that could account for this difference is the larger bulk of the astatine atom compared with iodine. Indeed, use of a stannyl precursor with smaller alkyl substituents, N-succinimidyl 3-(trimethylstannyl)be-nzoate, instead of its tri-n-butyl analog increased radiochemical yields signifi-cantly (82).

The current procedure for labeling mAbs with ^{211}At is as follows: to the chloroform trap containing the ^{211}At activity distilled from the cyclotron target are added t-butylhydroperoxide and N-succinimidyl 3-(trimethylstannyl)ben-zoate. After a 15-min reaction, the SAB is purified by HPLC and then incubated with the mAb in borate buffer on ice for 15 min. Utilizing these methods, ^{211}At-labeled mAbs have been produced in a 90-min total synthesis time at specific activities of up to 4 mCi/mg. Higher specific activities are certainly possible because of the larger quantities of ^{211}At that now can be produced using our internal cyclotron target. However, at least with one mAb, radiation self-dose to the ^{211}At-labeled mAb should be kept <1000 Gy in order to maximize mAb immunoreactivity (83).

2. In Vitro Cytotoxicity of ^{211}At-Labeled mAbs

Because of the short range of ^{211}At α particles, the degree of cell kill is highly dependent on the geometry in which the assay is performed. The cytotoxicity measured under single-cell conditions, monolayer, and spheroids will be different due to variation in crossfire irradiation and the contribution of free ^{211}At-labeled mAb in the incubation medium to tumor cell killing.

The in vitro cytotoxicity of an ^{211}At-labeled TP-3, a mAb reactive with an osteosarcoma-associated antigen, has been investigated both under single-cell conditions and in a microcolony assay. The clonogenic potential of three human

osteosarcoma cell lines was determined under single-cell conditions after incubation with ^{211}At-labeled TP-3 IgG, and to control for nonspecific cell kill, ^{211}At-
labeled bovine serum albumin (BSA), and [^{211}At]astatide (84). At higher specific
activities, the cytotoxicity of ^{211}At-labeled TP-3 was 3 to 80 times higher than
that of ^{211}At-labeled BSA. With specific mAb, reduction in survival to 37% (D_{37})
required about 40 ^{211}At atoms bound per cell. In this micro colony assay, cells
grew as 10 to 15 cell planar arrays, replicating the geometry which might be
present for tumor spread on a cavity surface such as in ovarian carcinoma or
neoplastic meningitis. Osteosarcoma cell microcolonies were treated with ^{211}At-
labeled TP-3 and BSA and the therapeutic gain factor, defined as the ^{211}At-labeled
BSA activity divided by the ^{211}At-labeled TP-3 activity required to reduce microcolony survival to a given level, was calculated (85). The therapeutic gain factor
was about 4, 2, and 1 on antigen-rich, antigen-poor, and antigen-negative cell
lines, respectively. Even more favorable results would have been possible if
higher specific activity preparations had been used. Nonetheless, both of these
studies confirm the exquisite and specific cytotoxicity of ^{211}At-labeled mAbs, and
their comparison shows the importance of considering assay geometry in the
interpretation of experiments of this type.

3. Immunoreactivity and Tissue Distribution of ^{211}At-Labeled mAbs and Fragments

The potential utility of SAB for labeling the F(ab')$_2$ fragment of Mel-14, a mAb
reactive with a chondroitin sulfate proteoglycan found in melanomas and glioma,
has been investigated (82). Immunoreactivity for binding to human glioma homogenate as well as the affinity constant for binding to antigen-positive TE-671
human rhabdomyosarcoma cells for ^{211}At-labeled Mel-14 F(ab')$_2$ were identical
to those seen when this fragment was radioiodinated using the analogous reagent,
SIB. The tissue distribution of ^{211}At-labeled Mel-14 F(ab')$_2$ was evaluated in
athymic mice bearing subcutaneous D-54 MG human glioma xenografts (82).
Tumor retention of ^{211}At and ^{131}I after injection of Mel-14 F(ab')$_2$ labeled using
SAB and SIB were not significantly different until 24 hr, at which time ^{211}At
already had decayed to 10% of initial activity levels. The localization index (ratio
between tissue/blood activity concentration ratios for specific and nonspecific
mAb) was determined by comparing the distribution of ^{211}At-labeled Mel-14 and
isotype-matched nonspecific RPC-5 F(ab')$_2$ in separate groups of mice. The tumor
localization index increased from 1.7 ± 0.3 at 3 hr to 11 ± 1 at 24 hr, while
normal tissue localization indices were near unity at all time points. These results
confirmed that the uptake of ^{211}At-labeled Mel-14 F(ab')$_2$ in these human glioma
xenografts was specific.

Recently, we have evaluated the tissue distribution of ^{211}At-labeled human/
mouse chimeric anti-tenascin mAb 81C6 (86). High coupling efficiencies

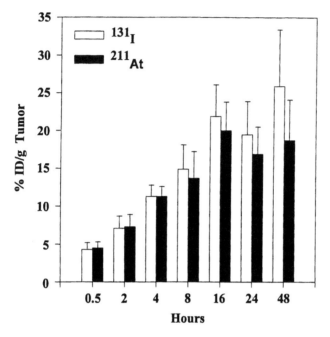

Figure 3 Paired-label tissue distribution of ^{211}At- and ^{131}I-labeled human/mouse chimeric 81C6 antitenascin antibody in athymic mice; retention of ^{211}At and ^{131}I activity in D-54 MG human glioma xenografts as a function of time.

(>70%) of SAB to the mAb were achieved and the specific binding of the ^{211}At-labeled 81C6 to glioma homogenate was 81 ± 8%. A paired-label experiment performed in D-54 MG-bearing athymic mice demonstrated a high degree of similarity in the tissue distribution of mAb labeled using SAB and SIB. As shown in Figure 3, tumor accumulation of ^{211}At and ^{131}I were nearly identical for most of the 48-hr experimental period. Higher retention of ^{211}At in spleen and stomach was observed at some time points; however, ^{211}At/^{131}I tissue activity ratios were less than those seen with the two radiohalogenated Me1-14 F(ab')$_2$ fragments in the same animal model (87).

The in vitro properties and tissue distribution of several other ^{211}At-labeled mAbs and mAb fragments have been determined in athymic mouse human tumor xenograft models. In general, the immunoreactivity and peak tumor uptake observed with SAB labeling were similar to those encountered when the same mAb or fragment was labeled with SIB (88–90). However, with F(ab')$_2$ and Fab fragments, levels of ^{211}At were significantly higher than those of ^{125}I in spleen, stomach, and lungs.

In interpreting these differences in normal tissue behavior, it is necessary to examine the distribution of likely catabolites of mAbs and mAb fragments labeled by these methods. Paired-label comparisons of [^{211}At]astatide and [^{131}I]iodide distribution in normal mice demonstrated that the levels of ^{211}At were higher than ^{131}I in most normal tissue, particularly in the spleen, stomach, and lungs (91). Similar divergent behavior was noted for m-[^{211}At]astatobenzoic and m-[^{131}I]iodobenzoic acids. Given that free halides and halobenzoic acids are catabolites which are anticipated from mAbs labeled using SAB and SIB, the same degree of mAb catabolism would lead to higher normal tissue levels for ^{211}At than for ^{131}I. It appears that the stability of intact mAbs labeled with ^{211}At using SAB may be acceptable for patient studies, particularly in settings where nonintravenous application could be utilized to minimize absorbed dose to normal tissues. On the other hand, alternative methods for labeling mAb fragments with ^{211}At probably will be needed for mAb fragments, particularly when intravenous administration is contemplated.

4. Radioimmunotherapy

The therapeutic potential of ^{211}At-labeled mAbs has not been investigated in solid tumor models because it is unlikely that α-particle-emitting endoradiotherapeutic agents will be effective in this context due to slow diffusion of mAb into the tumor. For this reason, a rat model of neoplastic meningitis was selected for initial evaluation of the radioimmunotherapeutic efficacy of ^{211}At-labeled mAbs (92). Neoplastic meningitis is characterized by free-floating tumor cells in the cerebrospinal fluid and formation of a thin sheet of tumor around the subarachnoid space; thus, its geometry would seem compatible with ^{211}At-labeled mAb therapy. The development of more specific treatments for neoplastic meningitis is an important goal from a clinical perspective because the mean survival for patients with neural primary and extra cranial primary malignancies is only 12 to 13 and 2 to 3 months, respectively.

Neoplastic meningitis was created by giving athymic rats intrathecal injections of TE-671 human rhabdomyosarcoma cells via an indwelling catheter inserted into the subarachnoid space and therapeutic trials were begun 4 to 8 days later, respectively. Histological analyses of selected animals confirmed that tumor had been well established at the time of therapy and had spread from the base of the brain to the caudate equina.

Survival prolongation following treatment with ^{211}At-labeled murine 81C6 and an isotype-matched nonspecific mAb, 45.6, was measured. In an initial dose-finding experiment, groups of rats received intrathecal injections of saline or ^{211}At-labeled 81C6 (3 mCi/mg) at doses of 4, 7, and 13 μCi. The median survival measured for the control animals was 22.5 days and a significant, 33% increase in median survival was seen even at 4 μCi. Two of the rats receiving 13 μCi survived for 6 months at which time they were killed for histopathological analysis. The specificity of this therapeutic response was demonstrated in the next experiment; 12 μCi of ^{211}At-labeled 45.6 mAb did not increase survival significantly compared with saline while ^{211}At-labeled 81C6 prolonged survival by 113% with three apparent cures. Finally, 6 of 10 rats receiving 18 μCi of ^{211}At-labeled 81C6 remained alive with no evidence of disease 10 months after treatment. The neuraxis of all the animals in these experiments were examined for the presence of tumor, hemorrhage, necrosis, peripheral demyelination, edema, and inflammation (92). No toxicities were seen in the 11 long-term survivors from both experiments except for focal edema in one rat. It is worth noting that no statistically significant prolongation in median survival was seen in the same model with 150 μCi of an ^{131}I-labeled mAb fragment (93). Clinical protocols for the evaluation of ^{211}At-labeled mAbs administered by nonintravenous routes in patients with central nervous system malignancies are under way.

ACKNOWLEDGMENTS

Research performed in the author's laboratory was supported by Grants CA42324 and NS20023 from the National Institutes of Health and by Grants DE-FG02-96ER62148 and DE-FG-05-95ER62021 from the Department of Energy.

REFERENCES

1. Wikstrand CJ, Hale LP, Batra SK, Hill ML, Humphrey PA, Kurpad SN, McLendon RE, Moscatello D, Pegram CN, Reist CJ, Traweek ST, Wong AJ, Zalutsky MR, Bigner DD. Monoclonal antibodies against EGFRvIII are tumor specific and react with breast and lung carcinomas and malignant gliomas. Cancer Res 1995; 55:3140–3148.
2. Adams GP, McCartney JE, Tai M-S, Oppermann H, Huston JS, Stafford WF III, Bookman MA, Fand I, Houston LL, Weiner LM. Highly specific in vivo tumor targeting by monovalent and divalent forms of 741F8 anti-c-erbB-2 single-chain Fv. Cancer Res 1993; 53:4026–4034.
3. Hu S-Z, Shively L, Raubitschek A, Sherman M, Williams LE, Wong JYC, Shively JE, Wu AM. Minibody: a novel engineered anti-carcinoembryonic antigen antibody fragment (single-chain Fv-C$_H$3) which exhibits rapid, high-level targeting of xenografts. Cancer Res 1996; 56:3055–3061.
4. Hauck ML, Dewhirst MW, Bigner DD, Zalutsky MR. Local hyperthermia improves uptake of a chimeric monoclonal antibody in a subcutaneous xenograft model. Clin Cancer Res 1997; 3:63–70.
5. Bast RC Jr, Zalutsky MR, Frankel A. Monoclonal Serotherapy. In: Holland JF, Frei

E III, Bast RC Jr, Kufe DW, Morton DL, Weichselbaum RR, eds. Cancer Medicine, 4th ed. Baltimore: Williams and Wilkins, 1996:1245–1262.

6. Kairemo KJA. Radioimmunotherapy of solid cancers. Acta Oncol 1996; 35:345–355.

7. Kozak RW, Raubitschek A, Mirzadeh S, Brechbiel MW, Junghaus R, Gansow OA, Waldmann TA. Nature of the bifunctional chelating agent used for radioimmunotherapy with yttrium-90 monoclonal antibodies: critical factors in determining in vivo survival and organ toxicity. Cancer Res 1989; 49:2639–2644.

8. Schold SC Jr, Zalutsky MR, Coleman RE, Glantz MJ, Friedman AH, Jaszczak RJ, Bigner SH, Bigner DD. Distribution and dosimetry of I-123-labeled monoclonal antibody 81C6 in patients with anaplastic glioma. Invest Radiol 1993; 28:488–496.

9. Larson SM, Pentlow KS, Volkow ND, Wolf AP, Finn RD, Lambrecht RM, Graham MC, Resta GD, Bendriem B, Daghighian F, Yeh SDJ, Wang GJ, Cheung N-KV. PET scanning of iodine-124-3F9 as an approach to tumor dosimetry during treatment planning for radioimmunotherapy in a child with neuroblastoma. J Nucl Med 1992; 33:2020–2023.

10. Daghighian F, Pentlow KS, Larson SM, Graham MC, DiResta GR, Yeh SDJ, Macapinlac H, Finn RD, Arbit E, Cheung N-KV. Development of a method to measure kinetics of radiolabelled monoclonal antibody in human tumour with applications to microdosimetry: positron emission tomography studies of iodine-124 labelled 3F8 monoclonal antibody in glioma. Eur J Nucl Med 1993; 20:402–409.

11. O'Donoghue JA, Bardies M, Wheldon TE. Relationships between tumor size and curability for uniformly targeted therapy with beta-emitting radionuclides. J Nucl Med 1995; 36:1902–1909.

12. Nahum AE. Microdosimetry and radiocurability: modelling targeted therapy with β-emitters. Phys Med Biol 1996; 41:1957–1972.

13. Millar WT, Barrett A. Dosimetric model for antibody targeted radionuclide therapy of tumor cells in cerebrospinal fluid. Cancer Res 1990; 50(suppl):1043s–1048s.

14. Sharkey RM, Motta-Hennessy C, Pawlyk D, Siegel JA, Goldenberg DM. Biodistribution and radiation dose estimates for yttrium- and iodine-labeled monoclonal antibody IgG and fragments in nude mice bearing human colonic tumor xenografts. Cancer Res 1990; 50:2330–2336.

15. Buchsbaum DJ, Lawrence TS, Roberson PL, Heidorn DB, Ten Haken RK, Steplewski Z. Comparison of ^{131}I- and ^{90}Y-labeled monoclonal antibody 17-1A for treatment of human colon cancer xenografts. Int J Radiat Oncol Biol Phys 1993; 25:629–638.

16. Bloomer WD, Adelstein SJ. 5-(^{125}I)-Iododeoxyuridine and the Auger effect: biological consequences and implications for therapy. In: Ioachim HL, ed. Pathobiology Annual 1978. New York: Raven Press, 1978:407–421.

17. Bender H, Takahashi H, Adachi K, Belser P, Liang S, Prewett M, Schrappe M, Sutter A, Rodeck U, Herlyn D. Immunotherapy of human glioma xenografts with unlabeled, ^{131}I-, or ^{125}I-labeled monoclonal antibody 425 to epidermal growth factor receptor. Cancer Res 1992; 52:121–126.

18. Howell RW. Radiation spectra for Auger-electron emitting radionuclides: Report No. 2 of AAPM Nuclear Medicine Task Group No. 6a. Med Phys 1992; 19:1371–1383.

19. Humm JL, Bagshawe KD, Sharma SK, Boxer G. Tissue dose estimates following the

selective uptake of [125]IUdR and other radiolabelled thymidine precursors in resistant tumours. Br J Radiol 1991; 64:45–49.

20. Makrigiorgos GM, Kassis AI, Baranowska-Kortylewicz J, McElvany KD, Welch MJ, Sastry KSR, Adelstein SJ. Radiotoxicity of 5-[123]iodo-2'-deoxyuridine in V79 cells: a comparison with 5-[125]iodo-2'-deoxyuridine. Radiat Res 1989; 118:532–544.

21. Rogoeczi, E. Reactivities of amino acids and proteins with iodine. In: Iodine-Labeled Plasma Proteins. Vol. 1. New York: CRC Press, 1984:127–213.

22. Hunter WM, Greenwood FC. Preparation of iodine-131 labelled human growth hormone of high specific activity. Nature 1962; 194:495–496.

23. Fraker PJ, Speck JC. Protein and cell membrane iodinations with a sparingly soluble chloramide 1,3,4,5-tetrachloro-3α-6α-diphenylglycouril. Biochem Biophys Res Commun 1978; 80:849–857.

24. Shechter Y, Burstein Y, Patchornik A. Selective oxidation of methionine residues in proteins. Biochemistry 1975; 14:4497–4503.

25. Hayes DF, Noska M, Kufe D, Zalutsky M. Effect of radioiodination on the binding of monoclonal antibody DF3 to breast carcinoma cells. Nucl Med Biol 1988; 15: 235–241.

26. Zalutsky MR, Colcher D, Kaplan W, Kufe D. Radioiodinated B6.2 monoclonal antibody: further characterization of a potential radiopharmaceutical for the identification of breast tumors. Int J Nucl Med Biol 1985; 12:227–233.

27. Hayes DF, Zalutsky MR, Kaplan W, Noska M, Thor A, Colcher D, Schlom J, Kufe D. Pharmacokinetics of radiolabeled monoclonal antibody B6.2 in patients with breast cancer. Cancer Res 1986; 46:3157–3163.

28. Garg PK, Alston KL, Zalutsky MR. Catabolism of radioiodinated murine monoclonal antibody F(ab')₂ fragment labeled using N-succinimidyl 3-iodobenzoate and Iodogen methods. Bioconjugate Chem 1995; 6:493–501.

29. Dumas P. Deshalogenation de divers derives iodes phenoliques chez le rat normal et thyroidectomise. Biochem Pharmacol 1973; 22:1599–1605.

30. Leonard JL, Rosenbert IN. Subcellular distribution of thyroxine 5'-deiodinase in the rat kidney: a plasma membrane location. Endocrinology 1977; 103:274–280.

31. Smallridge RC, Burman KD, Ward KE, Wartofsky L, Dimond RC, Wright FD, Latham KR. 3',5'-diiodothyronine to 3'-monoiodothyronine conversion in the fed and fasted rat: enzyme characteristics and evidence for two distinct 5'-deiodinases. Endocrinology 1981; 108:2336–2345.

32. Ong ML, Kellen JA, Malkin DG, Malkin A. 3,5,3'-triiodothyronine (T3) and 3,3'-triiodothyronine (rT3) synthesis in rats hosting the R3230AC mammary tumour. Tumour Biol 1986; 7:105–113.

33. Lee JK, Gordon PR, Stall GM, Gilchrest BA, Kaplan MM. Phenolic and tyrosyl ring iodothyronine deiodination by the caco-2 human colon carcinoma cell line. Metabolism 1989; 38:1154–1161.

34. Itagaki Y, Yoshida K, Ikeda H, Kaise K, Kaise N, Yamamoto M, Sakurada T, Yoshinaga K. Thyroxine 5'-deiodinase in human anterior pituitary tumors. J Clin Endocrinol Metab 1990; 71:340–344.

35. LeBron BA, Pekary AE, Mirell C, Hahn TJ, Hershman JM. Thyroid hormone 5'-deiodinase activity, nuclear binding, and effects on mitogenesis in UMR-106 osteoblastic osteosarcoma cells. J Bone Miner Res 1989; 4:173–178.

36. Zalutsky MR, Narula AS. A method for the radiohalogenation of proteins resulting in decreased thyroid uptake of radioiodine. Appl Radiat Isot 1987; 38:1051–1055.
37. Wilbur DS, Hadley SW, Hylarides MD, Abrams PG, Beaumier PA, Morgan AC, Reno JM, Fritzberg AR. Development of a stable radioiodinating reagent to label monoclonal antibodies for radiotherapy of cancer. J Nucl Med 1989; 30:216–226.
38. Vaidyanathan G, Zalutsky MR. Radioiodination of antibodies via N-succinimidyl-2,4-dimethoxy-3-(trialkylstannyl)benzoates. Bioconjugate Chem 1990; 1:387–393.
39. Garg PK, Garg S, Zalutsky MR. N-Succinimidyl-4-methyl-3-(tri-n-butylstannyl)benzoate synthesis, radioiodination and potential untility for the radioiodination of monoclonal antibodies. Nucl Med Biol 1993; 20:379–388.
40. Hadley, SW, Wilbur DS. Evaluation of iodovinyl antibody conjugates: comparison with a p-iodobenzoyl conjugate and direct radioiodination. Bioconjugate Chem 1990; 1:154–161.
41. Garg S, Garg PK, Zalutsky MR. N-Succinimidyl-5-(trialkylstannyl)-3-pyridinecarboxylates: a new class of reagents for protein radioiodination. Bioconjugate Chem 1991; 2:50–56.
42. Garg S, Garg PK, Zhao X-G, Friedman HS, Bigner DD, Zalutsky MR. Radioiodination of a monoclonal antibody using N-succinimidyl 5-iodo-3-pyridinecarboxylate. Nucl Med Biol 1993; 20:835–842.
43. Wilbur DS. Radiohalogenation of proteins: an overview of radionuclides, labeling methods, and reagents for conjugate labeling. Bioconjugate Chem 1992; 3:433–470.
44. Bolton AM, Hunter RM. The labeling of proteins to high specific radioactivities by conjugation to a I-125 containing acylating agent. Biochem J 1973; 133:529–539.
45. Vaidyanathan G, Zalutsky MR. Protein radiohalogenation: observations on the design of N-succinimidyl ester acylation agents. Bioconjugate Chem 1990; 1:269–273.
46. Zalutsky MR, Narula AS. Radiohalogenation of a monoclonal antibody using an N-succinimidyl 3-(tri-n-butylstannyl) benzoate intermediate. Cancer Res 1988; 48:1446–1450.
47. Vaidyanathan G, Affleck DJ, Zalutsky MR. Radioiodination of proteins using N-succinimidyl 4-hydroxy-3-iodobenzoate. Bioconjugate Chem 1993; 4:78–84.
48. Zalutsky MR, Noska MA, Colapinto EV, Garg PK, Bigner DD. Enhanced tumor localization and in vivo stability of a monoclonal antibody radioiodinated using N-succinimidyl-3-(tri-n-butylstannyl)benzoate (ATE). Cancer Res 1989; 49:5543–5549.
49. Schuster JM, Garg PK, Bigner DD, Zalutsky MR. Improved therapeutic efficacy of a monoclonal antibody radioiodinated using N-succinimidyl-3-(tri-n-butylstannyl)-benzoate. Cancer Res 1991; 51:4164–4169.
50. Press OW, Howell-Clark J, Anderson S, Bernstein I. Retention of B-cell-specific monoclonal antibodies by human lymphoma cells. Blood 1994; 83:1390–1397.
51. Geissler F, Anderson SK, Press O. Intracellular catabolism of radiolabeled anti-CD3 antibodies by leukemic T cells. Cell Immunol 1991; 137:96–110.
52. Novak-Hofer I, Amstutz HP, Morgenthaler JJ, Schubiger PA. Internalization and degradation of monoclonal antibody chCE7 by human neuroblastoma cells. Int J Cancer 1994; 57:427–432.
53. Slamon DJ, Godolphin W, Jones LA, Holt JA, Wong SG, Keith DE, Levin WJ,

Stuart SG, Udove J, Ullrich A, Press MF. Studies of the HER-2/neu proto-oncogene in human breast and ovarian cancer. Science 1989; 244:707–712.

54. Daghighian F, Barendswaard E, Welt S, Humm J, Scott A, Willingham MC, McGuffie E, Old LJ, Larson SM. Enhancement of radiation dose to the nucleus by vesicular internalization of iodine-125-labeled A33 monoclonal antibody. J Nucl Med 1996; 37:1052–1057.

55. Press OW, DeSantes K, Anderson SK, Geissler F. Inhibition of catabolism of radiolabeled antibodies by tumor cells using lysosomotropic amines and carboxylic ionophores. Cancer Res 1990; 50:1243–1250.

56. Reist CJ, Garg PK, Alston KL, Bigner DD, Zalutsky MR. Radioiodination of internalizing monoclonal antibodies using N-succinimidyl 5-iodo-3-pyridinecarboxylate. Cancer Res 1996; 56:4970–4977.

57. Thorpe SR, Baynes JW, Chroneos ZC. The design and application of residualizing labels for studies of protein catabolism. FASEB J 1993; 7:399–405.

58. Ali SA, Eary JF, Warren SD, Badger CC, Krohn KA. Synthesis and radioiodination of tyramine cellobiose for labeling monoclonal antibodies. Nucl Med Biol 1988; 15: 557–561.

59. Ali SA, Warren SD, Richter KY, Badger CC, Eary JF, Press OW, Krohn KA, Bernstein ED, Nelp WB. Improving the tumor retention of radioiodinated antibody: aryl carbohydrate adducts. Cancer Res 1990; 50(suppl):783s–788s.

60. Reist CJ, Archer GA, Kurpad SN, Wikstrand CJ, Vaidyanathan G, Willingham MC, Wong AJ, Bigner DD, Zalutsky MR. Tumor-specific anti-epidermal growth factor receptor variant III monoclonal antibodies: use of the tyramine-cellobiose radioiodination method enhances cellular retention and uptake in tumor xenografts. Cancer Res 1995; 55:4375–4382.

61. Schilling U, Friedrach EA, Sinn H, Schrenk HH, Clorius JH, Maier-Borst W. Design of compounds having enhanced tumor uptake, using serum albumin as a carrier-part II. In vivo studies. Nucl Med Biol 1992; 19:685–695.

62. Stein R, Goldenberg DM, Thorpe SR, Basu A, Mattes MJ. Effects of radiolabeling monoclonal antibodies with a residualizing iodine radiolabel on the accretion of radioisotope in tumors. Cancer Res 1995; 55:3132–3139.

63. Stein R, Goldenberg DM, Thorpe SR, Mattes MJ. Advantage of a residualizing iodine radiolabel for radioimmunotherapy of xenografts of human non-small-cell carcinoma of the lung. J Nucl Med 1997; 38:391–395.

64. Reist CJ, Archer GE, Wikstrand CJ, Bigner DD, Zalutsky MR. Improved targeting of an anti-epidermal growth factor receptor variant III monoclonal antibody in tumor xenografts after labeling using N-succinimidyl 5-iodo-3-pyridinecarboxylate. Cancer Res 1997; 57:1510–1515.

65. Kassis AI, Adelstein SJ. Lethality of Auger Electrons from the decay of bromine-77 in the DNA of mammalian cells. Radiat Res 1982; 90:362–373.

66. Lövqvist A, Sundin A, Ahlström H, Carlsson J, Lundqvist H. 76-Br-labeled monoclonal anti-CEA antibodies for radioimmuno positron emission tomography. Nucl Med Biol 1995; 22:125–133.

67. Wilbur DS, Hylarides MD. Radiolabeling of a monoclonal antibody with N-succinimidyl para-[^{77}Br]bromobenzoate. Nucl Med Biol 1991; 18:363–365.

68. Lövqvist A, Sundin A, Ahlström H, Carlsson J, Lundqvist H. Pharmacokinetics and

experimental PET Imaging of a bromine-76-labeled monoclonal anti-CEA antibody. J Nucl Med 1997; 38:395–401.

69. Geissler F, Anderson SK, Venkatsesan P, Press O. Intracellular catabolism of radio-labeled anti-μ antibodies by malignant B-cells. Cancer Res 1992; 52:2907–2915.

70. Turkington TG, Zalutsky MR, Jaszczak RJ, Garg P, Vaidyanathan G, Coleman RE. Measuring astatine-211 distributions with SPECT. Physics Med Biol 1993; 38:1121–1130.

71. Johnson EL, Turkington TG, Jaszczak RJ, Vaidyanathan G, Green KL, Coleman RE, Zalutsky MR. Quantitation of ^{211}At in small volumes for evaluation of targeted radiotherapy in animal models. Nucl Med Biol 1995; 22:45–54.

72. Larsen RH, Wieland BW, Zalutsky MR. Evaluation of an internal cyclotron target for the production of astatine-211 via the ^{209}Bi$(\alpha,2n)^{211}$At reaction. Nucl Med Biol 1996; 47:135–143.

73. Humm JL. Dosimetric aspects of radiolabeled antibodies for tumor therapy. J Nucl Med 1986; 27:1490–1497.

74. Humm, JL. A microdosimetric model of astatine-211 labeled antibodies for radioimmunotherapy. Int J Radiat Oncol Biol Phys 1987; 13:1767–1773.

75. Roeske JC, Chen GTY. A dosimetry model for intracavitary radioimmunotherapy of cystic brain tumors. Antibody Immunoconj Radiopharm 1991; 4:637–647.

76. Roeske JC, Chen GTY, Atcher RW, Pelizzari CA, Rotmensch J, Haraf D, Montag A, Weichselbaum RR. Modeling of dose to tumor and normal tissue from intraperitoneal radioimmunotherapy with alpha and beta emitters. Int J Radiat Oncol Biol Phys 1990; 19:1539–1548.

77. Hall EJ. Radiobiology for the Radiologist. Philadelphia: Lippincott, 1994.

78. Kampf G. Induction of DNA double-strand breaks by ionizing radiation of different quality and their relevance for cell inactivation. Radiobiol Radiother 1988; 29:631–658.

79. Aaij C, Tschroots WRJM, Lindner L, Feltkamp TEW. The preparation of astatine labelled proteins. Int J Appl Radiat Isot 1975; 26:25–30.

80. Friedman AM, Zalutsky MR, Wung W, Buckinham F, Harper PVJ, Scherr GH, Wainer B, Hunter RL, Appelman EH, Rothberg RM, Fitch FW, Stuart FP, Simonian SJ. Preparation of a biologically stable and immunogenically competent astatinated protein. Int J Nucl Med Biol 1977; 4:219–224.

81. Zalutsky MR, Narula AS. Astatination of proteins using an N-succinimidyl tri-n-butylstannyl benzoate intermediate. Int J Radiat Appl Instrum [A] 1988; 39:227–232.

82. Zalutsky MR, Garg PK, Friedman HS, Bigner DD. Labeling monoclonal antibodies and F(ab')$_2$ fragments with the alpha particle emitting nuclide astatine-211 preservation of immunoreactivity and in vivo localizing capacity. Proc Natl Acad Sci USA 1989; 86:7149–7153.

83. Larsen RH, Bruland ØS. Radiolysis of radioimmunoconjugates. Reduction in antigen-binding ability by α-particle radiation. J Labelled Compd Radiopharm 1995; 36:1009–1018.

84. Larsen RH, Bruland ØS, Hoff P, Alstad J, Lindmo T, Rofstad EK. Inactivation of human osteosarcoma cells in vitro by ^{211}At-TP-3 monoclonal antibody: comparison

with astatine-211-labeled bovine serum albumin, free astatine-211 and external-beam x-rays. Radiat Res 1994; 139:178–184.

85. Larsen RH, Bruland ØS, Hoff P, Alstad J, Rofstad EK. Analysis of the therapeutic gain in the treatment of human osteosarcoma microcolonies in vitro with [211]At-labelled monoclonal antibody. Br J Cancer 1994; 69:1000–1005.

86. Zalutsky MR, Stabin M, Larsen RH, Bigner DD. Tissue distribution and radiation dosimetry of astatine-211-labeled chimeric 81C6, an α-particle emitting immunoconjugate. Nucl Med Biol 1997; 24:255–262.

87. Garg PK, Bigner DD, Zalutsky, MR. Tumor dose enhancement via improved antibody radiohalogenation. In: Epenetos AA, ed. Monoclonal Antibodies—Applications in Clinical Oncology. New York: Chapman and Hall, 1991:103–114.

88. Larsen RH, Hoff P, Alstad J, Bruland ØS. Preparation and quality control of [211]At-labelled and ^{125}I-labelled monoclonal antibodies. Biodistribution in mice carrying human osteosarcoma xenografts. J Labelled Compd Radiopharm 1994; 34:773–785.

89. Hadley SW, Wilbur DS, Gray MA, Atcher RW. Astatine-211 labeling of an antimelanoma antibody and its Fab fragment using N-succinimidyl p-astatobenzoate: comparisons in vivo with the p-^{125}I]iodobenzoyl conjugate. Bioconjugate Chem 1991; 2:171–179.

90. Wilbur DS, Vessella RL, Stray JE, Goffe DK, Blouke KA, Atcher RW. Preparation and evaluation of para[211]At]-astatobenzoyl labeled anti–renal cell carcinoma antibody A6H F(ab')₂. In vivo distribution comparison with para[125]I]-iodobenzoyl labeled A6H F(ab')₂. Nucl Med Biol 1993; 20:917–927.

91. Garg PK, Harrison CL, Zalutsky MR. Comparative tissue distribution of the alpha emitter [211]At and ^{131}I as labels of a monoclonal antibody and F(ab')₂ fragment. Cancer Res 1990; 50:3514–3520.

92. Zalutsky MR, McLendon R, Garg PK, Archer GE, Schuster JM, Bigner DD. Radioimmunotherapy of neoplastic meningitis in rats using an α-particle-emitting immunoconjugate. Cancer Res 1994; 54:4719–4725.

93. Zalutsky MR, Schuster JM, Garg PK, Archer GE Jr, Dewhirst MW, Bigner DD. Two approaches for enhancing radioimmunotherapy: alpha emitters and hyperthermia. Recent Results Cancer Res 1996; 141:101–121.

5

Tumor Architecture and Targeted Delivery

Harold F. Dvorak, Janice A. Nagy, Dian Feng, and Ann M. Dvorak
*Beth Israel Deaconess Medical Center and Harvard Medical School,
Boston, Massachusetts*

I. INTRODUCTION

Despite tremendous advances over the past several decades, current therapies—
surgery, radiation, and chemotherapy—fail to cure many of the most important
human cancers. So much is this the case that some have argued that the "war
on cancer" has not only not been won—it is being lost (1,2). The reasons for
this pessimism are many. Some tumors are not surgically resectable, because of
either their location or their prior spread into vital structures. Many tumors have
already metastasized by the time of diagnosis; therefore, although the primary
tumor can be removed, metastases, which tend to be multiple and widespread,
do not lend themselves to surgical excision. Radiation is often helpful for the
treatment of localized tumors but cancers vary widely in their sensitivity, and
radiation is not generally useful for metastatic disease. In recent years several
promising new chemotherapeutic agents have been introduced (e.g., cis-platinum,
taxol derivatives). Nonetheless, with notable exceptions (e.g., choriocarcinoma,
many cancers of childhood, etc.), chemotherapy usually serves only as an adjunct
to delay recurrence, reduce tumor bulk, or afford palliation; it seldom cures cancer
in adult patients. However, even if radiation and chemotherapy were more widely
effective against tumors, they would not be ideal treatments because of their lack
of specificity and the severe morbidity that commonly results from their use.
Because of their relatively low therapeutic ratios, they can be toxic to many
normal tissues when used at the levels that are necessary to kill tumor cells.

It is not surprising, therefore, that investigators have searched for entirely new approaches to tumor therapy that are more specifically lethal for cancer cells and less toxic for normal cells. The development of monoclonal antibody technology and the potential of antibodies to carry radionuclides has greatly stimulated this search, reawakening once again the hope for a "magic bullet" that could destroy cancer cells selectively without harming normal cells (3–6). However, this approach introduces a new level of complexity and an additional problem, that of delivering therapeutic macromolecules in effective quantities to tumor cells as they exist in the context of solid tumors. It is important that investigators who are developing new antibodies or improved radionuclides have some knowledge of tumor architecture in order that they may appreciate the barriers that confront them and that may limit the delivery of antibodies or other circulating macromolecules to target tumor cells.

II. STRUCTURE OF SOLID TUMORS

Tumors are usually classified on the basis of their origin from normal cells. The majority of malignant tumors that develop in adults are *carcinomas*. Carcinomas arise from epithelial cells and account for ~80% of all human cancers. The remaining 20% include *sarcomas*, which arise from mesenchymal cells (e.g., bone or muscle cells), *leukemias* (tumors arising from hematopoietic cells), or *lymphomas* (tumors of lymphoid origin).

Generally speaking, tumors are comprised of two distinct but interdependent compartments: the malignant cells (parenchyma) and the supporting connective tissue (stroma) that they induce and in which they are dispersed (7,8) (Fig. 1). This discrete separation of parenchymal cells from stroma is not unique to tumors. Normal tissues are organized in a similar fashion and are also comprised of avascular parenchymal compartments that abut on vascularized connective tissue stroma. For example, the epidermis of the skin and the epithelial lining of the gastrointestinal tract and bronchi, skeletal muscle, and lymphoid tissues represent parenchymal elements, all of which are supported by connective tissue stroma. As in normal tissues, a basement membrane may envelop the neoplastic cell compartment, demarcating it from stroma (Fig. 1B); however, the basement membrane is often incomplete, especially when tumors are invasive and/or poorly differentiated (Fig. 1C). Tumors may also arise from stromal cells such as fibroblasts, pericytes or vascular endothelium but even in such instances parenchyma and stroma can generally be distinguished.

A. Tumor Cell Compartment (Parenchyma)

The tumor cells that comprise carcinomas and other types of solid tumors in animals and man are organized into "units" that consist of sheets or nests of

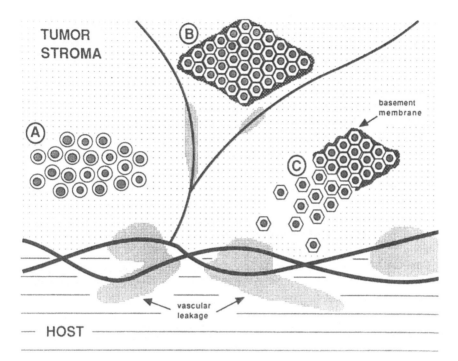

Figure 1 Schematic representation of solid tumor structure. Solid tumors consist of parenchymal (tumor cell) units (A,B, and C) enveloped in stroma. Blood vessels and focal sites of vascular leakage from hyperpermeable blood vessels are concentrated at the tumor-host interface but also traverse tumor stroma. Parenchymal units may consist of (A) loosely packed tumor cells, typical of lymphomas, melanomas, and poorly differentiated carcinomas, or (B) tightly packed tumor cells linked together by occlusive intercellular junctions and an enveloping basement membrane, typical of well-differentiated carcinomas. In (C), a well differentiated carcinoma with occlusive junctions exhibits focal invasion at a site of basement membrane dissolution.

malignant cells (Fig. 1). Together, many individual tumor cell units, along with accompanying stroma, form the tumor mass that is visible to the naked eye. Tumor cell units vary widely in size from clusters of a few cells (or even single cells) to nodules that may measure hundreds of micrometers in diameter. Individual tumor cell units are separated from each other by stroma which may be abundant or scant but which in every case provides the vascular supply necessary for tumor cell nutrition and waste disposal.

The cells within tumor islands are neither structurally nor functionally homogeneous. Like normal tissues, tumors are comprised of a hierarchy of cells that result from the differentiation and division of a relatively small number of stem cells (9). Stem cells are the least differentiated cells in a tumor and, for lack of appropriate markers, may be difficult to recognize by morphological or biochemical features. They are defined by two functional properties, *self renewal* and *population renewal*. Thus, a stem cell divides asymmetrically into two daughter cells. One daughter cell remains a stem cell, whereas the other enters into the process of differentiation. In normal tissues, differentiation proceeds to cell maturity (terminal differentiation) and, subsequently, to death, either by shedding or apoptosis. However, in tumors differentiation may be arrested at any step along the line and full maturity may never be achieved.

Stem cells are also characterized by a second property, that of population renewal. They are the only cells in a tumor that can generate new tumors. Therefore, it is essential that they be eliminated if treatment is to be successful. Elimination of large numbers of differentiating or differentiated tumor cells may significantly reduce tumor bulk but will not prevent the tumor from reestablishing itself if stem cells are not also destroyed. While this type of thinking may seem obvious, it has received remarkably little emphasis. As a result, many monoclonal antibodies have been prepared against antigenic markers that are represented on differentiating or mature cells but not on tumor stem cells; even if their delivery to tumor cells was not a problem, such antibodies would not be expected to effect cures if every cell must be targeted as in drug and toxin immunoconjugates. However, the "crossfire" of beta particle radioimmunoconjugates does provide for bystander killing.

B. Tumor Stroma Compartment

Tumor stroma is connective tissue of host origin that is induced by tumor cells. It is essential for tumor growth. All solid tumors, regardless of their type or cellular origin, require new blood vessels if they are to grow beyond a minimal size of 1 to 2 mm (10). New blood vessels are necessary for tumors to obtain nutrients, for gas exchange, and for waste disposal. However, blood vessels are but one component of stroma. Stroma as a whole may be regarded as a three-dimensional sieve that regulates the passage of small molecules (including drugs), macromolecules, and inflammatory, mesenchymal, and tumor cells. Stroma, therefore, provides a necessary lifeline for tumors and also imposes a barrier that must be breached if monoclonal antibodies or other macromolecular medicines are to reach tumor cells in sufficient quantity to be therapeutically effective. Additional barriers may be interposed by the parenchymal compartment (see below) and by a basement membrane, if present.

Tumors differ markedly from each other in stroma content. Sometimes these differences are primarily *quantitative*. For example, desmoplastic carcinomas arising in the breast or gastrointestinal tract are characterized by abundant dense fibrous connective tissue stroma that may comprise an overwhelming (>80%) proportion of the tumor mass. In other tumors, including some that develop in the same organs (e.g., medullary carcinoma of the breast), connective tissue stroma may be minimal, accounting for only a small percentage of the tumor mass. The differences in stromal composition between different tumors may also be *qualitative*. Whereas desmoplastic cancers elicit abundant connective tissue stroma, others induce a lymphocytic response or deposit specialized connective tissue elements such as elastin, cartilage, or even bone.

While tumors arising in the same organ in different patients may differ from each other markedly in both the quality and quantity of stroma they elicit, individual tumors tend to "breed true." Thus, despite tumor "progression," distant metastases generally resemble the primary tumor from which they were derived, even if they develop many years after the primary tumor was resected. Points of resemblance include not only the morphology of individual tumor cells and their arrangements but also the composition and extent of tumor stroma. The structure of many transplantable animal tumors also tends to remain remarkably constant over many years and after hundreds of passages.

C. Origin, Organization, and Composition of Tumor Stroma

As previously mentioned, tumors induce their stroma from host elements. Interstitial fluid and inflammatory cells are derived by extravasation from local blood vessels; other components, such as fibroblasts and new blood vessels, arise from the local proliferation and inward migration of cells from adjacent connective tissue. Still others, such as interstitial collagens, hyaluronan, and proteoglycans, are produced locally by immigrant connective tissue cells.

Just as the malignant cells that comprise carcinomas resemble but nonetheless differ significantly from normal epithelium, so tumor stroma, though generally not itself malignant (but see Ref. 11), is readily distinguished from normal connective tissue. One major difference is that of *organization*. The stroma of normal tissues includes differentiated blood vessels and supporting elements that in number, type, and distribution are especially arranged to meet the nutritional and waste disposal needs of the epithelia which they supply. Furthermore, normal blood vessels respond rapidly to changes in tissue metabolism by increasing or decreasing blood flow locally as may be required for optimal function of individual tissues and of the host as a whole. In contrast, tumor stroma is poorly organized and functionally deficient, resembling more closely the connective tissue of healing wounds than the corresponding normal tissue of which it is a caricature. In fact, wound healing is a useful paradigm for understanding tumor stroma and its generation (12).

Tumor stroma also differs from normal tissues with respect to its *composi-*

tion. Thus, tumor stroma lacks both lymphatics* and nerves. Moreover, although virtually any other component found in normal connective tissues may also be represented in tumor stroma, additional components are present that normally are found in the fetus and in healing wounds but not in normal adult tissues. Thus, in some respects oncogenesis mimics both ontogeny and the wound healing response. Also, some components are found in tumor stroma in much greater quantities than in normal adult connective tissues. An example is the structural protein fibronectin. Fibronectin is an adhesive protein that circulates in the blood and is present at low levels in normal adult connective tissue; it contains an arg-gly-asp (RGD) sequence that provides a binding site for cell-surface integrins and thereby facilitates cell adherence and migration (14). Fibronectin is much more abundant in tumor stroma than in normal adult connective tissues. Also, the fibronectin expressed locally in tumor stroma differs from that present in plasma or normal tissues in that, as the result of alternative splicing, it includes elements (EIIIa, EIIIb) that characterize fetal forms of fibronectin (15–17). The significance of "fetal fibronectins" in tumors is not well understood but is thought to facilitate cell adhesion and migration.

Tenascin is another RGD-containing structural protein that is synthesized locally in tumor stroma by fibroblasts; normally absent from adult connective tissues, it, like alternatively spliced fibronectins, is prominent in fetal connective tissues and is associated with cell migration (18–26). Other RGD-containing structural proteins that are newly synthesized or synthesized in increased amounts in tumor stroma are osteopontin and thrombospondin (21,27,28).

Hyaluronan and various proteoglycans (PGs)† are also prominent components of tumor stroma and merit more interest than they have received (29–33). A chondroitin sulfate containing PG, resembling versican, is greatly increased in the stroma of a number of human and animal tumors (32). In normal adult tissues this PG is confined to a thin rim enveloping blood vessels, hair follicles, etc., but is diffusely distributed throughout the stroma of many animal and human tumors (32). In these same tumors, another proteoglycan, decorin, itself a major component of normal stroma, is often increased further in tumor stroma and may differ from normal decorin by possessing abnormally long glycosaminoglycan (GAG) side chains (32). Other workers have also called attention to hypomethylation of the decorin gene in human colon cancers (34).

New blood vessels are an important component of tumor stroma. Vascular

---

* Tumor cells commonly metastasize via lymphatics. These are thought to be preexisting and to belong to the surrounding host tissue which the tumor invades rather than being a part of tumor-induced stroma. However, it has recently been discovered that some tumors overexpress VEGF-C, a cytokine that selectively generates the formation of new lymphatics (13). Therefore, it is possible that some tumors do in fact initiate the formation of new lymphatic vessels.

† Proteoglycans are composed of a protein core with one or more glycosaminoglycan (GAG) side

density varies widely from tumor to tumor and also within different portions of the same tumor (35), a finding of some significance for drug and antibody delivery and one that we will consider in great detail later.

Perhaps the most overlooked feature of tumor stroma is its high concentration of protein-rich interstitial fluid (36). This fluid represents a plasma filtrate and includes plasma proteins at concentrations that approach those of plasma (36,37). Among these extravasated plasma proteins are several that possess RGD sequences. The most prominent of these, because of its relatively high concentration in normal plasma ($\sim$3 mg/mL), is the clotting protein fibrinogen. Fibrinogen clots to form fibrin which serves as a major component of provisional tumor stroma before being replaced eventually by durable, mature connective tissue stroma. However, several other RGD-containing proteins, present in plasma at much lower concentrations, also extravasate into tumor stroma. These include fibronectin, vitronectin, osteopontin, and thrombospondin, all proteins that may also be synthesized locally in tumor stroma.

III. GENERATION OF TUMOR STROMA

Tumor stroma is generated as the result of a series of complex interactions between tumor cells and surrounding host tissues. Efforts to elucidate these interactions over the past 20 years have provided a framework for understanding tumor stroma generation in terms of wound healing, inflammation, and other fundamental responses of the host to injury (12,38,39). One early clue to understanding the pathogenesis of tumor stroma generation was the finding that tumor stroma contains greatly increased amounts of plasma protein-rich interstitial fluid and particularly fibrin, the insoluble clotted form of plasma fibrinogen (7,8,12,40–43). For fibrin to be deposited outside of the blood vasculature in tumor stroma, two important criteria must be met: 1) Blood vessels must be leaky so as to allow the extravasation of fibrinogen (and other plasma proteins), and 2) mechanisms must exist for clotting extravasated fibrinogen to fibrin. Both of these criteria are met in tumors.

A. Hyperpermeability of Tumor Blood Vessels: Role of Vascular Permeability Factor/Vascular Endothelial Growth Factor (VPF/VEGF)

Tumor blood vessels differ from those of normal tissues in important aspects of structure and function (44–46). Particularly relevant to the present discussion

---

chains. PGs differ from glycoproteins in several respects, the most obvious of which are the length, complexity, and degree of sulfation of the carbohydrate moieties comprising the GAG side chains.

is their hyperpermeability to plasma and plasma proteins, including fibrinogen (7,12,37,40–42,46–50). Measurements of different types made on a variety of tumors have shown that tumor blood vessels are ~4–10 times more permeable to circulating macromolecules than are normal blood vessels. As a consequence, plasma and plasma proteins that normally are retained within the vasculature extravasate extensively into the surrounding connective tissues. Such extravasation has profound consequences, which will be discussed in greater detail below.

Although other mechanisms may contribute, it is generally thought that the most important single factor responsible for tumor vessel hyperpermeability is the secretion by tumor cells of a multifunctional angiogenic cytokine, vascular permeability factor (VPF, also known as vascular endothelial growth factor, VEGF, or VEGF-A) (12,38–41,51–60) (Table 1). VPF/VEGF is consistently overexpressed by the great majority of human and animal tumors. With equal consistency, both of VPF/VEGF's high affinity receptors, flt-1 (VEGFR-1) and KDR/flk-1 (VEGFR-2), are overexpressed by the endothelial cells that line tumor-supplying blood vessels.

VPF/VEGF is a dimeric protein of molecular weight 34 to 43 kD whose structure is extensively conserved in species as diverse as mouse and man (58,60). Several VPF/VEGF isoforms are synthesized as the result of alternative splicing of a single gene but, as far as is known, all have the same biological functions (60). Within a matter of minutes after local injection, VPF/VEGF renders venules and small veins hyperpermeable to circulating macromolecules and does so with a potency some 50,000 times that of histamine (58). VPF/VEGF increases micro-

Table 1 VPF/VEGF Is a Multifunctional Cytokine that Interacts with High–Affinity Receptor Tyrosine Kinases (VEGFR-1, VEGFR-2) that are Selectively Expressed on Vascular Endothelium to Exert a Number of Time-Dependent Functions

Seconds to a few minutes
  Induces calcium transients, protein phosphorylations, activates phospholipase C, generates IP3, releases von Willebrand factor
  Potently (50,000 × histamine) increases microvessel permeability to plasma, thereby altering the native extracellular matrix and rendering it proangiogenic and prostromagenic
  Increases NO synthesis

Hours to days to weeks
  Alters endothelial cell gene expression, leading to overexpression of the following proteins: uPA, tPA, PAI-1, uPAR, collagenase, tissue factor, GLUT-1, integrins and others
  Alters endothelial cell shape and initiates endothelial cell migration and division
  Angiogenesis
  Protects against endothelial cell apoptosis and senescence

vascular permeability by increasing the hydraulic conductivity of venular endo-thelium (61) (Table 2).

An immediate consequence of increased microvascular permeability is ex-travasation of plasma and plasma proteins into the surrounding connective tissue (12,39–42). VPF/VEGF exerts a number of additional effects on vascular endo-thelium in a time-dependent manner (Table 1). These include the induction of transient accumulations of cytoplasmic calcium (59) and endothelial cell shape change, division, and migration (55,59,60,62). VPF/VEGF also alters the pattern of endothelial cell gene expression, leading to increased synthesis of clotting (63) and fibrinolysis-related proteins (64), matrix metalloproteases (65), GLUT-1 (66), osteopontin, and different integrins (28,67,68). Finally, VPF/VEGF is an endo-thelial cell survival factor that prevents apoptosis and delays and even reverses endothelial cell senescence (69,70).

B. Clotting of Extravasated Fibrinogen to Form a Provisional Stromal Matrix

The vascular hyperpermeability induced by VPF/VEGF is relatively non-dis-criminatory over a broad range of molecular sizes and shapes; as a result, plasma proteins extravasate along with water and low-molecular-weight solutes. Among the former are fibrinogen and clotting factors V, VII, X, and XIII and prothrom-bin, proteins that participate at various steps in the clotting cascade. Within min-utes of increased vessel permeability, plasma proteins leak, the coagulation sys-tem is activated, and extravasated fibrinogen is clotted to fibrin (71). Clotting is initiated in tumors by activation of the extrinsic clotting system as factor VII, extravasated from plasma, comes into contact with tissue factor, a procoagulant expressed on the surface of many cells in normal tissues. Tissue factor is also expressed by many tumor cells and is thought to be the principal initiator of extravascular coagulation (72,73). However, several other procoagulants have been described that may initiate clotting in specific tumors. Once initiated, succes-sive steps in the extrinsic and common coagulation pathways follow pari passu.

Tumor cells also participate in at least one later stage of the clotting cascade in that they provide a surface that supports the assembly of prothrombinase, the enzyme that generates thrombin from prothrombin (74). Thrombin, in turn, cleaves the A and B fibrinopeptides from fibrinogen to generate fibrin. In addition to clotting fibrinogen, thrombin also activates clotting factor XIII, a transglutami-nase which covalently crosslinks fibrin α and γ chains, thereby stabilizing its structure. Thus, so far as has been determined, the fibrin deposited in tumors is identical to that which forms when blood is clotted in wounds or in vitro in a test tube (42,48).

The fibrin-rich provisional matrix that is deposited in tumors inserts itself into the interstices of surrounding tissue, entrapping extravasated fluid and solu-

Table 2 Parameters that Regulate Blood Flow and the Passage of Molecules Within the Circulation and Across Blood Vessel Walls, Stroma, and Parenchyma

1. Blood flow rate (86):

$$\text{Blood flow rate} = q = \frac{\Delta p}{\eta z}$$

where q is blood perfusion (flow) rate (cm³/h/g tissue), Δp is arteriovenous pressure drop (mm Hg), η is apparent blood viscosity (g/cm³) where 1 g/m/s = 2.08 × 10⁻⁹ mmHg · h = 1 centipoise, and z is extrinsic geometric resistance (g/cm³).

2. Transport across the vascular wall. This is governed by equations which reflect the respective contributions of convection and diffusion (82):

$$\text{Convective flux} = L_p S[(P_v - P_i) - \sigma(\pi_v - \pi_i)]$$

where L_p = vessel hydraulic conductivity (cm⁴/sec × mm Hg), S = surface area per unit volume (cm²/cm³), P_v and P_i = vascular and interstitial pressures (mm Hg), and π_v and π_i = vascular and interstitial osmotic pressures (mm Hg), and σ = osmotic reflection coefficient.

$$\text{Diffusive flux} = PS(C_v - C_i)$$

where P = vascular permeabiltiy (cm/sec), S = surface area per unit volume (cm²/cm³), C_v and C_i = concentrations (mole/cm³) in the vascular and interstitial spaces, respectively.

3. Transport in stroma and parenchyma. These are governed by equations which reflect the respective contributions of convection and diffusion (131):

$$\text{Convective flux} = -CR_f K \frac{\partial p}{\partial x}$$

where C is concentration, R_f is the retardation factor (solute convective velocity/ solvent convective velocity), K is the tissue hydraulic conductivity for convective flow of solvent through the medium, and the fraction is the the pressure gradient (p minus hydrostatic pressure).

$$\text{Diffusive flux} = -D \frac{\partial C}{\partial x}$$

where D is the diffusion constant of the solute in the medium, and the second term expresses the concentration gradient (C is concentration and x is distance).

ble plasma proteins and providing a provisional stroma. Other leaked plasma proteins such as fibronectin may be incorporated into fibrin by factor XIII–mediated crosslinking. The fibrin matrix is not a permanent structure but one that forms continually and that simultaneously undergoes continuing modulation by proteases. One of these proteases is plasmin, generated locally from another leaked plasma protein, plasminogen, by the action of plasminogen activators that are expressed both by tumor cells and by VPF/VEGF-activated vascular endothelium (40,42,64,75,76). Plasmin also activates matrix metalloproteases (MMPs) which are secreted as proenzymes; once activated, MMPs degrade collagen, proteoglycans, and other matrix elements including fibrin and fibronectin. As a result, the fibrin found in tumor stroma at any point in time reflects a balance between coagulation and fibrinolysis, a balance that is determined individually for each tumor by quantitative differences in vascular hyperpermeability, clotting, and fibrinolysis.

C. Transformation of Provisional Stroma into Mature Stroma

The native connective tissue stroma found in normal adult tissues is designed for the steady state in which turnover of vascular endothelium and other stromal cells is extremely low. In contrast, the fibrin provisional matrix of tumors is highly supportive of mesenchymal cell adhesion and migration; i.e., it is *proangiogenic and prostromagenic*. For this reason, deposition of a fibrin- and fibronectin-rich provisional matrix is an important preliminary step in angiogenesis and new stroma generation.

Each tumor has a characteristic amount of provisional fibrin stroma associated with it which is thought to be predictive of the amount of mature stroma that will eventually replace the provisional matrix. In some as yet poorly understood manner, provisional matrix incites the ingrowth of endothelial cells and fibroblasts as well as varying numbers of inflammatory cells. This pro-angiogenic, pro-mature matrix-generating effect is mediated, in part, by the favorable surface that fibrin, fibronectin, and other components of provisional stroma provide for cell attachment and migration (77). Endothelial cells migrate into the fibrin gel and organize to form blood vessels; immigrating fibroblasts synthesize and secrete the matrix proteins, proteoglycans, and hyaluronan that constitute mature tumor stroma. In parallel with these events, the provisional fibrin-rich matrix undergoes proteolytic degradation and is replaced by mature stromal elements.

Independent evidence for this model of tumor stroma generation comes from in vitro studies which have provided direct evidence that crosslinked fibrin of the type deposited in tumors provides a matrix that supports and favors inflammatory and mesenchymal cell migration (77–79). Furthermore, implantation of crosslinked fibrin in guinea pigs, in the absence of tumor cells, induces the progressive ingrowth of new blood vessels and fibroblasts which together generate vascularized stroma of the type found in many tumors (41,80).

IV. BARRIERS TO THE TARGETED DELIVERY OF MACROMOLECULES TO SOLID TUMORS

An understanding of tumor stroma generation and the structure of solid tumors provides a helpful background for appreciating some of the opportunities and difficulties that are encountered in delivering monoclonal antibodies or other therapeutic macromolecules to tumors. Effective delivery of a molecule of any size to a tumor (or for that matter to any other tissue by the blood vascular route) requires that the tissue have adequate vascular supply and blood flow, that the molecule is able to cross the microvascular wall, and that, once outside of the vasculature, it can pass through the connective tissue stroma to reach target parenchymal cells in therapeutically effective concentrations. Each of these steps needs to be considered in turn as it relates to the delivery of macromolecular medicines to solid tumors. (For a more detailed discussion, see Refs. 81–84).

A. Intravascular Transport: Tumor Blood Supply and Blood Flow

The microvessels comprising the vascular beds of normal tissues form a regular hierarchy of arteries, arterioles, capillaries, postcapillary venules, and small veins that feed into larger veins. Each of these vessel subtypes proceeds in a relatively straight line for at least a short distance and has a characteristic, tissue-specific structure, branching pattern, and size range. Moreover, each vessel subtype is configured to perform certain specialized functions, including pressure regulation (muscular arteries and arterioles); exchange of gases, ions, vitamins and other small molecules (capillaries); increased permeability in response to vasoactive mediators such as histamine or VPF/VEGF (venules, small veins); inflammatory cell extravasation (venules, small veins), etc. In addition, the blood vessels supplying normal tissues are distributed at regular and closely spaced intervals (e.g., 100 μm) and as a result are able to provide adequate tissue nutrition and effective waste removal.

Blood flow (Table 2) is proportional to the *drop in blood pressure* across a vascular bed and is inversely proportional to blood *viscosity* and to *extrinsic geometric resistance*, a complex function of vascular morphology dependent on vessel number and types, their branching pattern, diameter, and length (85–87). Blood viscosity depends on hematocrit and shear rate. With regard to the former, blood viscosity increases with rising hematocrit. As blood vessel diameter falls below ~500 μm, the cell-free marginal layer constitutes a larger portion of microvessel blood volume with a resulting lowering of hematocrit (Fahraeus effect) that results in reduced blood viscosity. *Shear rate* also affects blood viscosity. At low shear rates, red blood cells form rouleaux, causing blood viscosity to increase.

The blood vessels supplying solid tumors differ markedly from this normal pattern with respect to their *organization, structure* and *function*; together these alterations result in disturbed blood flow.

1. Tumor Vessel Organization

Unlike the vessels that supply normal tissues, tumor vessels commonly exhibit a serpentine course, branch irregularly, and form arteriovenous shunts. Moreover, tumor vessels are distributed nonuniformly and, on average, at intervals considerably greater than in normal tissues; i.e., the tumor vasculature exhibits *spatial heterogeneity*. As a result, some portions of a tumor receive relatively normal amounts of blood, whereas other areas are underperfused and become hypoxic (45,88,89); not uncommonly, prolonged hypoxia leads to tumor necrosis. Tissue hypoxia has additional significance in that it potently upregulates VPF/VEGF expression in many cell types (90–92). As a consequence, tumor cells in hypoxic areas commonly overexpress VPF/VEGF to an even greater extent than their counterparts in better oxygenated portions of the same tumor (93).

2. Tumor Vessel Structure

Tumor vessels do not conform to the hierarchical pattern of normal vascular beds and are often difficult to classify as arterioles, capillaries, and venules (88). Individual tumor microvessels often assume a sinusoidal morphology, forming large, thin-walled, tortuous, endothelium-lined but pericyte-poor, channels. Unlike the vessels supplying normal tissues, tumor vessels lack innervation.

3. Tumor Vessel Function

Not unexpectedly, abnormal function follows from abnormal structure. Tumor vessels lack vasomotion, and, lacking appropriate receptors, are unresponsive to a number of vasoactive agents (e.g., histamine) that regulate diameter (and so blood flow) of normal microvessels. However, as was already mentioned, the vascular endothelial cells lining tumor vessels overexpress the two high-affinity VPF/VEGF receptors, VEGFR-1 and -2, thereby allowing tumor vessels to respond to VPF/VEGF with all of the consequences listed in Table 1.

Another functional abnormality of tumor vessels is that blood flow is not constant over time; i.e., there is *temporal heterogeneity* (89). In some areas, blood flow may become sluggish and stop altogether for a time; blood flow may also reverse direction locally.

4. Tumor Blood Flow

For many years it was thought that tumors had a more extensive blood supply than that of normal tissues. However, in now classic studies, Gullino (94) demonstrated that blood perfusion rates in animal tumors were actually lower than those of the normal tissue from which they arose. Moreover, as tumors grew in size, their average perfusion rate decreased further as an increasingly inadequate blood supply leads to foci of necrosis (36). Subsequent studies by many investigators have confirmed and generalized these observations.

What accounts for the relatively reduced blood flow found in tumors? Although all of the reasons responsible are not fully understood, measurements by many investigators and particularly by the Jain laboratory have shown that all of the variables in Eq. 1, Table 2, are altered in experimental tumors (95). Whereas pressures in the arteries supplying normal and tumor vessels are quite similar, *microvascular pressures* within tumors are actually elevated due to venous compression while venous pressures are significantly reduced. Also, tumor blood vessels exhibit greater resistance to flow than do the vessels supplying normal tissues. Because of their serpentine course, thin walls, exposure to increased interstitial pressure, and other local factors, *extrinsic geometric resistance* is also increased in experimental tumors, frequently by more than an order of magnitude (87). Finally, the *viscosity* of the blood within tumor vessels is increased because of elevated hematocrit (tumor vessels are hyperpermeable and leak plasma) and increased mean vessel diameter (46,86). Blood viscosity is also increased by sluggish blood flow which reduces shear rate, leading to rouleaux formation. As noted, however, nearly all measurements of blood flow have been made in animal systems and measurements on human tumors are needed to confirm and extend these observations (95).

B. Transport Across the Microvascular Wall in Normal Tissues and in Tumors

1. Normal Tissues

Following entry into a vascular bed, a therapeutic molecule must cross the walls of "exchange vessels" to reach parenchymal cells or other extravascular targets. In normal tissues molecules can cross this barrier passively, through existing endothelial pores by convection and/or diffusion (Eq. 2, Table 2), or, alternatively, by mechanisms that require active participation of vascular endothelial cells (96–102).

For the most part, water, glucose, ions, and other small molecules are thought to cross vascular endothelium by passing between adjacent endothelial cells (81,103,104)*. The interendothelial space can accommodate molecules of diameter up to ~2 nm but larger solutes such as most proteins are too large to employ this route. Instead, plasma proteins and other macromolecules are thought to exit capillaries by means of transcytosis (103,104), a process in which uncoated vesicles (caveolae) bud off from the luminal endothelial surface, containing as cargo quanta of plasma, and cross the endothelium to the abluminal surface where they discharge their contents into the extravascular space.

Exposure of normal vascular beds to vasoactive agents such as histamine, serotonin or VPF/VEGF greatly increases microvascular permeability to both plasma and plasma proteins. Majno and coworkers (105,106) demonstrated that this increase in permeability was localized to venules, not capillaries. Moreover, they proposed that increased permeability resulted from a pulling apart of adjacent endothelial cells, leading to the formation of large (≥ 1 μm in diameter) gaps that allowed the free passage of soluble proteins and particulates, even including occasional erythrocytes and other cellular elements. At present there is controversy as to whether these openings in fact represent interendothelial cell "*gaps*" (99,107) or are instead membrane-lined "*pores*" that pass through endothelial cell cytoplasm (98,100–102,108); possibly both types of opening may develop.

Another mechanism of transendothelial transport involves a recently described organelle, the vesiculo-vacuolar organelle or VVO (96,97,109). VVOs are grapelike clusters of linked, uncoated vesicles and vacuoles, sometimes numbering more than one hundred, that cluster in the peripheral cytoplasm of venular endothelium (Fig. 2). VVOs extend across endothelial cells from lumen to ablumen, also interfacing with the lateral plasma membranes (interendothelial cell clefts) above or below tight junctions. The individual vesicles and vacuoles that comprise VVOs are interconnected to each other (and to the endothelial cell plasma membrane) by stomata (fenestrae) that may be open or that are closed by thin diaphragms. These structures resemble the stomata and diaphragms of caveolae; although smaller in diameter, they also resemble the fenestrae and diaphragms of fenestrated endothelium.

Circulating macromolecular tracers such as ferritin or other plasma proteins enter VVOs luminally and percolate through linked vesicles and vacuoles to reach the abluminal surface. In normal venules this process is slow and likely of only modest quantitative significance compared with transcytotic transport of plasma

---

* In some specialized vascular beds (central nervous system) the endothelium is unusually impermeable and even small molecules are transported across microvessels by receptor-mediated transport. Some other vascular beds (e.g., kidney, adrenal gland) are lined by *fenestrated* endothelium, which is relatively more permeable to water and small solutes than continuous endothelium. Finally, the microvasculature supplying liver, spleen, and bone marrow is *discontinuous*, exhibiting obvious spaces between adjacent endothelial cells.

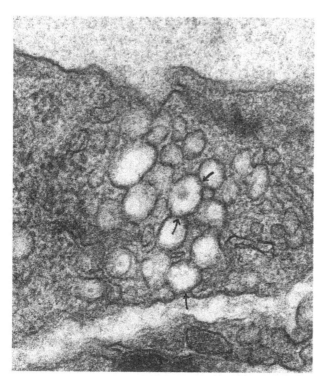

Figure 2 Electron micrograph illustrating a VVO in the endothelium of a venule from normal mouse skin. Note cluster of interconnected, uncoated vesicles and vacuoles that span the cytoplasm from lumen (top) to ablumen. Individual vesicles and vacuoles are connected to each other and to the luminal and abluminal plasma membrane by thin diaphragms (arrows). (×110,000.)

proteins across capillaries. However, when stimulated by vasoactive agents, soluble circulating macromolecules extravasate readily across endothelium by way of VVOs. Transendothelial cell transport by way of VVOs apparently requires opening of the diaphragms that normally guard the stomatae that join individual vesicles and vacuoles with each other and with the plasma membrane. However, the precise structural and biochemical changes responsible for opening diaphragms are not understood. VVO stomatae are generally not large enough to allow the passage of particulates such as colloidal carbon or of cells. However, images have been captured that appear to be intermediate between VVOs and transendothelial "pores" (39,108). It is possible that at least some of these result from a rearrangement of VVO vesicle and vacuole membranes into transendothelial channels; ''pore'' formation was greatly increased when foreign particulates (such as colloidal carbon) are injected into the circulation (98).

2. Solid Tumors

As was noted earlier, one of the striking properties of tumor microvessels is their hyperpermeability to circulating macromolecules. What accounts for this hyperpermeability and what is its structural basis? One explanation commonly offered is that newly formed blood vessels, such as those that are induced to form in tumors, are lined by endothelial cells that fail initially to form proper tight junctions, leaving gaps between endothelial cells that allow plasma to escape. Alternatively, openings could develop as a result of immune damage or ischemic injury to individual endothelial cells. While such openings have been described (110), it has not been shown convincingly that they are important sites of vascular leakage, i.e., that circulating tracers actually leak through them. Endothelial openings in vessels that supply unperfused or underperfused tumor (necrotic and hypoxic zones) will obviously not contribute importantly to plasma leakage.

Another possible explanation for tumor vessel hyperpermeability is that tumor vessels are of a different structural type than corresponding normal vessels, e.g., lined by fenestrated rather than by continuous endothelium. This possibility has some merit in that fenestrated endothelium is relatively more permeable than continuous endothelium to water and small solutes, and some tumors (like some normal tissues) are supplied by vessels with fenestrated endothelium (46,110– 112). Moreover, VPF/VEGF, a product of many tumor cells, is reported to induce the generation of new vessels with fenestrated endothelium (108,112,113). However, fenestration cannot explain the hyperpermeability demonstrated by the large number of human and animal tumors that are supplied by vessels with continuous endothelium (46,109,113; Dvorak AM, unpublished data).

The discovery of VPF/VEGF as an important tumor product suggested that this cytokine might have an important role in tumor vessel hyperpermeability and there is now considerable evidence supporting this thesis (38,39,58). As noted above, a sizable majority of important human cancers overexpress VPF/VEGF and the endothelial cells lining the blood vessels that supply these tumors regularly overexpress both of the high-affinity VPF/VEGF receptors. The question remains as to how VPF/VEGF renders tumor vessels hyperpermeable. Earlier it was said that VPF/VEGF acts on venules to increase their hydraulic conductivity (61) (Table 2). However, what does this mean in anatomic terms, i.e., in terms of the actual pathways that protein solutes will follow in crossing vascular endothelium? Based on studies of the microvasculature supplying several normal tissues, VPF/VEGF could increase tumor vessel permeability by activating VVOs, by inducing transendothelial pores or interendothelial cell gaps, or by inducing endothelial cell fenestration. Studies of this problem are still at an early stage, but our experience with several animal tumors indicates that VVOs account for the bulk of increased permeability to circulating soluble macromolecules such as plasma proteins (96,109). Fenestrae also play an important role when they are present. However, because fenestrae are not normally permeable to macromolecules (111,114,115), it is necessary to postulate that VPF/VEGF opens fenestrae to the passage of macromolecules in much the same manner it opens VVOs. This has not yet been proved formally. We ourselves have not observed gaps or holes in the endothelium of microvessels supplying animal or human tumors but these have been documented by others (110). Taken together, it is likely that different pathways are followed in different tumors.

C. Transport Across Stroma

Having extravasated from hyperpermeable blood vessels, therapeutic molecules must next make their way across tumor stroma before they can engage tumor cell targets. Many common human carcinomas have extensive stroma; as noted earlier, upwards of 80% of the mass of some carcinomas is comprised of stroma. It is therefore important to consider how molecules pass through stroma or other living tissues. According to the laws of physics, molecules move through space by *convection* and/or *diffusion* (Eq. 3, Table 2).

Convection describes the movement of molecules down a pressure gradient and is thought to contribute importantly to the passage of circulating macromolecules across normal microvessels as well as to their movement in extravascular connective tissues (81). Intravascular pressures within microvessels normally approximate 40 mm Hg whereas the hydrodynamic pressure of normal interstitial tissues is close to zero, resulting in a significant transvascular pressure gradient. However, these relationships are very different in tumors where interstitial pressures are greatly increased because of the hyperpermeability of tumor blood vessels with leakage of plasma proteins and the lack of lymphatics that in normal tissues relieve tissue pressure by draining excess extravasated fluid and protein. Interstitial pressures are relatively uniformly elevated throughout solid tumors and fall abruptly and precipitously to normal at the tumor-host interface (116–120). Interstitial pressures within tumors may be sufficiently high so as to balance intravascular pressures, thus preventing effective extravasation of circulating therapeutic molecules on the basis of convection. Indeed, because molecules flow down a pressure gradient, the high interstitial pressure of tumors directs convective flow away from the tumor center toward the periphery (121), i.e., in the opposite direction desired for the entry of therapeutic molecules delivered from the blood.

In contrast to convection, *diffusion* is driven by solute concentration gradients and these may be expected to favor the passage of blood-delivered molecules across stroma. However, movement of large molecules across significant distances by diffusion is extremely slow. Jain has estimated that a macromolecule such as IgG can diffuse a distance of $\sim 100\ \mu m$ in the course of 1 hour but would require some days to cover a distance of ~ 1 mm (83). These times are likely to be underestimates because many molecules bind at least weakly to stromal components, thus impairing diffusion further. Taken together, it would seem that diffusion would not permit therapeutic macromolecules to reach tumor cells in a timely fashion, although it is a useful mechanism for the delivery of small molecules which diffuse much more rapidly.

D. Transport Across Parenchyma

The movement of molecules in parenchyma, like that in stroma, is governed by the physical laws of diffusion and convection. However, the parenchyma may offer an additional barrier, that provided by intercellular junctions between tumor cells. Some tumors, such as lymphomas and malignant melanomas, arise from cells that do not form specialized junctions with each other, and the malignant cells comprising such tumors also do not form intercellular junctions (Fig. 1A), though they may be tightly packed together. On the other hand, carcinomas are derived from epithelial cells which normally form complex intercellular junctions with each other. Not unexpectedly, therefore, depending on the particular cell type and the degree of tumor differentiation, carcinoma cells form numerous strong attachments with each other whereas lymphoma and melanoma cells do not. Typically, intercellular junctions are prominent in well-differentiated carcinomas; for example, well-differentiated squamous cell carcinomas exhibit desmosomal junctions of the type found in normal epidermis. On the other hand, desmosomes may be infrequent or altogether absent in poorly differentiated tumors. When present (Fig. 1B,C), interepithelial cell junctions, unlike those joining endothelial cells, may limit the passage of even small molecules such as salts or water and totally restrict the passage of macromolecules. To make matters still more difficult, it is common to find that different regions of the same tumor vary extensively in their level of differentiation and therefore in the complexity of tumor cell junctions. This heterogeneity suggests that, like blood flow, the passage of large and small molecules will also vary considerably from one region to another within the same tumor.

V. DELIVERING THERAPEUTIC MACROMOLECULES TO SOLID TUMORS

This chapter has described a formidable set of barriers that are likely to limit the delivery of circulating therapeutic macromolecules to tumors. The barriers we have cited apply primarily to solid tumors with connective tissue stroma; tumor cells growing as loosely joined masses or as cell suspensions (e.g., leukemias, tumors growing in ascites form in the peritoneal or other body cavities) may be exempt from these barriers and could be good candidates for therapy with macromolecular medicines. For most solid tumors, however, the barriers present a formidable obstacle. Thus, even if an antibody-toxin complex of ideal tumor cell specificity were available, it might be of little practical use because of the difficulties of delivering it in effective concentration to tumor sites scattered throughout the body.

Are there strategies that might reduce these barriers and allow circulating macromolecular therapeutics more rapid access to their targets in solid tumors? Among the possibilities that have been proposed, several seem worthy of further consideration:

1. To the extent that the passage of molecular medicines across tumor vessels, stroma and parenchyma depends primarily on diffusion, it is advantageous to reduce the size of therapeutic macromolecules. Progress has been made in this regard, for example by the engineering of various small antibody fragments. Perhaps still smaller fragments can be designed that retain specificity and avidity for tumor antigen targets. Of course, small size has a downside: shorter circulation time, more extensive extravasation across normal microvessels, and hence higher concentrations of potentially toxic molecules in normal tissues.

2. The relative hyperpermeability to macromolecules of tumor vessels as compared with normal vessels is likely responsible for such success as has been achieved in the therapy of solid tumors with monoclonal antibodies. It may be possible to further augment the innate hyperpermeability of tumor vessels (122). Additional increases in vessel permeability would be expected to increase the effectiveness of therapeutic macromolecules in solid tumors as long as interstitial pressures do not rise concomitantly.

3. The high interstitial pressures within solid tumors direct convective currents away from the tumor center and thereby inhibit the entry of therapeutic macromolecules. Approaches that reduced tumor interstitial pressure would be expected to enhance the effectiveness of tumor therapy with macromolecular medicines.

4. Most current strategies seek to target tumor cells. Difficulties of delivery would be reduced greatly if the tumor vasculature, and particularly the endothelial cells lining tumor vessels, were targeted instead (123–125). Indeed, the effectiveness of this approach has already been demonstrated in principle (126,127). The difficulty has been to find a marker that is uniquely expressed on tumor as compared with normal vascular endothelium. VPF/VEGF may itself be such a marker in that it has been shown to accumulate in quantity on tumor blood vessel endothelium (38,128,129) and can be successfully targeted there (126). A number of groups are searching for other targets (130). The advantages of this general approach are obvious: delivery of a therapeutic macromolecule without

the need to cross vessels, stroma, or parenchyma; a multiplier effect in that destruction of a single blood vessel will result in the destruction of the many tumor cells it supplies; the likelihood that a single antibody would recognize the endothelium of many different tumors (i.e., tumor vessel endothelial cell antigens are not likely to be specific for a single tumor), etc. Presumably such macromolecular medicines would need to be supplemented by currently available chemotherapeutic drugs which would mop up residual malignant cells at the periphery of solid tumors that are not dependent for survival on a new vascular supply.

ACKNOWLEDGMENTS

This work was supported by USPHS NIH grants CA-50453 and AI-33372, by the BIH Pathology Foundation, Inc., and under terms of a contract with the National Foundation for Cancer Research.

REFERENCES

1. Bailar JC, Smith EM. Progress against cancer? N Engl J Med 1986; 314:1226–1232.
2. Sporn MB. The war on cancer. Lancet 1996; 347:1377–1381.
3. Frankel AE, FitzGerald D, Siegall C, Press OW. Advances in immunotoxin biology and therapy: a summary of the Fourth International Symposium on Immunotoxins. Cancer Res 1996; 56:926–932.
4. Pai LH, Wittes R, Setser A, Willingham MC, Pastan I. Treatment of advanced solid tumors with immunotoxin LMB-1: an antibody linked to Pseudomonas exotoxin. Nat Med 1996; 2:350–353.
5. Thrush GR, Lark LR, Clinchy BC, Vitetta ES. Immunotoxins: an update. Annu Rev Immunol 1996; 14:49–71.
6. Goldenberg D. Seventh conference on radioimmunodetection and radioimmunotherapy of cancer. Clinical Cancer Research 1999; 5:2991s–3344s.
7. Nagy JA, Brown LF, Senger DR, Lanir N, Van De Water L, Dvorak AM, Dvorak HF. Pathogenesis of tumor stroma generation: a critical role for leaky blood vessels and fibrin deposition. Biochim Biophys Acta 1988; 948:305–326.
8. Yeo T-K, Dvorak HF. Tumor stroma. In: Colvin R, Bhan A, McCluskey R, eds. Diagnostic Immunopathology. New York: Raven Press, 1995:685–697.
9. Knudson AG. Stem cell regulation, tissue ontogeny, and oncogenic events. Semin Cancer Biol 1992; 3:99–106.
10. Folkman J. Tumor angiogenesis. Adv Cancer Res 1985; 43:175–203.
11. Pritchard-Jones K. Malignant origin of the stromal component of Wilms' tumor. J Natl Cancer Inst 1997; 89:1089–1091.
12. Dvorak HF. Tumors: wounds that do not heal. similarities between tumor stroma generation and wound healing. N Engl J Med 1986; 315:1650–1659.

13. Tsurusaki T, Kanda S, Sakai H, Kanetake H, Saito Y, Alitalo K, Koji T. Vascular endothelial growth factor-C expression in human prostatic carcinoma and its relationship to lymph node metastasis. Br J Cancer 1999; 80:309–313.

14. Yamada K. Fibronectin and other cell interactive glycoproteins. In: Hay E, ed. Cell Biology of Extracellular Matrix. New York: Plenum Press, 1991:111–146.

15. Ffrench-Constant C, Van de Water L, Dvorak HF, Hynes RO. Reappearance of an embryonic pattern of fibronectin splicing during wound healing in the adult rat. J Cell Biol 1989; 109:903–914.

16. Grimwood RE, Huff JC, Harbell JW, Clark RAF. Fibronectin in basal cell epithelioma: sources and significance. J Invest Dermatol 1984; 82:145–149.

17. Kornblihtt AR, Pesce CG, Alonso CR, Cramer P, Srebrow A, Werbajh S, Muro AF. The fibronectin gene as a model for splicing and transcription studies. FASEB J 1996; 10:248–257.

18. Chiquet-Ehrismann R. Tenascin and other adhesion-modulating proteins in cancer. Semin Cancer Biol 1993; 4:301–310.

19. Leprini A, Querze G, Zardi L. Tenascin isoforms: possible targets for diagnosis and therapy of cancer and mechanisms regulating their expression. Perspect Dev Neurobiol 1994; 2:117–123.

20. Iskaros BF, Tanaka KE, Hu X, Kadish AS, Steinberg JJ. Morphologic pattern of tenascin as a diagnostic biomarker in colon cancer. J Surg Oncol 1997; 64:98–101.

21. Iruela-Arispe M, Hasselaar P, Sage H. Differential expression of extracellular proteins is correlated with angiogenesis in vitro. Lab Invest 1991; 64:174–186.

22. Gladson CL. The extracellular matrix of gliomas: modulation of cell function. J Neuropathol Exp Neurol 1999; 58:1029–1040.

23. Pilch H, Schaffer U, Schlenger K, Lautz A, Tanner B, Hockel M, Knapstein PG. Expression of tenascin in human cervical cancer—association of tenascin expression with clinicopathological parameters. Gynecol Oncol 1999; 73:415–421.

24. Matsumoto E, Yoshida T, Kawarada Y, Sakakura T. Expression of fibronectin isoforms in human breast tissue: production of extra domain A+/extra domain B+ by cancer cells and extra domain A+ by stromal cells. Jpn J Cancer Res 1999; 90:320–325.

25. Talts JF, Wirl G, Dictor M, Muller WJ, Fassler R. Tenascin-C modulates tumor stroma and monocyte/macrophage recruitment but not tumor growth or metastasis in a mouse strain with spontaneous mammary cancer. J Cell Sci 1999; 112:1855–1864.

26. Ishihara A, Yoshida T, Tamaki H, Sakakura T. Tenascin expression in cancer cells and stroma of human breast cancer and its prognostic significance. Clin Cancer Res 1995; 1:1035–1041, 1995.

27. Iruela-Arispe ML, Dvorak HF. Angiogenesis: a dynamic balance of stimulators and inhibitors. Thromb Haemost 1997; 78:672–677.

28. Senger DR. Molecular framework for angiogenesis: a complex web of interactions between extravasated plasma proteins and endothelial cell proteins induced by angiogenic cytokines [comment]. Am J Pathol 1996; 149:1–7.

29. Takeuchi J, Sobue M, Sato E, Shamoto M, Miura K. Variation in glycosaminoglycan components of breast tumors. Cancer Res 1976; 36:2133–2139.

30. Horai T, Nakamura N, Tateishi R, Hattori S. Glycosaminoglycans in human lung cancer. Cancer 1981; 48:2016–2021.
31. De Klerk DP, Lee DV, Human HJ. Glycosaminoglycans of human prostatic cancer. J Urol 1984; 131:1008–1012.
32. Yeo TK, Brown L, Dvorak HF. Alterations in proteoglycan synthesis common to healing wounds and tumors. Am J Pathol 1991; 138:1437–1450.
33. Yeo TK, Nagy JA, Yeo KT, Dvorak HF, Toole BP. Increased hyaluronan at sites of attachment to mesentery by CD44-positive mouse ovarian and breast tumor cells. Am J Pathol 1996; 148:1733–1740.
34. Adany R, Iozzo RV. Hypomethylation of the decorin proteoglycan gene in human colon cancer. Biochem J 1991; 276:301–306.
35. Weidner N, Folkman J. Tumoral vascularity as a prognostic factor in cancer. In: De Vita VT HS, Rosenberg SA, ed. Important Advances in Oncology 1996. 1996: 167–190.
36. Gullino PM. Extracellular compartments of solid tumors. In: Becker FF, ed. Cancer: A Comprehensive Treatise. New York: Plenum Press, 1975:327–354.
37. Nagy JA, Herzberg KT, Dvorak JM, Dvorak HF. Pathogenesis of malignant ascites formation: Initiating events that lead to fluid accumulation. Cancer Res 1993; 53: 2631–2643.
38. Dvorak HF, Brown LF, Detmar M, Dvorak AM. Vascular permeability factor/vascular endothelial growth factor, microvascular hyperpermeability, and angiogenesis. Am J Pathol 1995; 146:1029–1039.
39. Dvorak HF, Nagy JA, Feng D, Brown LF, Dvorak AM. Vascular permeability factor/vascular endothelial growth factor and the significance of microvascular hyperpermeability in angiogenesis. Curr Top Microbiol Immunol 1999; 237:97–132.
40. Dvorak HF, Orenstein NS, Carvalho AC, Churchill WH, Dvorak AM, Galli SJ, Feder J, Bitzer AM, Rypysc J, Giovinco P. Induction of a fibrin-gel investment: an early event in line 10 hepatocarcinoma growth mediated by tumor-secreted products. J Immunol 1979; 122:166–174.
41. Dvorak HF, Dvorak AM, Manseau EJ, Wiberg L, Churchill WH. Fibrin gel investment associated with line 1 and line 10 solid tumor growth, angiogenesis, and fibroplasia in guinea pigs: role of cellular immunity, myofibroblasts, microvascular damage, and infarction in line 1 tumor regression. J Natl Cancer Inst 1979; 62: 1459 -1472.
42. Dvorak HF, Harvey VS, McDonagh J. Quantitation of fibrinogen influx and fibrin deposition and turnover in line 1 and line 10 guinea pig carcinomas. Cancer Res 1984; 44:3348–3354.
43. Nagy JA, Meyers MS, Masse EM, Herzberg KT, Dvorak HF. Pathogenesis of ascites tumor growth: fibrinogen influx and fibrin accumulation in tissues lining the peritoneal cavity. Cancer Res 1995; 55:369–375.
44. Warren BA. The vascular morphology of tumors. In: Peterson H-I, ed. Tumor Blood Circulation: Angiogenesis, Vascular Morphology and Blood Flow of Experimental and Human Tumors. Boca Raton, FL: CRC Press, 1979:1–47.
45. Vaupel P, Kallinowski F, Okunieff P. Blood flow, oxygen and nutrient supply, and metabolic microenvironment of human tumors: a review. Cancer Res 1989; 49: 6449–6465.

46. Dvorak HF, Nagy JA, Dvorak JT, Dvorak AM. Identification and characterization of the blood vessels of solid tumors that are leaky to circulating macromolecules. Am J Pathol 1988; 133:95–109.

47. Brown LF, Chester JF, Malt RA, Dvorak HF. Fibrin deposition in autochthonous Syrian hamster pancreatic adenocarcinomas induced by the chemical carcinogen N-nitroso-bis(2-oxopropyl)amine. J Natl Cancer Inst 1987; 78:979–986.

48. Brown LF, Van De Water L, Harvey VS, Dvorak HF. Fibrinogen influx and accumulation of cross-linked fibrin in healing wounds and in tumor stroma. Am J Pathol 1988; 130:455–465.

49. O'Connor SW, Bale WF. Accessibility of circulating immunoglobulin G to the extravascular compartment of solid rat tumors. Cancer Res 1984; 44:3719–3723.

50. Nagy JA, Masse EM, Herzberg KT, Meyers MS, Yeo K-T, Yeo T-K, Sioussat TM, Dvorak HF. Pathogenesis of ascites tumor growth: vascular permeability factor, vascular hyperpermeability and ascites fluid accumulation. Cancer Res 1995; 55: 360–368.

51. Senger DR, Galli SJ, Dvorak AM, Perruzzi CA, Harvey VS, Dvorak HF. Tumor cells secrete a vascular permeability factor that promotes accumulation of ascites fluid. Science 1983; 219:983–985.

52. Senger DR, Perruzzi CA, Feder J, Dvorak HF. A highly conserved vascular permeability factor secreted by a variety of human and rodent tumor cell lines. Cancer Res 1986; 46:5629–5632.

53. Senger DR, Connolly D, Perruzzi CA, Alsup D, Nelson R, Leimgruber R, Feder J, Dvorak HF. Purification of a vascular permeability factor (VPF) from tumor cell conditioned medium. Fed Proc 1987; 46:2102.

54. Senger DR, Connolly DT, Van de Water L, Feder J, Dvorak HF. Purification and NH_2-terminal amino acid sequence of guinea pig tumor-secreted vascular permeability factor. Cancer Res 1990; 50:1774–1778.

55. Connolly DT, Heuvelman DM, Nelson R, Olander JV, Eppley BL, Delfino JJ, Siegel NR, Leimgruber RM, Feder J. Tumor vascular permeability factor stimulates endothelial cell growth and angiogenesis. J Clin Invest 1989; 84:1470–1478.

56. Leung DW, Cachianes G, Kuang W-J, Goeddel DV, Ferrara N. Vascular endothelial growth factor is a secreted angiogenic mitogen. Science 1989; 246:1306–1309.

57. Park J, Keller G-A, Ferrara N. The vascular endothelial growth factor (VEGF) isoforms: differential deposition into the subepithelial extracellular matrix and bioactivity of extracellular matrix-bound VEGF. Mol Biol Cell 1993; 4:1317–1326.

58. Brown L, Detmar M, Claffey K, Nagy J, Feng D, Dvorak A, Dvorak H. Vascular permeability factor/vascular endothelial growth factor: a multifunctional angiogenic cytokine. In: Goldberg I, Rosen E, eds. Regulation of Angiogenesis. Basel: Birkhauser Verlag, 1997.

59. Brock TA, Dvorak HF, Senger DR. Tumor-secreted vascular permeability factor increases cytosolic Ca^{2+} and von Willebrand factor release in human endothelial cells. Am J Pathol 1991; 138:213–221.

60. Ferrara N. Vascular endothelial growth factor: molecular and biological aspects. Curr Top Microbiol Immunol 1999; 237:1–30.

61. Bates DO, Curry FE. Vascular endothelial growth factor increases hydraulic conductivity of isolated perfused microvessels. Am J Physiol 1996; 271:H2520–H2528.

62. Tischer E, Mitchell R, Hartman T, Silva M, Gospodarowicz D, Fiddes JC, Abraham JA. The human gene for vascular endothelial growth factor. Multiple protein forms are encoded through alternative exon splicing. J Biol Chem 1991; 266:11947–11954.

63. Clauss M, Gerlach M, Gerlach H, Brett J, Wang F, Familletti PC, Pan Y-CE, Olander JV, Connolly DT, Stern D. Vascular permeability factor: A tumor-derived polypeptide that induces endothelial cell and monocyte procoagulant activity, and promotes monocyte migration. J Exp Med 1990; 172:1535–1545.

64. Pepper MS, Ferrara N, Orci L, Montesano R. Vascular endothelial growth factor (VEGF) induces plasminogen activators and plasminogen activator inhibitor-1 in microvascular endothelial cells. BBRC 1991; 181:902–906.

65. Unemori EN, Ferrara N, Bauer EA, Amento EP. Vascular endothelial growth factor induces interstitial collagenase expression in human endothelial cells. J Cell Physiol 1992; 153:557–562.

66. Pekala P, Marlow M, Heuvelman D, Connolly D. Regulation of hexose transport in aortic endothelial cells by vascular permeability factor and tumor necrosis factor-alpha, but not by insulin. J Biol Chem 1990; 265:18051–18054.

67. Senger DR, Ledbetter SR, Claffey KP, Papadopoulos-Sergiou A, Peruzzi CA, Detmar M. Stimulation of endothelial cell migration by vascular permeability factor/vascular endothelial growth factor through cooperative mechanisms involving the alphavbeta3 integrin, osteopontin, and thrombin. Am J Pathol 1996; 149:293–305.

68. Varner JA, Cheresh DA. Tumor angiogenesis and the role of vascular cell integrin alphavbeta3. Important Adv Oncol 1996:69–87.

69. Alon T, Hemo I, Itin A, Pe'er J, Stone J, Keshet E. Vascular endothelial growth factor acts as a survival factor for newly formed retinal vessels and has implications for retinopathy of prematurity. Nature Medicine 1995; 1:1024–1028.

70. Watanabe Y, Lee SW, Detmar M, Ajioka I, Dvorak HF. Vascular permeability factor/vascular endothelial growth factor (VPF/VEGF) delays and induces escape from senescence in human dermal microvascular endothelial cells. Oncogene 1997; 14:2025–2032.

71. Dvorak HF, Senger DS, Dvorak AM, Harvey VS, McDonagh J. Regulation of extravascular coagulation by microvascular permeability. Science 1985; 227:1059–1061.

72. Dvorak HF, Quay SC, Orenstein NS, Dvorak AM, Hahn P, Bitzer AM, Carvalho AC. Tumor shedding and coagulation. Science 1981; 212:923–924.

73. Dvorak HF, Senger DR, Dvorak AM. Fibrin as a component of the tumor stroma: Origins and biological significance. Cancer Metastasis Rev 1983; 2:41–73.

74. Van de Water L, Tracy PB, Aronson D, Mann KG, Dvorak HF. Tumor cell generation of thrombin via functional prothrombinase assembly. Cancer Res 1985; 45:5521–5525.

75. Dvorak HF, Galli SJ, Dvorak AM. Cellular and vascular manifestations of cell-mediated immunity. Hum Pathol 1986; 17:122–137.

76. Danø K, Andreasen PA, Grøndahl-Hansen J, Kristensen P, Nielsen LS, Skriver L. Plasminogen activators, tissue degradation, and cancer. In: Klein G, Weinhouse S, eds. Advances in Cancer Research. Vol. 44, Orlando, FL: Academic Press, 1985: 139–266.

77. Brown LF, Lanir N, McDonagh J, Czarnecki K, Estrella P, Dvorak AM, Dvorak HF. Fibroblast migration in fibrin gel matrices. Am J Pathol 1993; 142:273–283.

78. Ciano PS, Colvin RB, Dvorak AM, McDonagh J, Dvorak HF. Macrophage migration in fibrin gel matrices. Lab Invest 1986; 54:62–70.

79. Lanir N, Ciano PS, Van De Water L, McDonagh J, Dvorak AM, Dvorak HF. Macrophage migration in fibrin gel matrices. II. Effects of clotting factor XIII, fibronectin, and glycosaminoglycan content on cell migration. J Immunol 1988; 140:2340–2349.

80. Dvorak HF, Harvey VS, Estrella P, Brown LF, McDonagh J, Dvorak AM. Fibrin containing gels induce angiogenesis: implications for tumor stroma generation and wound healing. Lab Invest 1987; 57:673–686.

81. Rippe B, Haraldsson B. Transport of macromolecules across microvascular walls: the two-pore theory. Physiol Rev 1994; 74:163–219.

82. Jain R. Transport of molecules across tumor vasculature. Cancer Metastasis Rev 1987; 6:559–593.

83. Jain RK. Delivery of novel therapeutic agents in tumors: physiological barriers and strategies. J Natl Cancer Inst 1989; 81:570–576.

84. Jain RK. Physiological barriers to delivery of monoclonal antibodies and other macromolecules in tumors. Cancer Res 1990; 50:814s–819s.

85. Zweifach B, Lipowsky H. Pressure-flow relations in blood and lymph microcirculation. In: Renkin E, Michel C, eds. Handbook of Physiology. Vol. Sect. 2, Vol. 4, Chap. 7. Bethesda, MD: American Physiological Society, 1984:251–308.

86. Sevick EM, Jain RK. Viscous resistance to blood flow in solid tumors: effect of hematocrit on intratumor blood viscosity. Cancer Res 1989; 49:3513–3519.

87. Sevick EM, Jain RK. Geometric resistance to blood flow in solid tumors perfused ex vivo: effects of tumor size and perfusion pressure. Cancer Res 1989; 49:3506–3512.

88. Peterson H-I. Tumor Blood Circulation: Angiogenesis, Vascular Morphology and Blood Flow of Experimental and Human Tumors. Boca Raton, FL: CRC Press, 1979:229.

89. Chaplin DJ, Olive PL, Durand RE. Intermittent blood flow in a murine tumor: radiobiological effects. Cancer Res 1987; 47:597–601.

90. Shweiki D, Itin A, Soffer D, Keshet E. Vascular endothelial growth factor induced by hypoxia may mediate hypoxia-initiated angiogenesis. Nature 1992; 359:843–845.

91. Goldberg M, Schneider T. Similarities between the oxygen sensing mechanisms regulating the expression of vascular endothelial growth factor and erythropoietin. J Biol Chem 1994; 269:4355–4359.

92. Claffey KP, Brown LF, del Aguila LF, Tognazzi K, Yeo KT, Manseau EJ, Dvorak HF. Expression of vascular permeability factor/vascular endothelial growth factor by melanoma cells increases tumor growth, angiogenesis, and experimental metastasis. Cancer Res 1996; 56:172–181.

93. Plate KH, Breier G, Weich HA, Risau W. Vascular endothelial growth factor is a potential tumour angiogenesis factor in human gliomas in vivo. Nature 1992; 359:845–848.

94. Gullino P, Grantham F. Studies on the exchange of fluids between host and tumor.

II. The blood flow of hepatomas and other tumors in rats and mice. The Journal Of The National Cancer Institute 1961; 27:1465–1491.

95. Jain RK. Determinants of tumor blood flow: a review. Cancer Res 1988; 48:2641–2658.

96. Dvorak AM, Kohn S, Morgan ES, Fox P, Nagy JA, Dvorak HF. The vesiculo-vacuolar organelle (VVO): A distinct endothelial cell structure that provides a trans-cellular pathway for macromolecular extravasation. J Leukoc Biol 1996; 59:100–115.

97. Feng D, Nagy J, Hipp J, Dvorak H. Dvorak A. Vesiculo-vacuolar organelles and the regulation of venule permeability to macromolecules by vascular permeability factor, histamine and serotonin. J Exp Med 1996; 183:1981–1986.

98. Feng D, Nagy J, Hipp J, Pyne K, Dvorak H, Dvorak A. Reinterpretation of endothe-lial cell gaps induced by vasoactive mediators in guinea-pig, mouse and rat: many are transcellular pores. J Physiology (London) 1997; 504(3):747–761.

99. McDonald DM, Thurston G, Baluk P. Endothelial gaps as sites for plasma leakage in inflammation. Microcirculation 1999; 6:7–22.

100. Michel CC, Neal CR. Openings through endothelial cells associated with increased microvascular permeability. Microcirculation 1999; 6:45–54.

101. Neal CR, Michel CC. Transcellular gaps in microvascular walls of frog and rat when permeability is increased by perfusion with the ionophore A23187. J Physiol (Lond) 1995; 488:427–437.

102. Neal C, Michel C. Openings in frog microvascular endothelium induced by high intravascular pressure. J Physiol (Lond) 1996; 492:39–52.

103. Simionescu N. Cellular aspects of transcapillary exchange. Physiol Rev 1983; 63:1536–1579.

104. Palade GE. The microvascular endothelium revisited. In: Simionescu N, Simi-onescu M, eds. Endothelial Cell Biology in Health and Disease. New York: Plenum Press, 1988:3–22.

105. Majno G, Gilmore V, Leventhal M. On the mechanism of vascular leakage caused by histamine type mediators. A microscopic study in vivo. Circ Res 1967; 21:833–847.

106. Majno G, Shea SM, Leventhal M. Endothelial contraction induced by histamine-type mediators: an electron microscopic study. J Cell Biol 1969; 42:647–672.

107. Baluk P, Hirata A, Thurston G, Fujiwara T, Neal CR, Michel CC, McDonald DM. Endothelial gaps: time course of formation and closure in inflamed venules of rats. Am J Physiol 1997; 272:L155–L170.

108. Feng D, Nagy JA, Pyne K, Hammel I, Dvorak HF, Dvorak AM. Pathways of macro-molecular extravasation across microvascular endothelium in response to VPF/VEGF and other vasoactive mediators. Microcirculation 1999; 6:23–44.

109. Kohn S, Nagy JA, Dvorak HF, Dvorak AM. Pathways of macromolecular tracer transport across venules and small veins: structural basis for the hyperpermeability of tumor blood vessels. Lab Invest 1992; 67:596–607.

110. Roberts WG, Palade GE. Neovasculature induced by vascular endothelial growth factor is fenestrated. Cancer Res 1997; 57:765–772.

111. Clementi F, Palade GE. Intestinal capillaries. I. Permeability to peroxidase and ferritin. J Cell Biol 1969; 41:33–58.

112. Roberts WG, Palade GE. Increased microvascular permeability and endothelial fenestration induced by vascular endothelial growth factor. J Cell Sci 1995; 108:2369–2379.

113. Feng D, Nagy J, Dvorak A, Dvorak H. Different pathways of macromolecule extravasation from hyperpermeable tumor vessels. Microvasc Res. In press.

114. Milici AJ, Bankston PW. Fetal and neonatal rat intestinal capillaries: permeability to carbon, ferritin, hemoglobin, and myoglobin. Am J Anat 1982; 165:165–186.

115. Levick JR, Smaje LH. An analysis of the permeability of a fenestra. Microvasc Res 1987; 33:233–256.

116. Young J, Lumsden C, Stalker A. The significance of the "tissue pressure" of normal testicular and of neoplastic (Brown-Pearce carcinoma) tissue in the rabbit. J Pathol Bacteriol 1950; 62:313–333.

117. Jain RK, Baxter LT. Mechanisms of heterogeneous distribution of monoclonal antibodies and other macromolecules in tumors: significance of elevated interstitial pressure. Cancer Res 1988; 48:7022–7032.

118. Boucher Y, Baxter LT, Jain RK. Interstitial pressure gradients in tissue-isolated and subcutaneous tumors: implications for therapy. Cancer Res 1990; 50:4478–4484.

119. Baxter LT, Zhu H, Mackensen DG, Jain RK. Physiologically based pharmacokinetic model for specific and nonspecific monoclonal antibodies and fragments in normal tissues and human tumor xenografts in nude mice. Cancer Res 1994; 54:1517–1528.

120. Baxter LT, Jain RK. Pharmacokinetic analysis of the microscopic distribution of enzyme-conjugated antibodies and prodrugs: comparison with experimental data. Br J Cancer 1996; 73:447–456.

121. Butler TP, Grantham FH, Gullino PM. Bulk transfer of fluid in the interstitial compartment of mammary tumors. Cancer Res 1975; 35:3084–3088.

122. Monsky WL, Fukumura D, Gohongi T, Ancukiewcz M, Weich HA, Torchilin VP, Yuan F, Jain RK. Augmentation of transvascular transport of macromolecules and nanoparticles in tumors using vascular endothelial growth factor. Cancer Res 1999; 59:4129–4135.

123. Denekamp J. Vascular attack as a therapeutic strategy for cancer. Cancer Metastasis Rev 1990; 9:267–282.

124. Dvorak HF, Nagy JA, Dvorak AM. Structure of solid tumors and their vasculature: implications for therapy with monoclonal antibodies. Cancer Cells 1991; 3:77–85.

125. Kerbel RS. Inhibition of tumor angiogenesis as a strategy to circumvent acquired resistance to anti-cancer therapeutic agents. Bioessays 1991; 13:31–36.

126. Ke-Lin, Qu-Hong, Nagy JA, Eckelhoefer IA, Masse EM, Dvorak AM, Dvorak HF. Vascular targeting of solid and ascites tumours with antibodies to vascular endothelial growth factor. Eur J Cancer 1996; 32A:2467–2473.

127. Huang X, Molema G, King S, Watkins L, Edgington TS, Thorpe PE. Tumor infarction in mice by antibody-directed targeting of tissue factor to tumor vasculature. Science 1997; 275:547–550.

128. Dvorak HF, Sioussat TM, Brown LF, Nagy JA, Sotrel A, Manseau, E., Van De Water L, Senger DR. Distribution of vascular permeability factor (vascular endo-

thelial growth factor) in tumors: concentration in tumor blood vessels. J Exp Med 1991; 174:1275–1278.

129. Qu-Hong, Nagy JA, Senger DR, Dvorak HF, Dvorak AM. Ultrastructural localization of vascular permeability factor/vascular endothelial growth factor (VPF/ VEGF) to the abluminal plasma membrane and vesicuolo-vacuolar organelles of tumor microvascular endothelium. J Histochem Cytochem 1995; 43:381–389.

130. Jacobson BS, Stolz DB, Schnitzer JE. Identification of endothelial cell-surface proteins as targets for diagnosis and treatment of disease. Nat Med 1996; 2:482–484.

131. Jain RK. Transport of molecules in the tumor interstitium: a review. Cancer Res 1987; 47:3039–3051.

6

Antibodies and Novel Constructs for Tumor Targeting

Dale C. Slavin-Chiorini, Patricia Horan Hand,*
and John W. Greiner
National Cancer Institute, National Institutes of Health,
Bethesda, Maryland

I. INTRODUCTION

Since the seminal work of Kohler and Milstein (1) ushered in the monoclonal antibody (MAb) era 20 years ago, developments in MAb technology have led to the identification of numerous new human tumor-associated antigens (TAAs). Monoclonal antibody technology has had a significant impact on our understanding of basic cancer biology and has also become an important component in the evolution of the immunodiagnosis and immunotherapy of cancer. The unique properties of MAbs including their antigenic specificity, internalization by the cell, and their clearance and excretion from the body have been capitalized upon in both preclinical and clinical studies of cancer.

Thus far, MAb therapy has been most successful for patients with B-cell malignancies (2–4). In fact, therapy using multiple doses or one large dose of a radiolabeled MAb has been effective in a large percentage of patients with non-Hodgkin's lymphoma (5,6). The information from these MAb studies and those directed at carcinomas has elucidated the difficulties that need to be overcome for MAbs to be a more successful therapeutic venue for all cancer patients. Defining more successful diagnostic and therapeutic clinical MAb protocols requires an understanding of the physical properties of a MAb as well as the biology of the human tumor cell, including those factors which govern the expression of a given TAA. Within this chapter, we will discuss current efforts to apply ge-

*Current affiliation: Center for Scientific Review, National Institutes of Health, Bethesda, Maryland.

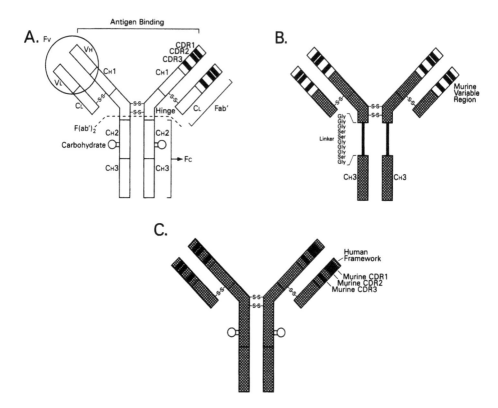

Figure 1 Schematic diagram of immunoglobulin forms. (A) Intact murine immunoglobulin (IgG1) illustrated within the diagram are the different fragments and domains of the
antibody. (B) A chimeric (mouse variable regions/human constant regions) CH2 domain-
deleted IgG1 with the 10 amino acid linker bridging the hinge and CH3 regions. (C) An
intact humanized IgG1 antibody. It has human constant regions and murine complementar-
ity determining regions grafted onto human framework regions.

netic engineering techniques to murine MAbs to design novel MAb constructs
(Fig. 1). These "designer MAbs" may have altered physical and biological properties which should make them more amenable to specific clinical goals.

Concomitant with a rational approach to developing new MAbs, there needs
to be an understanding of the rationale behind engineering novel antibody constructs and the relationship of MAb targeting to the regulation of tumor antigen
expression. Numerous laboratories have shown that differentiation inducing
agents, particularly the interferons (IFNs), can enhance expression of TAAs which
leads to better tumor detection and therapy with radiolabeled MAbs in an experimental model. Current research on these elements of MAb technology to aid in

cancer diagnosis and therapy, and the regulation of tumor antigen expression to enhance MAb cancer diagnosis and therapy will be discussed within this chapter.

II. RADIOLABELED MAbs IN THE DIAGNOSIS AND TREATMENT OF CANCER

Numerous preclinical studies using human tumor xenografts and radiolabeled MAbs have demonstrated the utility of MAbs for immunodetection and immunotherapy of human TAAs (7–10). For example, significant regression of carcinoembryonic antigen (CEA)-expressing human tumor xenografts was observed after administration of an ^{131}I-labeled anti-CEA MAb, COL-1 (11). In other studies, an ^{131}I-radiolabeled anti-GD2 MAb targeting neuroblastoma xenografts effectively improved the neurological function of 100% of the tumor bearing rats (12). Furthermore, a ^{177}Lu-conjugated MAb CC49, reactive with the pancarcinoma antigen, tumor associated glycoprotein (TAG)-72, effectively eliminated human tumor xenográfts in 90% of treated mice (13). Preclinical studies have also suggested the advantage of dose fractionation of a radiolabeled MAb for therapeutic protocols. Studies in a murine tumor xenograft model demonstrated that 300 µCi of ^{131}I-B72.3, reactive with TAG-72, administered once per week for 3 weeks more effectively minimized the tumor growth and mortality than one administration of 900 µCi of ^{131}I-B72.3 (14).

The promising results of preclinical experiments led to the use of several radiolabeled MAbs in clinical trials for both radioimmunodiagnosis (RAID) and radioimmunotherapy (RAIT) of cancer (7,8,15). Clinical trials with anti-carcinoma MAbs, including 17-1A, BW431/26, 3F8, B72.3, and CC49 have demonstrated the successful localization of 50% to 90% of colon carcinoma lesions (16–18). Recently, successful RAID has also been demonstrated in five of five breast carcinoma patients receiving a ^{99m}Tc-labeled anti-CEA MAb and 5 of 7 patients receiving an ^{123}I-labeled antihuman milk fat globule (HMFG) MAb (19).

Comparative analyses of the success rate of radiolabeled MAbs versus more conventional methods of tumor detection have been reported. For example, clinical trials have demonstrated that the anti-TAG-72 MAb B72.3 detects a significantly higher percentage of patients' tumors than CT imaging (20,21). Radioimmunoguided surgery (RIGS) entails the use of a hand-held gamma detecting probe in combination with radiolabeled MAb for detection of tumors during surgical intervention. Several studies using the gamma detecting probe in conjunction with ^{131}I-B72.3 for RIGS have demonstrated the identification of tumor cells undetected by other methods (22). B72.3 was the first MAb to be approved by the FDA for the detection of colorectal and ovarian cancer. Clinical studies using the radiolabeled anti-TAG-72 MAb CC49, a MAb with a higher antigen affinity than B72.3, have shown that CC49 targeted >90% of patients' colorectal lesions

(23,24). Furthermore the use of ^{131}I-CC49 for RIGS led to altered management of over 40% of surgical cases (8).

Radiolabeled MAb therapy has been most successful for patients with B-cell malignancies (2–4). The results of one clinical trial showed that 10 of 12 B-cell lymphoma patients treated with anti-B1, an anti-CD20 MAb, had complete remissions and the remaining two had partial responses (25). Moreover, a Phase II clinical trial of patients with relapsed B-cell lymphomas resulted in complete responses in 16 of the 21 patients treated with therapeutic infusions of ^{131}I-anti-CD20 (B1) MAb (4).

Radiolabeled MAbs have also been used for RAIT of solid tumors. In Phase I studies in which increasing doses of [186]Re radiolabeled anti-CEA MAb were administered, two partial responses were observed (26). Radioimmunotherapy of ovarian and breast peritoneal effusions has also shown some success. The anti-ovarian carcinoma MAb NR-LU-10 was labeled with [186]Re and used to treat patients with peritoneal disease (27). Of the 17 patients treated, four had partial regression of their tumors. ^{131}I-B72.3 and ^{131}I-CC49 have also demonstrated some therapeutic efficacy in the treatment of ovarian carcinomas (28,29). Radiolabeled CC49 in combination with recombinant α interferon has elicited partial responses in a Phase II clinical trial for breast cancer (29) and has demonstrated some therapeutic efficacy in an ovarian cancer study (30).

The clinical utility of radiolabeled antibody fragments, $F(ab')_2$ and Fab', has also been explored. In comparison with intact MAbs, fragments clear the plasma faster (31); however, substantial uptake in normal tissues (32) and human antimurine antibody responses (HAMA) (33) have both been documented. In an attempt to reduce immunoglobulin (Ig) clearance rate and HAMA response (34), genetically engineered single-chain Fv (sFv) antibodies have also been developed. sFvs clear more rapidly from the plasma (31) and exhibit faster tumor localization (35) than Fab', $F(ab')_2$ or intact MAb. sFvs have also demonstrated greater tumor penetration than intact Ig (36); however, therapeutic efficacy may be compromised by the significantly lower uptake of an sFv to tumor relative to that of an intact MAb. Divalent sFvs have been engineered with significantly better tumor-targeting properties than the monovalent sFvs described above (37,38). Further studies will be required to delineate the therapeutic efficacy of these new Ig forms.

III. LIMITATIONS OF RADIOLABELED MAbs IN THE CLINICAL SETTING

Although MAbs have shown clinical promise, some obstacles need to be overcome to increase their success in RAID and RAIT. Murine MAbs may elicit HAMA in approximately 40% to 50% of patients after a single injection of MAb and, with repeated administrations, the number of patients developing HAMA may increase to as much as 90% (39–41). However, the extent and nature of patients' HAMA response may differ with the MAb administered (40). One of the possible effects of a HAMA response is complex formation between the murine MAb and the patients' human antimouse Ig, which may decrease MAb localization to the tumor site thereby undermining the efficacy of RAID or RAIT. A patient may also develop an anaphylactic response to the administered murine MAb. These potential difficulties may necessitate termination of further treatment with the murine monoclonal (42).

Another observation from early clinical trials is that the prolonged clearance time of an intact Ig may necessitate an increase in the time between administration of a MAb and the initiation of clinical treatment. For example, in diagnostic imaging, 7 to 10 days are required to have a reduction of radiolabeled MAb in the blood pool and thus have a clear image of the tumor (43). And when RIGS is the chosen diagnostic modality, 2 to 3 weeks are required between injection of radiolabeled MAb and surgery for optimal MAb clearance (44). In therapy protocols using radiolabeled MAbs, the dose-limiting toxicity is myelotoxicity, which appears to be caused primarily by the long clearance time of the radiolabeled MAb from the blood pool (45).

IV. GENETICALLY ENGINEERED ANTIBODIES

Results of early clinical trials confirmed the central hypothesis of using MAb-based protocols for tumor diagnosis and treatment. That is, MAbs which recognize specific human tumor antigens are capable of selectively targeting radionuclides, toxins, and other potential cytolytic agents to the tumor. In fact, as stated previously, MAb B72.3, which recognizes TAG-72, was the first murine MAb to receive FDA approval for clinical use as an immunodiagnostic agent. More recent clinical success has been reported for murine 17-1A which recognizes a 37-kD glycoprotein associated with carcinomas of the gastrointestinal tract (46). 17-1A was administered to patients diagnosed with Dukes' stage C colorectal carcinoma who had undergone curative surgery and were free of residual tumor. Adjuvant antibody treatment was associated with a reduced overall death rate and rate of recurrence. Despite those successes, the early clinical trials also underscored the need to implement molecular biology–based approaches to specifically design new antibody constructs. The specific goal was to alter the physical makeup of the antibody in order to reduce the immune response to the mouse Ig, referred to as HAMA. That change would possibly permit multiple administrations of a conjugated Ig which may be required to elicit any sustained therapeutic effect. Later, more sophisticated hypotheses were developed which required the design of other altered Ig constructs in order to exploit the resultant changes in their biological properties (e.g., pharmacokinetics). As shown below, those constructs might not only further reduce the HAMA response, but also dampen the second organ (i.e., bone marrow) toxicity which is often dose limiting for a radioimmunoconjugate. The following section will summarize several studies designed to generate and characterize chimeric, aglycosylated, domain-deleted, and, finally, humanized antibodies.

A. Chimeric Monoclonal Antibodies

Using molecular biology techniques, mouse/human chimeric MAbs (cMAbs) have been developed which consist of variable regions derived from their native murine molecule and human constant regions (47) (Fig. 1B). Thus, cMAbs may maintain the antigenic recognition of their native murine antibody molecules while decreasing their potential antigenicity in patients.

To develop cIgs, the native murine Ig DNA is cloned as genomic or cDNA and the V_H and V_L regions are excised from the DNA and ligated to human constant regions (48–50). Polymerase chain reaction (PCR) has been used to increase the efficiency of cloning variable region DNA (51). The cIg heavy- or light-chain DNA is then inserted into appropriate expression vectors which contain a bacterial drug resistance gene or selectable marker. The expression vectors containing either the heavy or light chain can then be introduced sequentially into non-Ig-secreting cell lines such as some clones of Chinese hamster ovary (CHO) cells or murine myeloma cells. Several methods including calcium phosphate precipitation, protoplast fusion, lipofection, and electroporation have been used for the transfection of Ig expression vectors (47). Single vectors are now available in which both the murine variable heavy and light chain may be cloned and expressed simultaneously. An anti-CEA cMAb and an anti-CA125 cMAb have been developed using this vector (52).

cMAbs have been developed, and tested for antigen specificity, effector function, and reduced immunogenicity as compared to their murine counterparts. Numerous studies have reported that the antigenic specificity of a cMAb is similar to that of its native MAb (53–56). In several cases, effector functions of the cMAb have been enhanced in comparison to the native MAb. As one example, an anti-renal-cell carcinoma cMAb, ch-G250, was reported to have potent antibody-dependent cell-mediated cytotoxicity (ADCC) function with IL-2-activated human peripheral blood mononuclear cells (PBMCs) against several renal carcinoma cell lines (57). In chromium release assays with human effector cells, the antiganglioside cMAb ch14.18 (human γ1) demonstrated 50- to 100-fold greater efficacy than native 14.18 (murine γ2a) in mediating ADCC against melanoma cell lines (53). Moreover, when compared to the native Ig (murine γ3), the KM871 (human γ1) cMAb demonstrated not only more efficient ADCC with human effector cells, but also more efficient mediation of human CDC against

GD3 expressing target cells (58). Other illustrations of increased effector function capability are afforded by the anti-CEA cMAb 30.6, the anticolorectal gp37 MAb, c17-1A, and the anti-TAG-72 cMAb B72.3 (γ1), which have also demonstrated more efficient mediation of ADCC than their respective native murine Ig counterparts (59–61).

The development of cMAb technology has also allowed comparative analyses of plasma clearance rates of Ig subclasses. In one study, cB72.3 IgG4 had a significantly longer plasma clearance in nonhuman primates than the cIgG1B72.3. In contrast, no difference in plasma clearance was observed between these cMAbs in mice (54). The results of this study suggest that, although the murine tumor model system may be an important first step in characterizing a MAb, it may not always be an accurate indicator of the properties of a MAb in nonhuman primates or in humans. Recently, a dimeric IgA anti-CEA cMAb has been demonstrated to retain the specificity of its native MAb for CEA while exhibiting a novel function, i.e., the ability to translocate across kidney cells bound to membrane as a model for the interior and exterior lumenal surfaces (62). These studies suggest that the exchange of MAb isotypes may alter the biological function of a cMAb while maintaining its original affinity.

Clinical studies have been conducted to investigate the specificity, toxicity, and immunogenicity of cMAbs (8). Phase I clinical trials using the cL6 MAb for immunodetection of non-small-cell lung, colon, and breast cancer showed that the L6 cMAb had a similar clearance rate as the murine L6, and that patient antibody responses to the cL6 were directed to the murine variable region and were of low titer (63). Therapeutic responses have also been observed with high-dose administration of ^{131}I-cL6 (64) in which five of nine patients with metastatic breast cancer had a partial regression of their tumor. Other reports also demonstrated that cMAbs appear to be less immunogenic in patients after one administration than their murine counterparts, and that the immune response observed is anti-idiotypic (30,65,66). For example, after one administration of MOv18, a murine MAb directed against the human folate binding receptor, which is overexpressed on nonmucinous epithelial ovarian tumors, no antichimeric antibody response was observed in the ovarian carcinoma patients (67).

While the acquisition of specific effector functions by selectively choosing the appropriate human V_H variant was an important finding, an equally important goal was to generate a cMAb which could be administered multiple times with minimal immunogenicity. Chimeric B72.3, composed of the V regions of murine B72.3 and the constant regions of human IgG4 heavy and κ light chain, was administered as a radioimmunoconjugate to patients diagnosed with metastatic colon cancer. A transient radioimmunotherapeutic response was observed in one patient (68). The cB72.3 (γ4), unfortunately, retained immunogenicity which, in fact, was reminiscent of the antibody response (i.e., HAMA) for murine B72.3. The immunogenic response was directed at the murine V region, including epitopes in the antigen binding site (i.e., anti-idiotype specificity). The cB72.3 (γ4) also had a plasma retention time which was six to eight times longer than that of murine B72.3. A radiolabeled cB72.3(γ1) has also been used in radioimmunodiagnostic clinical trials for colon cancer. The cB72.3(γ1) localized well to the tumors, but also elicited variable antichimeric antibody responses in patients, although there was no appreciable toxic effect (66). However, in those patients who had a strong antibody response to one administration of cB72.3(γ1), subsequent administration of the cB72.3(γ1) led to decreased efficiency of tumor localization.

It was reasoned from the above studies that the immunogenicity of any Ig molecule depends on at least two characteristics: the inherent immunogenicity of its physical makeup, and its retention time in the blood. Those observations led to the development of a subsequent generation of new genetically engineered antibodies which were designed to further reduce their immunogenicity by incorporating additional human Ig sequences as well as intentionally deleting portions of the molecule in order to facilitate its blood and whole-body clearance.

B. Aglycosylated Chimeric MAbs

An increase in the plasma clearance rate of an Ig may minimize toxicity of the radiolabeled cMAb to normal tissues, as well as reduce the potential for eliciting an anti-Ig immune response in the patient. Several studies reported that carbohydrate residues are involved in plasma clearance of Igs (69) and their metabolism (70,71). These studies were done using enzymatic methods or growth of Ig-producing cells in tunicamycin to produce Igs with modified carbohydrate residues. Using site-directed mutagenesis, aglycosylated cMAbs have been developed including an anti-2-dimethyl-aminonapthalene-5-sulfonyl (DNS) chloride hapten aglycosylated cMAb, an aglycosylated anti-GD2 cMAb, and an aglycosylated anticarcinoma MAb, B72.3 (72–74). Aglycosylation resulted in loss of the major Ig glycosylation site at the CH2 domain and was predicted to affect the plasma clearance as well as effector functions of the resulting antibodies. The anti-DNS aglycosylated cMAb demonstrated a loss of CDC activity and FcγRI receptor binding whether a cIgG3 or a cIgG1 was aglycosylated (72). However, the effect of aglycosylation on plasma clearance was isotype dependent. The aglycosylated cIgG1 had similar pharmacokinetics in mice as the intact cIgG1, while the aglycosylated cIgG3 cleared faster than the intact cIgG3. In a separate study an aglycosylated ch14.18 cMAb retained its ability to bind complement, although at a decreased level, but lost all ADCC activity (73). In contrast to the results obtained with the aglycosylated anti-DNS IgG1 cMAb, the aglycosylated ch14.18 IgG1 cMAb had a faster rate of clearance in mice than the ch14.18. Aglycosylation of MAb cB72.3 did not affect its binding or affinity to TAG-72 in vitro, nor did it substantially affect antigen affinity or plasma clearance in mice after IV MAb administration (74). Aglycosylation of the cB72.3 at the CH2 domain did, however, eliminate ADCC activity. Thus, it appears that the major carbohydrate moiety on the CH2 region of a MAb is important for mediation of CDC and ADCC, and possibly for Fc or carbohydrate receptor-mediated clearance (75). These studies also suggest that the effects of aglycosylation on MAb plasma clearance may be unique for each antibody.

C. Domain-Deleted Chimeric MAbs

In continuing efforts to optimize the pharmacokinetics of plasma clearance and the efficiency of tumor localization and penetrance of cMAbs, domain-deleted Ig variants have been developed. A cDNA expression construct encoding an Ig heavy chain, composed of the variable region of murine MAb B72.3 and a human Ig constant region with a deletion of the CH2 domain, was designed and expressed with the appropriate chimeric light chain. The resulting antibody, cB72.3ΔCH2, has an intact hinge region and a linker peptide bridging the CH1 and CH3 constant regions (Fig. 1B) (76). The antigen-binding affinities of the cB72.3ΔCH2 and cB72.3 MAbs were similar; however, the pharmacokinetics of serum clearance of the two MAbs were significantly different. In athymic mice bearing human colon carcinoma xenografts, the cB72.3ΔCH2 essentially cleared the plasma by 24 h (1% ID/g), while 18% of the ID/g of the cB72.3 still remained at 72 h. The rapid clearance of the cB72.3ΔCH2 led to significantly higher tumor-to-normal-tissue ratios of the domain-deleted cMAb as compared with cB72.3.

The results of preclinical studies with the second-generation anti-TAG-72 MAb CC49 showed a higher affinity of binding of CC49 to TAG-72-positive tumor cells compared with B72.3 (77). MAb CC49 has also been chimerized and designed with a CH2 domain deletion (cCC49ΔCH2) and a CH1 deletion (cCC49ΔCH1) (78). That iodine-labeled cCC49ΔCH1 localized to the tumor and cleared at a rate similar to that of cCC49 was surprising, given that cCC49ΔCH1 is similar in size to cCC49ΔCH2. When compared with cCC49, cCC49ΔCH2 had faster serum kinetics in the mouse and in nonhuman primates (Fig. 2), and significantly higher tumor-to-normal-tissue ratios were observed for the blood, liver, spleen, kidney, and lung (78). An immunoscintigraphic scan of athymic mice bearing human colon carcinoma xenografts 24 h and 72 h after IV inoculation with MAb, demonstrates how rapidly the ^{125}I-cCC49ΔCH2 targets the tumor and clears from the blood pool as compared to ^{125}I-cCC49 (Fig. 3). A CH2 domain-deleted derivative of the cMAb ch14.18 has also been developed (79). The ch14.18ΔCH2 MAb has also demonstrated faster plasma clearance rates compared with its intact cMAb counterpart (80).

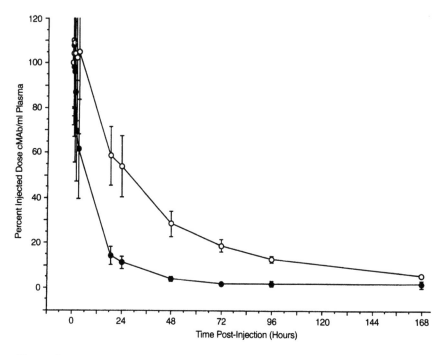

Figure 2 Plasma clearance of iodine-labeled cCC49 CH2 and cCC49 from the serum of juvenile rhesus primates. A mixture of ^{131}I-cCC49 CH2 (closed circles) and ^{125}I-cCC49 (open circles) was injected IV into four normal rhesus primates, and 1 mL of blood was removed from each at the indicated time points. Error bars indicate the SEM of four rhesus primates.

D.   Humanized MAbs

The mouse V region of mouse/human cMAbs is potentially immunogenic, and therefore, as described above, the development of an anti-idiotypic response among recipients is possible. One approach to minimizing this problem is to reshape human antibodies by transplanting antigen-binding sites from rodent MAbs onto human antibodies (Fig. 1C). The antigen binding sites are essentially composed of the Ig hypervariable loops supported by the β sheets of the framework region. Different methods have been used to develop these reshaped, humanized (Hu) MAbs. For example, in developing the CAMPATH-1H HuMAb, the hypervariable regions of the rat antibody reactive with the CAMPATH-1 antigen were grafted to a human Ig molecule resulting in a humanized antibody with similar affinity to the native MAb (81). Site-directed mutagenesis has also been used with mismatched primers encoding each of the rodent hypervariable

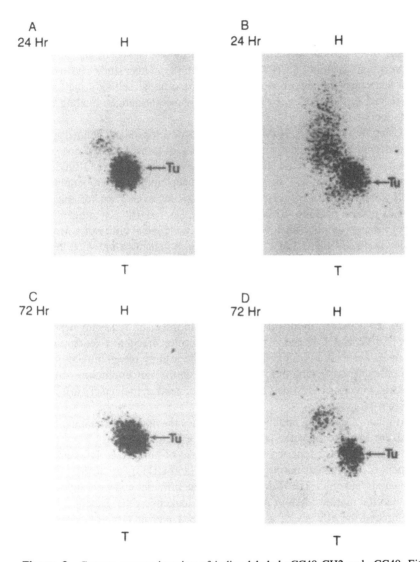

Figure 3 Gamma camera imaging of iodine labeled cCC49 CH2 and cCC49. Either ^{131}I-cCC49 CH2 (A and C) or ^{131}I-cCC49 (B and D) were injected into separate groups of LS-174T (a human colon carcinoma xenograft) tumor bearing athymic mice. Each mouse received either 48 µCi of ^{131}I-cCC49 CH2 or 12 µCi of ^{131}I-cCC49. Images of the mice were taken at 24 hours (A and B) and 72 hours (C and D). Letter designations indicate orientation of the mouse: head (H), tail (T); location of the tumor (Tu) is indicated by an arrow.

regions. In this approach, the 5′ and 3′ ends of the primers are complementary to the flanking framework regions (82). Results of initial studies to develop HuMAbs have demonstrated the importance of the choice of the human Ig framework for functional activity of the HuMAb (83). Other studies have demonstrated that some framework residues from the original antibody may need to be preserved in the humanized molecule if significant antigen-binding affinity is to be retained (84).

Using these methods, HuMAbs have been developed with defined specificity and decreased potential for immunogenicity in patients (82,85,86) in vitro studies have shown that some HuMAbs may have higher or lower affinities than their native MAbs (87–89). In some cases, lower binding affinity could be reversed by exchanging a few key framework residues to alter the variable region folding or residue packing (81,90,91). Moreover, a reduction in antigen affinity may not necessarily have an adverse effect on the clinical utility of a MAb. For example, a HuCC49 anti-TAG-72 MAb has been generated in which the MAb CC49 hypervariable regions were grafted onto the V_L and V_H frameworks of human MAbs while retaining those murine framework residues predicted to be required for the integrity of the antigen combining site (84). Although the relative affinity of the HuCC49 MAb was two- to three fold less than that of the chimeric and murine CC49 Igs, biodistribution studies in mice showed equivalent tumor targeting of the HuCC49 and cCC49 to human colon carcinoma xenografts (84). Thus, these observations suggest that while the affinity of an antibody plays a role in efficient tumor targeting, some decline in the antigen-binding affinity of a HuMAb, as compared to its parent molecule, need not adversely affect its in vivo tumor targeting.

Humanization of an antibody also provides the option of changing the isotype of the MAb to enhance affinity and/or effector functions. For example, Caron et al. (92) have reported the development of humanized IgG1 and IgG3 constructs of the IgG2a murine MAb M195 (anti-CD33) for therapy of acute myelogenous leukemia. The HuMAbs had higher affinities and were substantially better than the murine MAb in ADCC against leukemic cells. Hutchins in 1995 has compared the efficacy of a humanized IgG1 and IgG4 anti-CAMPATH-1 MAb (93). The IgG4 had better tumor targeting and a significantly decreased uptake in the spleen, bone marrow, and liver in a mouse xenograft model in comparison with the IgG1 HuMAb. And although the pharmacokinetics of the IgG4 was slower than that of the IgG1, a decrease in the mouse antihuman antibody response was observed with the humanized IgG4 (93). Thus, exploration of the biological function of different HuMAb isotypes may be useful in defining the course of HuMAb-based treatment for cancer patients.

Other HuMAbs have also demonstrated clinically relevant properties. For example, a humanized MAb 4D5-8 that binds the protooncogene HER-2 gene product p185[HER-2] has demonstrated a greater efficiency of tumor cell killing than the murine MAb, and inhibited tumor cell growth in vitro (90). In other studies, an anti-Tac MAb and an anti-CD18 HuMAb have both elicited a greatly decreased immune response in nonhuman primates (91,94). When coupled with a toxin, the humanized version of M195, which binds the CD33 antigen found on myeloid leukemias, demonstrated effective killing of $CD33^+$ HL60 cells in vitro (95).

To date, clinical trials of only a few HuMAbs have been reported. When two non-Hodgkin's lymphoma patients were treated with the humanized CAM-PATH-1H MAb, no antihuman antibody response was observed and both had remissions as demonstrated by clearance of lymphoma cells from the blood and bone marrow and resolution of splenomegaly (96). Administration of the Hu CAMPATH-1H MAb to 16 more patients with a variety of lymphoid malignancies also resulted in similar therapeutic effects on blood lymphocytes, marrow infiltration, and splenomegaly, although little improvement was detected in involved lymph nodes or extranodal masses (97). Initial clinical results with a humanized MAb (LL2) reactive against non-Hodgkin's lymphoma have shown that the HuMAb has similar targeting properties as the murine MAb (98). In a clinical study of adult T-cell leukemia treated with a radiolabeled anti-Tac HuMAb, 67% of the patients had either partial or complete remissions (99). In a separate clinical trial using the anti-Tac HuMAb, no measurable antibody response against the HuMAb was observed within the patient population (100). Recently, the HuMAb M195 has demonstrated targeting of leukemia cells without immunogenicity and reduction of large leukemic burdens when labeled with ^{131}I (101). Furthermore, therapeutic clinical trials using ^{131}I-labeled HuMAb M195 in combination with other agents for reduction of minimal residual disease and prolongation of remission in patients with relapsed acute promyelocytic leukemia have demonstrated few toxicities associated with the radiolabeled MAb and similar or better results as compared with other clinical approaches (101).

HuMAbs reactive with TAAs on solid tumors are also being evaluated clinically. Recently, the efficacy of a Hu anti-HER-2 MAb was assessed in a study of 46 patients with metastatic breast cancer that overexpressed the p185 HER-2 protooncogene product (102). Minimal toxicity and no antibody response against the HuMAb was detected. Furthermore, one complete remission and four partial remissions were observed in patients (102).

Antibody responses have been observed to some HuMAbs. In a comparison of the antibody response of patients to murine and humanized anti-B-cell lymphoma MAbs, patients treated with the murine MAb alone developed a HAMA response, while those treated with the HuMAb did not develop an immune response to the HuMAb. However, the patients treated with both murine and humanized MAbs developed an antibody response to both MAb forms (103). Similar results were observed in clinical studies evaluating an anticarcinoembryonic antigen (CEA) HuMAb, hMN-14 (103). In a pilot clinical trial, the hMN-14 and murine MN-14 MAbs showed similar biodistribution, tumor targeting, and pharmacokinetic behavior in patients with advanced CEA-producing tumors. As many as three doses of the hMN-14 MAb resulted in no human antihuman MAb response; however, patients treated with both MAbs developed an antibody response to the HuMAb. These results demonstrate the ability of HuMAbs to evoke anti-idiotypic responses (against murine idiotopes on the HuMAbs) in patients and suggest that radioimmunotherapy with HuMAbs may require a patient population with no prior exposure to murine MAbs.

V. TUMOR ANTIGEN AUGMENTATION

MAb technology has identified several novel human tumor antigens. The study of the biology of those tumor antigens has provided some important insights into their use as markers for the neoplastic process and as targets for MAb-based tumor diagnosis and therapy. Several tumor antigens share one characteristic— their heterogeneous expression within human tumor cell populations. Extensive tumor antigen heterogeneity, defined as the lack or attenuation of tumor antigen expression, is of concern when implementing MAb-based tumor studies. Tumor antigen-negative cells would escape MAb recognition, thereby negatively impacting on the efficiency of the MAb to detect and treat occult tumor. Indeed, experimental data supported the hypothesis that low antigen levels coincided with the tumor being refractory to the therapeutic effects of a radioimmunoconjugate.

In light of those results, several laboratories, including ours, designed and carried out in-depth studies to identify certain agents which augment tumor antigen expression. It was reasoned that identifying agents which could upregulate antigen expression on human carcinoma populations might be an important adjuvant for tumor targeting of anticarcinoma MAbs. Our research group carried out a series of studies focused on the regulation of TAG-72 and CEA using diverse differentiation agents, including interferon, interleukin-6, and selected cyclic AMP analogs. TAG-72 is a high-molecular-weight mucin expressed in a wide range of human carcinomas including gastrointestinal, breast, ovarian, non-small-cell lung, endometrial, pancreatic, prostate, etc. (104). Expression in normal tissues is limited to the transitional colonic mucosa and the secretory endometrium (105,106). CEA is an oncofetal antigen expressed on normal as well as malignant tissues (i.e., colorectal, breast, and lung carcinomas) (107).

Immunohistochemical studies clearly showed that the expression of both TAG-72 and CEA is highly heterogeneous as evidenced by a wide range of staining intensities as well as the presence of antigen negative cells within the human carcinoma populations (104,107). When studies were designed to identify agents which could upregulate TAG-72 and CEA expression, little was known about the regulation of tumor antigen expression. Since several interferons (IFN-α, -β, and -γ) had been reported to enhance major histocompatibility (MHC) antigen expression (108,109), they became the logical candidates for the initial study of TAG-72 and CEA regulation. Indeed, early reports showed that both type I (α and β) and type II (γ) interferons could upregulate the expression of TAG-72, CEA, and other human tumor antigens on the surface of human carcinoma and melanoma cells (110–120). Those studies established several important principles with respect to tumor antigen regulation: (a) unlike its ability to induce class II HLA expression de novo, IFN treatment did not de novo induce TAG-72 or CEA on tumor antigen negative cells (111,113,114); (b) clones from a carcinoma cell line responded differentially to the ability of either IFN-α or -γ to upregulate tumor antigen expression (112); and (c) 20% to 30% of human tumor lines were unresponsive to the ability of IFN-α or -γ to induce higher antigen levels.

Subsequent studies from different laboratories examined the molecular mechanisms involved in IFN-γ-mediated upregulation of CEA. Results found (a) that the increase of CEA expression following IFN-γ treatment coincided with an increased protein synthesis as evidenced by higher steady-state levels of CEA-specific mRNA transcripts (114), and (b) that posttranslational events also contribute to the increase in CEA expression following IFN-γ treatment (121). Those studies have provided important insights into the regulation of CEA and, perhaps, how interferon may affect the function of CEA as an homotypic adhesion molecule or a molecule capable of binding bacteria (122,123).

For the purpose of this chapter, discussion will focus on (a) the advantages gained by combining tumor antigen upregulation in experimental MAb-based tumor therapy/detection studies, and (b) some of the early clinical data illustrating the changes in TAG-72 and CEA expression following interferon administration. Complete details of these findings have been previously published (124–126).

A. Impact of IFN-γ TAG-72 Upregulation on Radioimmunotherapy

Initial in vivo studies showed that pretreatment of athymic mice with either IFN-α or IFN-γ increased MAb tumor localization (127,128). Subsequent studies demonstrated a delay in tumor growth in athymic mice treated with IFN-γ in combination with a MAb conjugated with ^{90}Y, chemotherapeutic drugs, or toxins (129–131). Our group carried out a study on the impact of IFN-γ-mediated TAG-72 upregulation on radioimmunotherapy. The experimental model was a human colorectal tumor cell, HT-29, grown as a subcutaneous tumor xenograft in athymic mice. Characteristics of the tumor model included: (a) constitutive TAG-72 levels that were similar to those in human colorectal tumor biopsies; (b) IFN-γ treatment increased tumor TAG-72 levels; and (c) higher TAG-72 levels coincided with better tumor uptake of the radioimmunoconjugate (124). We initially investigated whether differences in constitutive TAG-72 levels in colorectal tumors correlated with the antitumor effects observed following the administration of ^{131}I-CC49.

As explained earlier in this chapter, MAb CC49 recognizes a carbohydrate determinant on TAG-72. In addition, there is considerable clinical experience with CC49 and new research initiatives are aimed toward generating and characterizing novel recombinant forms of CC49 for future clinical protocols. In any case, mice bearing colorectal tumor xenografts which expressed different TAG-72 levels were injected with different doses of ^{131}I-CC49. A direct correlation between relative TAG-72 tumor levels and the antitumor effectiveness of the radioimmunoconjugate was observed. Tumor growth suppression was most dramatic in xenografts expressing the highest TAG-72 levels. Those results provided the rationale to use IFN-γ to increase tumor TAG-72 levels which should augment the antitumor effects of the radioimmunoconjugate. Dose and time-dependent studies with IFN-γ revealed that an 8-day treatment with 10^6 antiviral units IFN-γ/day significantly increased TAG-72 and CEA levels and enhanced tumor localization of anti-TAG-72 and CEA MAbs. Serum IFN-γ levels ranged from 90 to 150 units/mL, levels which are achievable and well tolerated levels in patients (132,133). ^{131}I-CC49 was administered on day 4 or 5 after the beginning of IFN-γ at a time of enhanced TAG-72 expression. Initial therapeutic studies were done in athymic mice bearing 7-day, palpable tumors with the administration of low doses of ^{131}I-CC49 ranging from 100 to 300 μCi alone or in combination with IFN-γ. Those mice treated with ^{131}I-CC49 alone exhibited transient reductions in their tumor volumes. However, by combining ^{131}I-CC49 with IFN-γ, complete, long-lasting tumor regression was achieved in 30–40% of mice. Those promising results with low tumor burden led us to design subsequent studies in mice bearing well-established tumors. Mice bearing large, well-established tumors (i.e., avg. tumor volume 350 mm^3) received repeat doses of ^{131}I-CC49 alone or in combination with IFN-γ. As before, treatment with ^{131}I-CC49 alone resulted in a transient tumor regression in a majority of mice (Fig. 4A). In contrast, complete, long-lasting tumor regression was observed in 90% of mice treated with the same dose of ^{131}I-CC49, but in combination with IFN-γ which enhanced tumor TAG-72 expression levels (Fig. 4B). Transient tumor regression was observed in other groups of mice treated with IFN-γ alone or ^{131}I-BL3, an irrelevant MAb alone or in combination with IFN-γ. These results clearly demonstrated that low, heterogeneous TAG-72 expression in tumors did impair the therapeutic effectiveness of a radioimmunoconjugate; IFN-γ increases tumor TAG-72 levels which resulted in better MAb tumor localization; inclusion of IFN-γ with ^{131}I-CC49 improved its therapeutic efficacy; and ^{131}I-CC49 in combination with IFN-γ-mediated complete regression of large, well-established tumors. The data supported the hypotheses that administration of a radiolabeled MAb with IFN-γ may not only be effective in an adjuvant setting, but also could impact patients diagnosed with primary and/or recurrent colorectal carcinoma.

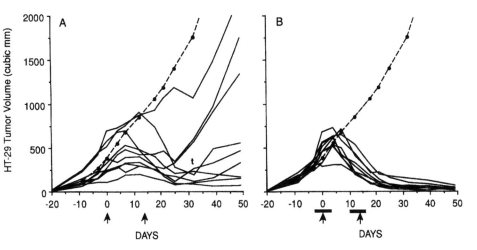

Figure 4 Antitumor effects of ^{131}I-CC49±IFN-γ in mice bearing well-established human tumor xenografts. IFN-γ was given to groups of tumor-bearing mice as indicated by the solid horizontal line in panel B. Mice were treated with 300 μCi ^{131}I-CC49 as indicated by the arrows (i.e., days 0 and 14). Tumor volumes for each individual mouse are indicated by solid lines. Average tumor volumes from saline-treated mice are represented by dashed lines.

B. Clinical Studies on Tumor Antigen Upregulation

Those experimental studies provided the rationale to design clinical trials to determine whether IFN treatment could, indeed, augment TAG-72 and/or CEA expression in carcinoma cell populations. Indirect evidence from early clinical studies supported that hypothesis. In a retrospective study (134), serum TAG-72 and CEA levels increased in patients diagnosed with various adenocarcinomas and treated with high doses of IFN-γ or IFN-β alone, or in combination. Another study reported improved tumor uptake of a radiolabeled antimelanoma MAb in patients pretreated with IFN-α (135). Direct evidence came in a study which was designed and carried out by investigators from this laboratory and the University of Wisconsin (125). IFN-γ was administered IP to patients with confirmed adenocarcinoma (G.I. and ovarian) and secondary malignant ascites. Intraperitoneal administration of IFN-γ would provide a pharmacokinetic advantage, while permitting multiple sampling of the malignant cells from the ascites for TAG-72 and CEA analysis. Tumor cells isolated from the ascites at different time intervals following IFN-γ treatment had significant increases in TAG-72/CEA expression as measured by flow cytometry and immunohistochemical staining. In some cases, the percentage of TAG-72-positive tumor cells increased from approximately 10% prior to IFN-γ to 90% after IFN-γ. The expression of other cell surface antigens, such as CA125 and cytokeratins, were unchanged (data not shown), indicating the selective nature by which IFN-γ upregulates TAG-72 and CEA expression.

The pharmacokinetic advantage gained by the intracavitary delivery of IFN-γ raised the question of whether systemic administration could effectively upregulate tumor antigen expression on primary and metastatic carcinomas. So in subsequent study (126), colorectal biopsies were taken from patients histologically confirmed to be carcinoma and stained to establish TAG-72/CEA baseline expression. Patients were then administered IFN-α2a at different schedules/doses. Immediately following IFN-α2a, surgical biopsies were found to express elevated TAG-72/CEA levels as measured by both immunostaining and quantitative analysis. The results in Table 1 illustrate changes in TAG-72/CEA expression in patients administered IFN-α2α. As shown, in some cases the percentage of tumor cells which expressed TAG-72 or CEA rose from 10% prior to IFN-α2a to 90–100% after IFN-α2a treatment. Staining intensity for each antigen was also significantly upregulated, indicating that IFN-α treatment not only increased the percentage of tumor cells expressing TAG-72/CEA, but also increased the amount of antigen per cell. The data also confirmed that a requirement for tumor antigen upregulation was the constitutive expression of that gene product since IFN-α failed to induce de novo TAG-72/CEA expression on tumor tissues which were constitutively negative for the tumor antigen(s). In retrospect, many of the results from the clinical studies were reminiscent of those initially observed in the preclinical, experimental studies. For instance, the most substantial increase of TAG-72/CEA expression occurred in those tumor samples which, prior to interferon treatment, expressed low to moderate tumor antigen levels. Temporal aspects (i.e., length of treatment) seem more important than dose for upregulating TAG-72 or CEA expression. The clinical data support the experimental hypothesis that the ability of IFN-α or -γ to enhance TAG-72/CEA expression selectively on the tumor cell surface can be exploited to enhance the tumor targeting of a radioimmunoconjugate. The findings reinforce the need to develop molecularly designed MAbs which permit multiple administrations in combination with an antigen upregulation regimen.

VI. FUTURE PROSPECTS

As described in this chapter, the development of MAb-based approaches for tumor diagnosis and treatment requires a multifaceted approach which includes the design of genetically engineered MAbs for tumor targeting as well as in depth knowledge of the biology of the tumor with respect to antigen expression. Experimental and clinical experience has led to the development of humanized MAbs.

Table 1 TAG-72 and CEA Expression in Tumor Biopsies Before and After IFN-α2a Administration to Patients with G.I. Carcinoma (Cohorts I-IV).

Cohort	IFN-α2a (dose/schedule)	Patients	Antigen expression/MAb reactivity[2]			
			TAG-72		CEA	
			Pre-IFN-α2a	Post-IFN-α2a	Pre-IFN-α2a	Post-IFN-α2a
I	3 × 10^8/2	1	40 (+++)[b]	40 (++)	50 (+)	80 (++)
		2	40 (++)	40 (++)	60 (+)	70 (+)
		3	40 (+)	40 (++)	70 (++)	80 (++)
		4	focal[b]	50 (+)	50 (+)	60 (+)
II	6 × 10^8/2	1	40 (++)	40 (++)	60 (++)	50 (++)
		2	focal	focal	100 (++)	90 (++)
		3	50 (+)	50 (+)	50 (+)	50 (+)
		4	70 (+)	80 (+)	focal	focal
III	3 × 10^8/3	1	focal	10 (++)	80 (++)	100 (++)
		2	10 (+)	80 (++)	neg	neg
		3	50 (+)	80 (++)	100 (+++)	100 (+++)
		4	10 (++)	100 (+++)	10 (+)	40 (++)
		5	30 (+)	60 (++)	50 (+)	70 (+)
IV	6 × 10^8/3	1	70 (+)	95 (++)	100 (++)	100 (+++)
		2	50 (++)	100 (+++)	10 (+)	50 (++)
		3	90 (+)	100 (+++)	focal	focal
		4	100 (++)	100 (++)	80 (+)	100 (+)
		5	10 (+)	40 (++)	40 (+)	70 (++)

[a] TAG-72 and CEA expression were defined using MAbs B72.3 and Col-1, respectively.

[b] Numbers represent percentage of TAG-72 or CEA-positive tumor cells; ( ) represents the relative MAb staining intensity. The term "focal" staining describes those samples in which <5% of the tumor cells were positive for MAb binding, yet there was moderate to strong levels of staining intensity.

The data suggest that by retaining only the CDRs of the native murine MAb, the potential for eliciting an immune response in patients will be minimal. Furthermore, the faster plasma clearance and efficient tumor-targeting properties observed with CH2 domain-deleted cMAbs should be advantageous for many diagnostic and therapeutic approaches. The results obtained thus far with humanized and domain-deleted Ig molecules provide a compelling argument for developing MAbs which combine the advantages of both molecules, i.e., humanized domain-deleted MAbs.

Historically, attempts to generate totally human antibodies using standard hybridoma technology have met with limited success (136,137). Recently, a major advance has been reported in the development of human MAbs, based on the ability to reconstruct large fragments of human DNA in yeast artificial chromosomes (YACs) and to incorporate them into the mouse germline. Mice, designated Xenomouse II (Abgenix Inc., Fremont, CA), have been genetically constructed with Ig loci coding for large subunits of the human heavy and light chains in place of the normal mouse Ig loci (138). These mice recognize human proteins as foreign and develop human antibodies in response to the foreign antigens. Recently, the Xenomouse II strain has been used to produce completely human high affinity antibodies reactive with IL-8, the epidermal growth factor receptor (EGFR), and tumor necrosis factor (TNF)-α (138).

Another novel approach, referred to as redirected T-cells, has emerged that combines the advantages of two diverse elements of the immune system: the MHC-unrestricted recognition of TAAs by an antibody, and the ability of T-cells to secrete cytokines and mediate other effector functions. In this approach, non-MHC-restricted T-cells with specificity for tumor cells are developed by genetic manipulation of T-cells to express chimeric receptors on their cell surface. The chimeric receptors consist of an extracellular antibody (or other antigen-binding) domain and an intracellular domain that initiates signal transduction pathways involved in T-cell activation and expansion. The binding of the antibody domain to the tumor cell surface sets into motion a cascade of T-cell biological functions including cytokine secretion and other effector cell functions. Recent advances in determining T-cell components important for target cell recognition and signal transduction have paved the way for initial attempts to determine the feasibility of this approach.

Chimeric receptors have been developed using MOv18, an antibody reactive to the folate binding protein overexpressed on the surface of human ovarian carcinomas, and the FcRγ chain. Tumor infiltrating lymphocytes (TILs) expressing the chimeric receptor produce cytokines and are cytolytically active against FBP-positive tumor cells (139,140). Adoptively transferred murine TILs expressing the MOv18-γ receptor have promoted increased survival of athymic mice bearing human ovarian carcinoma xenografts (141). Chimeric receptors have also been developed for redirection of the specificity of T-cells to the ERBB2 receptor, overproduced in many adenocarcinomas of the breast, ovary, lung, and stomach (142,143). The chimeric receptor is composed of an anti-ERBB2 receptor single chain antibody and the TCR zeta chain (143). In vitro studies showed CTL activity and ability to secrete IFN-γ after incubation of chimeric receptor positive T-cells with ERBB2 positive cells. Slower growth of murine NIH-3T3 cells transformed with human ERBB2 was observed in athymic mice after coadministration of the transformed cells with murine CTLs expressing the chimeric receptor (144).

A considerable amount of research interest continues in the study of the biology of the tumor target to identify novel approaches to augment MAb uptake. Tumor antigen augmentation studies are investigating the use of combinations of agents which can synergistically upregulate tumor antigen expression. Other researchers are utilizing novel approaches which include vasoactive immunoconjugates which can increase MAb tumor uptake and augment its therapeutic efficacy (145,146). A combined modality approach, which includes the rational design of a therapeutic Ig to permit multiple Ig administrations with the incorporation of proven agents which selectively increase target antigen expression and/ or tumor blood flow, may result in novel antibody-mediated approaches with greater potential for specific diagnostic and/or therapeutic applications for cancer.

REFERENCES

1. Kohler G, Milstein C. Continuous culture of fused cells secreting antibody of predefined specificity. Nature 1975; 256:495–497.
2. DeNardo GL, Kroger L, Mirick GR, Lamborn KR, DeNardo SJ. Analysis of anti-globulin (HAMA) response in a group of patients with B-lymphocytic malignancies treated with ^{131}I-Lym-1. Int J Biol Markers 1995; 10:67–74.
3. Kaminski MS, Zasadny KR, Fancis IR, Fenner MC, Ross CW, Milik AW, Estes J, Tuck M, Regan D, Fisher S, Glenn SD, Wahl RL. Iodine-131-anti-B1 radioimmunotherapy for B-cell lymphoma. J Clin Oncol 1996; 14:1974–1981.
4. Press OW, Eary JF, Appelbaum FR, Martin PJ, Nelp WB, Glenn S, Fisher DR, Porter B, Matthews DC, Gooley T. Phase II trial of ^{131}I-B1 (anti-CD20) antibody therapy with autologous stem cell transplantation for relapsed B cell lymphomas. Lancet 1995; 346:336–340.
5. DeNardo SJ, DeNardo GL, O'Grady LF, Macey DJ, Mills SL, Epstein AL, Peng JS, McGahan JP. Treatment of a patient with B cell lymphoma by I-131 LYM-1 monoclonal antibodies. Int J Biol Markers 1987; 2:49–53.
6. DeNardo GL, DeNardo SJ, O'Grady LF, Levy NB, Adams GP, Mills S. Fractionated radioimmunotherapy of B-cell malignancies with 131-I-Lym-1. Cancer Res 1990; 50(suppl):1014–1016.
7. Goldenberg DM. New developments in monoclonal antibodies for cancer detection and therapy. CA 1994; 44:43–64.

8. Schlom J. Monoclonal antibodies in cancer therapy. In: DeVita VT, Hellman S, Rosenberg SA, eds. Biologic Therapy of Cancer. Philadelphia: Lippincott, 1995: 180–220.

9. Buchsbaum DJ, Langmuir VK, Wessels BW. Experimental radioimmunotherapy. Med Phys 1993; 20:551–567.

10. Mach JP, Buchegger F, Pelegrin A, Ychou M, Lumbroso J, Rougier P, Lasser P, Elias D, Saccavini J, Eschewege F, Tubiana M, Parmentier C. Radioimmunotherapy of colon carcinoma with I-131 labeled antibodies successful experimental results and clinical dosimetry study. Pathol Biol 1990; 38:819–821.

11. Siler K, Eggensperger D, Hand PH, Milenic DE, Miller LS, Houchens DP, Hinkle G, Schlom J. Therapeutic efficacy of a high affinity anticarcinoembryonic antigen monoclonal antibody (COL-1). Biotechnol Ther 1993; 4:163–181.

12. Bergman I, Arbit E, Rosenblum M, Larson SM, Heller G, Cheung NKV. Treatment of spinal epidural neuroblastoma xenografts in rats using anti-GD2 monoclonal antibodies 3F8. J Neuro-Oncol 1993; 15:235–242.

13. Schlom J, Siler K, Milenic DE, Eggensperger D, Colcher D, Miller LS, Houchens D, Cheng R, Kaplan D, Goeckler W. Monoclonal antibody based therapy of a human tumor xenograft with a [177]lutetium-labeled immunoconjugate. Cancer Res 1991; 51:2889–2896.

14. Schlom J, Milenic DE, Roselli M, Colcher D, Bird R, Johnson S, Hardman KD, Guadagni F, Greiner JW. New concepts in monoclonal antibody based radioimmunodiagnosis and radioimmunotherapy of carcinoma. Nucl Med Biol 1991; 18:425–435.

15. Bruland OS. Cancer therapy with radiolabeled antibodies. An overview. Acta Oncol 1995; 34:1085–1094.

16. Behr TM, Becker WS, Bair HJ, Klein MW, Stühler CM, Cidlinsky KP, Wittekind CW, Scheele JR, Wolf FG. Comparison of complete versus fragmented technetium-99m-labeled anti-CEA monoclonal antibodies for immunoscintigraphy in colorectal cancer. J Nucl Med 1995; 36:430–441.

17. Baum RP, Hertel A, Lorenz M, Scharwz A, Encke A, Hor G. ^{99m}Tc-labelled anti-CEA monoclonal antibody for tumor immunoscintigraphy: first clinical results. Nucl Med Commun 1989; 10:345–352.

18. Mach J-P, Chatal J-F, Lumbroso J-D, Buchegger F, Forni M, Ritschard J, Berche C, Douillard J-Y, Carrel S, Herlyn M, Steplewski K, Koprowski H. Tumor localization in patients by radiolabeled monoclonal antibodies against colon carcinoma. Cancer Res 1983; 43:5593–5599.

19. Rosner D, Nabi H, Wild L, Ortman-Nabi J, Hreshchyshyn MM. Diagnosis of breast carcinoma with radiolabeled monoclonal antibodies (MoAbs) to carcinoembryonic antigen (CEA) and human milk fat globulin (HMFG). Cancer Invest 1995; 13:573–582.

20. Surwit EA, Childers JM, Krag DN, Katterhagen G, Gallion HH, Waggoner S, Mann WJJ. Clinical assessment of ^{111}In-Cyt-103 immunoscintigraphy in ovarian cancer. Gynecol Oncol 1993; 48:285–292.

21. Doerr RJ, Herrera L, Abdel-Nabi H. In-111 CYT-103 Monoclonal antibody imaging in patients with suspected recurrent colorectal cancer. Cancer 1993; 71(suppl):4241–4247.

22. Bell J, Mojzisik C, Hinkle G, Derman H, Schlom J, Martin E. Intraoperative radio-immunodetection of ovarian cancer using monoclonal antibody B72.3 and a portable gamma-detecting probe. Radioimmunoguided Surg Cancer 1990; 76:607–611.
23. Divgi CR, Scott AM, McDermott K, Fallone PS, Hilton S, Siler K, Carmichael N, Daghighian F, Finn RD, Cohen AM, Schlom J, Larson SM. Clinical comparison of radiolocalization of two monoclonal antibodies (mAbs) against the TAG-72 antigen. Nucl Med Biol 1994; 21:9–15.
24. Divgi CR, Scott AM, Dantis L, Capitelli P, Sgouros G, Siler K, Finn RD, Kemeny N, Kelsen D, Kostakoglu L, Schlom J, Larson SM. Phase I radioimmunotherapy trial with I-131 CC49 in metastatic colon carcinoma. J Nucl Med 1995; 36:586–592.
25. Press OW, Eary JF, Applebaum FR, Martin PJ, Badger CC, Nelp WB, Glenn S, Butchko G, Fisher D, Porter B, Mattews DC, Fisher LD, Bernstein ID. Radiolabeled-antibody therapy of B-cell lymphoma with autologous bone marrow support. N Engl J Med 1993; 329:1219–1224.
26. Schroff RW, Weiden PL, Appelbaum J, Fer MF, Breitz H, Vanderheyden J-L, Ratliff BA, Fisher D, Foisie D, Hanelin LG, Morgan AC, Fritzberg AR, Abrams PG. Rhenium-186 labeled antibody in patients with cancer: report of a pilot Phase I study. Antibody Immunoconj Radiopharm 1990; 3:99–111.
27. Jacobs AJ, Fer M, Su FM, Breitz H, Thompson J, Goodgold H, Cain J, Heaps J, Weiden P. A Phase I trial of a rhenium 186-labeled monoclonal antibody administered intraperitoneally in ovarian carcinoma: toxicity and clinical response. Obstet Gynecol 1993; 8:586–593.
28. Camera L, Del Vecchio S, Petrillo A, Esposito G, Frasci G, Iaffafioli RV, Bianco AR, Salvatore M. Evaluation of therapeutic response using iodine-131-B72.3 monoclonal antibody in patients with ovarian carcinoma. Eur J Nucl Med 1991; 18:269–273.
29. Murray JL, Macey DJ, Kasi LP, Rieger P, Cunningham J, Bhadkamkar V, Zhang H-Z, Schlom J, Rosenblum MG, Podoloff DA. Phase II radioimmunotherapy trial with ^{131}I-CC49 in colorectal cancer. Cancer 1994; 73(suppl):1057–1066.
30. Khazaeli MB, Saleh MN, Liu TP, Meredith RF, Wheeler RH, Baker TS, King D, Secher D, Allen L, Rogers K, Colcher D, Schlom J, Shochat D, LoBuglio A. Pharmacokinetics and immune response of ^{131}I-chimeric mouse/human B72.3 (human γ 4) monoclonal antibody in humans. Cancer Res 1991; 51:5461–5466.
31. Milenic DE, Yokota T, Filpula DR, Finkleman MAJ, Dodd SW, Wood JF, Whitlow M, Snoy P, Schlom J. Construction, binding properties, metabolism, and tumor targeting of a single-chain Fv derived from the pancarcinoma monoclonal antibody CC49. Cancer Res 1991; 51:6363–6371.
32. Buist MR, Kenemans P, den Hollander W, Vermorken JB, Molthoff CJM, Burger CW, Helmerhorst TJM, Baak JPA, Ross JC. Kinetics and tissue distribution of the radiolabeled chimeric monoclonal antibody MOv18 IgG and F(ab')$_2$ fragments in ovarian carcinoma patients. Cancer Res 1993; 53:5413–5418.
33. Breitz HB, Weiden PL, Vanderheyden JL, Appelbaum JW. Clinical experience with rhenium-186-labeled monoclonal antibodies for radioimmunotherapy: results of a Phase I trial. J Nucl Med 1992; 33:1110–1112.
34. Huston JS, McCartney J, Tai M-S, Mottala-Hartshorn C, Jin D, Warren F, Keck

P, Oppermann H. Medical applications of single-chain antibodies. Int Rev Immunol 1993; 10:195–217.

35. Schott ME, Milenic DE, Yokota T, Whitlow M, Wood JF, Fordyce WA, Cheng RC, Schlom J. Differential metabolic patterns of iodinated versus radiometal chelated anticarcinoma single-chain Fv molecules. Cancer Res 1992; 52:6413–6417.

36. Yokota T, Milenic DE, Whitlow M, Schlom J. Rapid tumor penetration of a single-chain Fv and comparison with other immunoglobulin forms. Cancer Res 1992; 52: 3402–3408.

37. Adams GP, McCartney JE, Wolf EJ, Eisenberg J, Tai MS, Huston JS, Stafford WFR, Bookman MA, Houston LL, Weiner LM. Optimization of in vivo targeting in SCID mice with divalent forms of 741F8 anti-c-erbB-2 single chain Fv: effects of dose escalation and repeated i.v. administration. Cancer Immunol Immunother 1995; 40:299–306.

38. Huston JS, Adams GP, McCartney JE, Tai MS, Hudziak RM, Opperman H, Stafford WFR, Liu S, Fand I, Apell G. Tumor targeting in a murine tumor xenograft model with the (sFv')₂ divalent form of anti-c-erbB-2 single chain Fv. Cell Biophys 1994; 24–25:267–278.

39. Dillman RO, Shawler DL, McCallister TJ, Halpern SE. Human anti-mouse antibody response in cancer patients following single low-dose injections of radiolabeled murine monoclonal antibodies. Cancer Biother 1994; 9:17–28.

40. Khazaeli MB, Conry RM, LoBuglio AF. Human immune response to monoclonal antibodies. J Immunother 1994; 15:42–52.

41. Reynolds JC, Del Vecchio S, Sakahara H, Lora ME, Carrasquillo JA, Neumann RD, Larson SM. Anti-murine response to mouse monoclonal antibodies: clinical findings and implications. Nucl Med Biol 1989; 16:121–125.

42. Oosterwijk E, Debruyne FM. Radiolabeled monoclonal antibody G250 in renal-cell carcinoma. World J Urol 1995; 13:186–190.

43. Colcher D, Esteban J, Carrasquillo JA, Sugarbaker P, Reynolds JC, Bryant G, Larson SM, Schlom J. Quantitative analyses of selective radiolabeled monoclonal antibody localization in metastatic lesions of colorectal cancer patients. Cancer Res 1987; 47:1185–1189.

44. Martin JEW, Mojzisik CM, Hinkle GH, Samsel J, Siddiqi MA, Tuttle SE, Sickle-Santanello BJ, Colcher D, Thurston MO, Bell JG, Farrar WB, Schlom J. Radioimmunoguided surgery using monoclonal antibody. Am J Surg 1988; 156:386–392.

45. Goldenberg DM. Imaging and therapy of gastrointestinal cancers with radiolabeled antibodies. Am J Gastroenterol 1991; 86:1392–1403.

46. Rietmuller G, Schneider-Gadicke E, Schlimok G, Schmiegel W, Raab W, Hoffken K, Gruber R, Pichlmaier H, Hirche H, Pichlmayer R, Buggisch P, Witte J. Group GCA-AS. Randomised trial of monoclonal antibody for adjuvant therapy of resected Dukes' C colorectal carcinoma. Lancet 1994; 343:1177–1183.

47. Morrison SL. Transfectomas provide novel chimeric antibodies. Science 1985; 229: 1202–1207.

48. Sun LK, Curtis P, Rakowicz-Szulczynska E, Ghrayeb J, Morrison SL, Chang N, Koprowski H. Chimeric antibodies with 17-1A derived variable and human constant regions. Hybridoma 1986; 5(suppl):S17–S20.

49. Liu AY, Robinson RR, Murray DJ, Ledbetter JA, Hellstroom I, Hellstrom KE.

Production of a mouse-human chimeric monoclonal antibody to CD20 with potent Fc-dependent biological activity. J Immunol 1987; 139:3521–3526.

50. Kashmiri SVS, Hand PH. Genetically engineered antitumor monoclonal antibodies. In: Garrett C, Sell S, eds. Cellular Cancer Markers. Totowa: Humana Press, 1995: 393–431.

51. Coloma MJ, Hastings A, Wims LA, Morrison SL. Novel vectors for the expression of antibody molecules using variable region generated by polymerase chain reaction. J Immunol Methods 1992; 152:89–104.

52. Kanda H, Mori K, Koga H, Taniguchi K, Kobayashi H, Sakahara H, Konishi J, Endo K, Watanabe T. Construction and expression of chimeric antibodies by a simple replacement of heavy and light chain V genes into a single cassette vector. Hybridoma 1994; 13:359–366.

53. Mueller BM, Romerdahl CA, Gillies SD, Reisfeld RA. Enhancement of antibody-dependent cytotoxicity with a chimeric anti-GD2 antibody. J Immunol 1990; 144: 1382–1386.

54. Hutzell P, Kashmiri S, Colcher D, Primus J, Horan Hand P, Roselli M, Yarranton G, Bodmer M, Whittle N, King D, Loullis CC, McCoy DW, Callahan R, Schlom J. Generation and characterization of a recombinant/chimeric B72.3 (human γ1). Cancer Res 1991; 46:850–857.

55. Orlandi R, Figini M, Tomassetti A, Canevari S, Colnaghi MI. Characterization of a mouse-human chimeric antibody to a cancer-associated antigen. Int J Cancer 1992; 52:588–593.

56. Naramura M, Gillies SD, Mendelsohn J, Reisfeld RA, Mueller BM. Therapeutic potential of chimeric and murine anti-(epidermal growth factor receptor) antibodies in a metastasis model for human melanoma. Cancer Immunol Immunother 1993; 37:343–349.

57. Surfus JE, Hank JA, Oosterwijk E, Welt S, Lindstrom MJ, Albertini MR, Schiller JH, Sondel PM. Anti-renal-cell carcinoma chimeric antibody G250 facilitates antibody-dependent cellular cytotoxicity with in vitro and in vivo interleukin-2-activated effectors. J Immunother Emphasis Tumor Immunol 1996; 19:184–191.

58. Shitara K, Kuwana Y, Nakamura K, Tokutake Y, Ohta S, Miyaji H, Hasegawa M, Hanai N. A mouse/human chimeric anti-(ganglioside GD3) antibody with enhanced antitumor activities. Cancer Immunol Immunother 1993; 36:373–380.

59. Mount PF, Sutton VR, Li W, Burgess J, McKenzie IFC, Pietersz GA, Trapani JA. Chimeric (mouse/human) anti-colon cancer antibody c30.6 inhibits the growth of human colorectal cancer xenografts in scid/scid mice. Cancer Res 1994; 54:6160–6166.

60. Pullyblank AM, Guillou PJ, Monson JRT. M17-1A-, c17-1A- and cSF25-mediated antibody-dependent cell-mediated cytotoxicity in patients with advanced cancer. Br J Cancer 1994; 70:753–758.

61. Primus FJ, Pendurthi TK, Hutzell P, Kashmiri S, Slavin DC, Callahan R, Schlom J. Chimeric B72.3 mouse/human (IgG1) antibody directs the lysis of tumor cells by lymphokine-activated killer cells. Cancer Immunol Immunother 1990; 31:349–357.

62. Terskikh A, Couty S, Pelegrin A, Hardman N, Hunziker W, Mach J-P. Dimeric

recombinant IgA directed against carcino-embryonic antigen, a novel tool for carcinoma localization. Mol Immunol 1994; 31:1313–1319.

63. Goodman GE, Hellstrom I, Yelton DE, Murray JL, O'Hara S, Meaker E, Zeigler L, Palazollo P, Nicaise C, Usakewicz J, Hellstrom KE. Phase I trial of chimeric (human-mouse) monoclonal antibody L6 in patients with non-small-cell lung, colon, and breast cancer. Cancer Immunol Immunother 1993; 36:267–273.

64. DeNardo SJ, Mirick GR, Kroger LA, O'Grady LF, Erickson KL, Yuan A, Lamborn KR, Hellstrom I, Hellstrom KE, DeNardo GL. The biologic window for chimeric L6 radioimmunotherapy. Cancer 1994; 73(suppl):1023–1032.

65. Saleh MN, Khazaeli MB, Wheeler RH, Allen LF, Tilden AB, Grizzle W, Reisfeld RA, Yu AL, Gillies SD, LoBuglio AF. Phase I trial of the chimeric anti-GD2 monoclonal antibody ch14.18 in patients with malignant melanoma. Hum Antibodies Hybrid 1992; 3:19–24.

66. Meredith RF, Khazaeli MB, Plott WE, Liu T, Russell C, Wheeler RH, LoBuglio AF. Effect of human immune response on repeat courses of 131-I-chimeric B72.3 antibody therapy. Antibodies Immunoconj Radiopharm 1993; 6:39–46.

67. Coney LR, Mezzanzanica D, Sanborn D, Casalini P, Colnaghi MI, Zurawski VRJ. Chimeric murine-human antibodies directed against folate binding receptor are efficient mediators of ovarian carcinoma cell killing. Cancer Res 1994; 54:2448–2455.

68. Meredith RF, Khazaeli MB, Liu T, Plott G, Wheeler RH, Russell C, Colcher D, Schlom J, Shocat D, LoBuglio AF. Dose fractionation of radiolabeled antibodies in patients with metastatic colon cancer. J Nucl Med 1992; 33:1648–1653.

69. Winkelhake JL, Nicolson GL. Aglycosylantibody: effects of exoglycosidase treatments on autochthonous antibody survival time in the circulation. J Biol Chem 1976; 251:1074–1080.

70. Leatherbarrow RJ, Rademacher TW, Dwek RA, Woof JM, Clark A, Burton DR, Richardson N, Feinstein A. Effector functions of a monoclonal aglycosylated mouse IgG2a: binding and activation of complement component C1 and interaction with human monocyte Fc receptor. Mol Immunol 1985; 22:407–415.

71. Koide N, Nose M, Muramatsu T. Recognition of IgG by Fc receptor and complement: effects of glycosidase digestion. Biochem Biophys Res Commun 1977; 75: 838–834.

72. Tao MH, Morrison SL. Studies of aglycosylated chimeric mouse-human IgG. J Immunol 1989; 143:2595–2601.

73. Dorai H, Mueller BM, Reisfeld RA, Gillies SD. Aglycosylated chimeric mouse/human IgG1 antibody retains some effector function. Hybridoma 1991; 10:211–217.

74. Horan Hand P, Calvo B, Milenic D, Yokota T, Finch M, Snoy P, Garmestani K, Gansow O, Schlom J. Comparative biologic properties of a recombinant chimeric anti-carcinoma MAb and a recombinant aglycosylated variant. Cancer Immunol Immunother 1992; 353:165–174.

75. Wright A, Morrison SL. Effect of altered C_H2-associated carbohydrate structure on the functional properties and in vivo fate of chimeric mouse-human immunoglobulin G1. J Exp Med 1994; 180:1087–1096.

76. Slavin-Chiorini DC, Horan Hand P, Kashmiri SVS, Calvo B, Zaremba S, Schlom

J. Biologic properties of a C_H2 domain-deleted recombinant immunoglobulin. Int J Cancer 1993; 53:97–103.

77. Muraro R, Kuroki M, Wunderlich D, Poole DJ, Colcher D, Thor A, Greiner JW, Simpson JF, Molinolo A, Noguchi P, Schlom J. Generation and characterization of B72.3 second generation monoclonal antibodies reactive with tumor-associated glycoprotein 72 antigen. Cancer Res 1988; 48:4588–4596.

78. Slavin-Chiorini DC, Kashmiri SVS, Schlom J, Calvo B, Shu LM, Schott ME, Milenic DE, Snoy P, Carrasquillo JA, Anderson K, Hand PH. Biologic properties of chimeric CH1 domain-deleted and CH2 domain-deleted anti-carcinoma immunoglobulins. Cancer Res 1995; 55(suppl):5957s–5967s.

79. Gillies SD, Wesolowski JS. Antigen binding and biological activities of engineered mutant chimeric antibodies with human tumor specificities. Hum Antibodies Hybrid 1990; 1:47–54.

80. Mueller BM, Reisfeld RA, Gillies SD. Serum half-life and tumor localization of a chimeric antibody deleted of the C_H2 domain and directed against the disialoganglioside GD2. Proc Natl Acad Sci USA 1990; 87:5702–5705.

81. Riechmann L, Clark M, Waldmann H, Winter G. Reshaping human antibodies for therapy. Nature 1988; 332:323–327.

82. Verhoeyen M, Milstein C, Winter G. Reshaping human antibodies: grafting an antilysozyme activity. Science 1988; 239:1534–1536.

83. Lewis GD, Figari I, Fendly B, Wong WL, Carter P, Gorman C, Shepard HM. Differential responses of human tumor cell lines to anti-p185HER2 monoclonal antibodies. Cancer Immunol Immunother 1991; 37:255–263.

84. Kashmiri SVS, Shu L, Padlan EA, Milenic DE, Schlom J, Horan Hand P. Generation, characterization and in vivo studies of humanized anticarcinoma antibody CC49. Hybridoma 1995; 14:461–473.

85. Winter G. Gene technologies for antibody engineering. Behring Inst Mitt 1990; 87: 10–20.

86. Padlan E. Anatomy of the antibody molecule. Mol Immunol 1993; 31:169–217.

87. Sha Y, Xiang J. A heavy-chain grafted antibody that recognizes the tumor-associated TAG72 antigen. Cancer Biother 1994; 9:341–349.

88. Caron PC, Co MS, Bull MK, Avdolivic NM, Queen C, Scheinberg DA. Biological and immunological features of humanized M195 (anti-CD33) monoclonal antibodies. Cancer Res 1992; 52:6761–6767.

89. Couto JR, Blank EW, Peterson JA, Kiwan R, Padlan EA, Ceriani RL. Engineering of antibodies for breast cancer therapy: construction of chimeric and humanized versions of the murine monoclonal antibody BrE-3. In: Ceriani RL, ed. Antigen and Antibody Molecular Engineering in Breast Cancer Diagnosis and Treatment, Vol. 353. New York: Plenum Press, 1992:55–59.

90. Carter P, Presta L, Gorman C, Ridgway JB, Henner D, Wong WLT, Rowland AM, Kotts C, Carver ME, Shepard HM. Humanization of an anti-p185[HER2] antibody for human cancer therapy. Immunology 1992; 89:4285–4289.

91. Singer II, Kawka DW, DeMartino JA, Daugherty BL, Elliston KO, Alves K, Bush BL, Cameron PM, Cuca GC, Davies P, Forrest MJ, Kazazis DM, Law M-F, Lenny AB, Macintyre DE, Meurer R, Padlan EA, Pandya S, Schmidt JA, Seamans TC, Scott S, Silberklang M, Willamson AR, Mark GE. Optimal humanization of 1B4,

an anti-CD18 murine monoclonal antibody, is achieved by correct choice of human V-region framework sequences. J Immunol 1993; 150:2844–2857.

92. Caron PC, Schwartz MA, Co MS, Queen C, Finn RD, Graham MC, Divgi C, Larson SM, Scheinberg DA. Murine and humanized constructs of monoclonal antibody M195 (anti-CD33) for the therapy of acute myelogenous leukemia. Cancer 1994; 73(suppl):1049–1056.

93. Hutchins JT, Kull FC, Bynum J, Knick VC, Thurmond LM, Ray P. Improved bio-distribution, tumor targeting, and reduced immunogenicity in mice with a gamma 4 variant of CAMPATH-1H. Proc Natl Acad Sci USA 1995; 92:11980–11984.

94. Hakimi J, Chizzonite R, Luke DR, Familletti PC, Bailon P, Kondas JA, Pilson RS, Lin P, Weber DV, Spence C, Mondini LJ, Tsien W-H, Levin JL, Gallati VH, Korn L, Waldmann TA, Queen C, Benjamin WR. Reduced immunogenicity and im-proved pharmacokinetics of humanized anti-Tac in cynomologus monkeys. J Im-munol 1991; 147:1352–1359.

95. McGraw KJ, Rosenblum MG, Cheung L, Scheinberg DA. Characterization of mu-rine and human anti-CD33, gelonin immunotoxins reactive against myeloid leuke-mias. Cancer Immunol Immunother 1994; 39:367–374.

96. Hale G, Clark MR, Marcus R, Winter G, Dyer MJS, Phillips JM, Riechmann L, Waldmann H. Remission induction in non-Hodgkin lymphoma with reshaped hu-man monoclonal antibody CAMPATH-1H. Lancet 1988; 1:1394–1399.

97. Dyer MJ, Hale G, Hayhoe FG, Waldmann H. Effects of CAMPATH-1 antibodies in vivo in patients with lymphoid malignancies: influence of antibody isotype. Blood 1989; 73:1431–1439.

98. Juweid M, Sharkey RM, Markowitz A, Behr T, Swayne LC, Dunn R, Hansen HJ, Shevitz J, Leung SO, Rubin AD, Goldenberg DM. Treatment of non-Hodgkin's lymphoma with radiolabeled murine, chimeric or humanized LL2, an anti-CD22 monoclonal antibody. Cancer Res 1995; 55(suppl):5899s–5907s.

99. Waldmann TA. Anti-IL-2 receptor monoclonal antibody (anti-Tac) treatment of T-cell lymphoma. In: Hellman S, DeVita VT, Rosenberg SA, eds. Important Ad-vances in Oncology. Philadelphia: Lippincott, 1994:131–141.

100. Anasetti C, Hansen JA, Waldmann TA, Appelbaum FR, Davis J, Deeg HJ, Doney K, Martin PJ, Nash R, Storb R. Treatment of acute graft versus host disease with humanized anti-Tac: an antibody that binds to the interleukin-2 receptor. Blood 1994; 84:1320–1327.

101. Jurcic JG, Caron PC, Nikula TK, Papadapoulos EB, Finn RD, Gansow OA, Miller WHJ, Geerlings MW, Warrell RPJ, Larson S. Radiolabeled anti-CD33 monoclonal antibody M195 for myeloid leukemias. Cancer Res 1995; 55(suppl):5908s–5910s.

102. Baselga J, Tripathy D, Mendelsohn J, Baughman S, Benz CC, Dontis L, Sklorin NT, Seidman AD, Hudis CA, Moore J, Rosen PP, Twaddell T, Henderson IC, Norton L. Phase II study of weekly intravenous recombinant humanized anti-p185HER2 monoclonal antibody in patients with HER2/neu-overexpressing meta-static breast cancer. J Clin Oncol 1996; 14:737–744.

103. Sharkey RM, Juweid M, Behr T, Shevitz J, Dunn R, Leung SO, Griffiths G, Hansen HJ, Goldenberg DM. Evaluation of a CDR-grafted (humanized) anti-carcinoembry-onic antigen (CEA) monoclonal antibody (MAb). J Nucl Med 1995; 36(suppl): 215P–216P.

104. Thor A, Ouchi N, Szpak CA, Johnston WW, Schlom J. Distribution of oncofetal

antigen tumor-associated glycoprotein-72 defined by monoclonal antibody B72.3. Cancer Res 1986; 46:3118–3124.

105. Wolf BC, D'Emilia JC, Salem RR, DeCoste D, Sears HF, Gottlieb LS, Steele GDJ. Detection of the tumor-associated glycoprotein antigen (TAG-72) in premalignant lesions of the colon. J Natl Cancer Inst 1989; 81:1913–1917.

106. Thor A, Viglione MJ, Muraro R, Ohuchi N, Schlom J, Gorstein F. Monoclonal antibody B72.3 reactivity with human endometrium: a study of normal and malignant tissues. Int J Gynecol Pathol 1987; 6:235–247.

107. Sikorska H, Shuster J, Gold P. Clinical applications of carcinoembryonic antigen. Cancer Detect Prev 1988; 12:321–355.

108. Wallach D, Fellous M, Revel M. Preferential effect of γ interferon on the synthesis of HLA antigens and their mRNAs in human cells. Nature 1982; 299:833–836.

109. Rosa F, Fellous M. Regulation of HLA-DR by IFN-γ. Transcription and post-transcriptional control. J Immunol 1988; 140:1660–1664.

110. Attallah AM, Needy CF, Noguchi PD, Elisberg BL. Enhancement of carcinoembryonic antigen expression by interferon. Int J Cancer 1979; 24:49–52.

111. Greiner JW, Horan Hand P, Noguchi P, Fisher PB, Pestka S, Schlom J. Enhanced expression of surface tumor-associated antigens on human breast and colon tumor cells after recombinant human leukocyte α-interferon. Cancer Res 1984; 44:3208–3214.

112. Greiner JW, Tobi M, Fisher PB, Langer JA, Pestka S. Differential responsiveness of cloned mammary carcinoma cell populations to human recombinant alpha interferon mediated enhancement of tumor antigen expression. Int J Cancer 1985; 36: 159–166.

113. Guadagni F, Schlom J, Johnston WW, Szpak CA, Goldstein D, Smalley R, Simpson JF, Borden EC, Pestka S, Greiner JW. Selective interferon-induced enhancement of tumor-associated antigen on a spectrum of freshly isolated human adenocarcinoma cells. J Natl Cancer Inst 1989; 81:502–511.

114. Kantor J, Tran R, Greiner JW, Pestka S, Fisher PB, Shively JE, Schlom J. Modulation of carcinoembryonic antigen messenger RNA levels in human colon carcinoma cells by recombinant human γ-interferon. Cancer Res 1989; 49:2651–2655.

115. Audette M, Carrel S, Hayoz D, Giuffre L, Mach J-P, Kuhn LC. A novel interferon-γ regulated human melanoma-associated antigen, gp33-38, defined by monoclonal antibody Me14-D12. Mol Immunol 1989; 26:515–522.

116. Clark S, McGuckin MA, Hurst T, Ward BG. Effect of interferon-γ and TNF-α on MUC1 mucin expression in ovarian carcinoma cell lines. Dis Markers 1994; 12: 43–50.

117. Giacomini P, Aguzzi A, Pestka S, Fisher PB, Ferrone S. Modulation of recombinant DNA leukocyte (α) and fibroblast (β) interferons of the expression and shedding of HLA- and tumor-associated antigens by human melanoma cells. J Immunol 1984; 133:1649–1655.

118. Iacobelli C, Scambia G, Natoli C, Panici PB, Biaocchi G, Perrone L, Mancuso S. Recombinant human leukocyte interferon-α2b stimulates the synthesis and release of a 90K tumor-associated antigen in human breast cancer cells. J Cancer 1988; 42:182–184.

119. Real FX, Carrato A, Schluessler MH, Welt S, Oettgen HE. IFN-γ-regulated expression of a differentiation antigen of human cells. J Immunol 1988; 140:1571–1576.

120. Gross N, Beck D, Favre S, Carrel S. In vitro antigenic modulation of human neuro-blastoma cells induced by IFN-γ, retinoic acid and dibutyryl cyclic AMP. Int J Cancer 1987; 39:521–529.
121. Hauck W, Stanners CP. Control of carcinoembryonic antigen gene family express-ing in differentiating colon carcinoma cell line, Caco-2. Cancer Res 1991; 51:3526–3533.
122. Benchimol S, Fuks A, Jothy S, Beauchemin N, Shirota K, Stanners CP. Carcinoem-bryonic antigen, a human tumor marker, functions as an intercellular adhesion mol-ecule. Cell 1989; 57:327–334.
123. Leusch H-G, Hefta SA, Drzeniek Z, Hummel K, Markos-Pusztai Z, Wagener C. Escherichia coli of human origin binds to carcinoembryonic antigen (CEA) and non-specific crossreacting antigen (NCA). FEBS Lett 1990; 261:405–409.
124. Greiner JW, Ulmann CD, Nieroda C, Qi C-F, Eggensperger D, Shimada S, Steinberg SM, Schlom J. Improved radioimmunotherapeutic efficacy of an anticar-cinoma monoclonal antibody (^{131}I-CC49) when given in combination with γ-inter-feron. Cancer Res 1993; 53:600–608.
125. Greiner JW, Guadagni F, Goldstein D, Smalley RV, Borden EC, Simpson JF, Moli-nolo A, Schlom J. Intraperitoneal administration of interferon-gamma to carcinoma patients enhances expression of tumor-associated glycoprotein-72 and carcinoem-bryonic antigen on malignant ascites cells. J Clin Oncol 1992; 10:735–746.
126. Roselli M, Guadagni F, Buonomo O, Belardi A, Vittorini V, Mariani-Constantini R, Greiner JW, Casciani CU, Schlom J. Systemic administration of recombinant interferon-α in carcinoma patients upregulates the expression of the carcinoma as-sociated antigens CEA and TAG-72. J Clin Oncol 1996; 10:2031–2042.
127. Greiner JW, Guadagni F, Noguchi P, Pestka S, Schlom J. Recombinant interferon enhanced monoclonal antibody-targeting of carcinoma lesions in vivo. Science 1987; 235:895–898.
128. Guadagni F, Greiner JW, Pothen S, Pestka S, Schlom J. Enhanced in vivo mono-clonal antibody localization to human carcinomas in athymic mice after recombi-nant interferon treatment. Cancer Immunol Immunother 1988; 26:222–230.
129. Yokota S, Hara H, Luo T, Seon BK. Synergistic potentiation of in vivo antitumor activity of anti-human T-leukemia immunotoxins by recombinant α-interferon and daunorubicin. Cancer Res 1990; 50:32–37.
130. Matsui M, Nakanishi T, Noguchi T, Ferrone S. Synergistic in vitro and in vivo anti-tumor effect of daunomycin-anti-96-kDa melanoma-associated antigen monoclonal antibody CL207 conjugate and recombinant IFN-γ. J Immunol 1988; 141:1410–1417.
131. Kuhn JA, Beatty BG, Wong JYC, Estaban JM, Wanek PM, Wall F, Buras RR, Williams LE, Beatty JD. Interferon enhancement of radioimmunotherapy for colon carcinoma. Cancer Res 1991; 51:2335–2339.
132. Kurzrock R, Rosenblum MG, Sherwin SA, Rios A, Talpaz M, Quesada JR, Gut-terman JU. Pharmacokinetics, single-dose tolerance, and the biological activity of recombinant γ-interferon in cancer patients. Cancer Res 1988; 45:2866–2872.
133. Maluish AE, Urba WJ, Longo DL, Overton WR, Coggin D, Crisp ER, Williams R, Sherwin SA, Gordon K, Steis RG. The determination of an immunologically active dose of interferon-γ in patients with melanoma. J Clin Oncol 1988; 6:434–445.

134. Greiner JW, Guadagni F, Goldstein D, Borden EC, Ritts REJ, LoBuglio AF, Suleh MN, Schlom J. Evidence for the elevation of serum carcinoembryonic antigen (CEA) and tumor-associated glycoprotein-72 (TAG-72) levels in patients administered interferon. Cancer Res 1991; 51:4155–4163.
135. Rosenblum MG, Lamki LM, Murray JL, Carlo DJ, Gutterman JU. Interferon-induced changes in pharmacokinetics and tumor uptake of ^{111}In-labeled antimelanoma antibody 96.5 in melanoma patients. J Natl Cancer Inst 1988; 80:160–165.
136. Bruggemann M, Williams GT, Caskey HM, Teale C, Spicer C, Surani MA, Neuberger MS. Construction, function and immunogenicity of recombinant monoclonal antibodies. Behring Inst Mitt 1990; 87:21–24.
137. Irie RF, Morton DL. Regression of cutaneous metastatic melanoma by intralesional injection with human monoclonal antibody to ganglioside GD2. Proc Natl Acad Sci USA 1986; 83:8694–8698.
138. Mendez MJ, Green LL, Corvalan RF, Jia X-C, Maynard-Currie CE, Yang X-D, Gallo ML, Louie DM, Lee DV, Erickson KL, Luna J, Roy CM-N, Abderrahim H, Kirschenbaum F, Noguchi M, Smith DH, Fukushima A, Hales JF, Finer MH, Davis CG, Zsebo KM, Jakobovits A. Functional transplant of megabase human immunoglobulin loci recapitulates human antibody response in mice. Nature Genet 1997; 15:146–156.
139. Hwu P, Shafer GE, Treisman J, Schindler DG, Grow G, Cowherd R, Rosenberg SA, Eshhar Z. Lysis of ovarian cancer cells by human lymphocytes redirected with a chimeric gene composed of an antibody variable region and the Fc receptor γ chain. J Exp Med 1993; 178:361–366.
140. Eshhar Z, Waks T, Gross G, Schindler D. Specific activation and targeting of cytotoxic lymphocytes through chimeric single chains consisting of antibody-binding domains and the γ or ζ subunits of the immunoglobulin and T-cell receptors. Proc Natl Acad Sci USA 1993; 90:720–724.
141. Hwu P, Yang C, Cowherd R, Treisman J, Shafer GE, Eshhar Z, Rosenberg SA. In vivo antitumor activity of T cells redirected with chimeric antibody/T-cell receptor genes. Cancer Res 1995; 55:3369–3373.
142. Moritz D, Wels W, Mattern J, Groner B. Cytotoxic T lymphocytes with a grafted recognition specificity of ERBB2-expressing tumor cells. Proc Natl Acad Sci USA 1994; 91:4318–4322.
143. Moritz D, Groner B. A spacer region between the single chain antibody and the CD3z-chain domain of chimeric T-cell receptor components is required for efficient ligand binding and signaling activity. Gene Ther 1995; 2:539–546.
144. Wels W, Moritz D, Schmidt M, Jeschke M, Hynes NE, Groner B. Biotechnological and gene therapeutic strategies in cancer treatment. Gene 1995; 159:73–80.
145. Khawli LA, Miller GK, Epstein AL. Effect of seven new vasoactive immunoconjugates on the enhancement of monoclonal antibody uptake in tumors. Cancer 1994; 73:824–831.
146. Huang X, Molema G, King S, Watkins L, Edgington TS, Thorpe PE. Tumor infarction in mice by antibody-directed targeting of tissue factor to tumor vasculature. Science 1997; 427:547–550.

7
Pretargeted Radioimmunotherapy of Cancer

**Marco Chinol, Chiara Grana, Roberto Gennari,
Marta Cremonesi, J. G. Geraghty,
and Giovanni Paganelli**
European Institute of Oncology, Milan, Italy

I. CONCEPTS OF PRETARGETING: VARIOUS SYSTEM TAGGING/EFFECTOR MOLECULES

A. Introduction

Strategies for treating most cancers usually employ surgical resection, chemotherapy, and/or radiation therapy. Although surgical resection can be very effective and sometimes curative in localized tumors, the presence of distant sites or inoperable tumors leaves the options of chemotherapy and/or radiotherapy. If chemotherapeutic drugs or radiotherapy could be selectively delivered to tumors, it would be possible to avoid, or at least reduce, unwanted toxicity and improve efficacy (1).

The utility of monoclonal antibodies (MoAbs) for targeting radioactive agents to tumor cells, for diagnostic and therapeutic purposes, has been extensively studied (2–5). The concept, which forms the basis of radioimmunoscintigraphy (ISG), radioimmunoguided surgery (RIGS), and radioimmunotherapy (RIT), has been an active area of research in various fields of oncology (6–9). Many investigations have focused on several parts of this process, including tumor antigen expression, tumor targeting vehicles, pharmacokinetic aspects and immunogenicity of these recognition units, radioisotopes, and nuclear imaging technology (10–14).

Although several studies have been carried out in this area for almost two decades, many limitations when using radiolabeled MoAbs for treating solid tumors in humans have been encountered.

B. Problems in Tumor Targeting

Tumors often display intrinsic heterogeneity in antigen density. This factor, together with the nonuniformity of tumor vascularization, capillary permeability, degree of tumor necrosis, and difference in interstitial pressure, accounts for the heterogeneous distribution of antibodies in targeted tumors (13).

Another problem with RIT is the relatively low tumor-to-normal-tissue radioactivity ratio and the small dose of radioactivity that consequently reaches the target tumor. Accumulation of up to 20% to 30% of the injected dose per gram tumor has been observed in mouse tumor models, whereas 0.001% to 0.1% injected dose per gram is more common in humans (15).

Other physical and physiological barriers prevent large quantities of MoAb from penetrating into solid masses (15–17), resulting in tumor-to-blood ratios in the range of 1:5. A low tumor-to-background ratio remains the main problem of radioimmunodetection.

C. Pretargeting Systems

In an attempt to overcome the low uptake of label by the tumor and improve the tumor-to-blood ratio, various studies have examined the concept of tumor pretargeting based on the separate administration of MoAbs and radiolabeled isotopes (18–23). Such systems require the use of a modified MoAb (*first* conjugates) that permits a second component (*second* conjugates) to bind specifically to it. Conceptually, the modified MoAb is administered first and allowed to distribute throughout the body, to bind to the tissues expressing antigen, and to clear substantially from other tissues. Then the radiolabeled second component is administered and, ideally, it localizes at sites where the modified MoAb has accumulated. If the second component has higher permeation, clearance, and diffusion rates than those of MoAb, more rapid radionuclide localization to the tumor and higher tumor selectivity are possible. Injection of the radiolabeled component can be delayed to a time when most of the primary MoAb has been cleared from the blood and normal tissues, thereby decreasing nontumor binding and achieving higher tumor-to-nontumor ratios (24).

1. First Conjugates

The first molecules to target a tumor are referred to as targeting vehicles, or first conjugates, since a specific tag is carried by them. Four different types of tagged targeting vehicles for the pretargeting system have been described in the literature: biotin-conjugated or biotinylated antibodies (25); streptavidin-conjugated or streptavidin antibodies (23); bifunctional MoAbs (Bs-MoAbs) (26); and monoclonal antibody-oligonucleotide conjugates (22). These vehicles require recognition by a second molecule. This tagging requires specific properties: (a) attachment of any agent to a MoAb must be achieved without changing the antibody's immune specificity; (b) tagged MoAbs must retain their antigen-binding affinity without causing premature shedding or internalization; (c) the tagged MoAb needs to display a selective and high affinity for the second recognition molecule.

The biotinylation of MoAbs is easily accomplished, and two or three biotin molecules can be incorporated per antibody molecule without loss of immunoreactivity (27). The biotinylation of MoAb increases the molecular weight only minimally, and has no effect on either plasma kinetics or rates of antibody permeation and diffusion (28). In addition, the use of a long spacer arm between the protein binding site and biotin reduces steric hindrance of the subsequent avidin-biotin reaction (27).

Conjugation of streptavidin to a MoAb will significantly increase its size (approximately 40% for an IgG) and thereby alter its pharmacokinetics, possibly reducing tumor uptake. However, in at least one study where streptavidin-MoAb conjugates were administered prior to radiolabeled biotin in rabbits, better images were obtained as compared to radiolabeled MoAb alone, suggesting that decreases in tumor uptake may be compensated by lower systemic levels and a higher tumor-to-blood ratio (29). Streptavidin is made up of four identical subunits, only one of which is presumed to attach to the MoAb.

An alternative approach for tumor targeting is to employ a multistage delivery system using bispecific MoAb. Bs-MoAbs made by chemical coupling of two different antibody fragments (Fab') (30) or by producing hybrid hybridomas (31) of two different antigen-specific binding sites, one for the tumor-associated antigen and the other for the radioactive effector compound. The Bs-MoAb is first targeted to the tumor and, after a suitable period of time has elapsed for the nonspecifically bound to be cleared, the radiolabeled hapten is then injected separately, resulting in its specific localization in the tumor. However, because of the univalency of Bs-MoAbs for the tumor antigen, as well as mismatched association of parental chains, tumor-binding affinity is generally deficient.

Another way to increase the tumor-to-blood ratio includes carbohydrate modifications of the target MoAb, which are able to effect the pharmacokinetics of these molecules. The attachment of oligonucleotides to MoAb typically binds three to five oligonucleotides per antibody molecule preserving the specificity and reducing the immunoreactivity to an average of 50% normal. The terminal sialic acids normally present on MoAb carbohydrates help retain them in circulation (31). Being DNA based conjugates, these targeting structures also need more careful preservation than other MoAb conjugates to avoid the rapid serum metabolism (32).

2. Second Conjugates

Second conjugates are most often radiolabeled avidin, streptavidin, or biotin molecules directed at the biotinylated or avidinylated MoAb (33). It is important that the second molecules exhibit low immunogenicity, a wide distribution, and a high selectivity for the tagged MoAb. It is also very important that this conjugate be cleared rapidly from the normal tissue and blood after achieving its highest concentration on tumor-bound antibodies. This pretargeting technique thus takes advantage of the avidin-biotin system, which has long and widely been used for in vitro applications (34).

3. The Avidin-Biotin System

The avidin-biotin system is widely used for in vitro applications, in immunohisto-chemistry, ELISA and molecular biology, for the stepwise construction of macro-molecular complex onto specific target molecules in order to make them detectable by chemical or physical methods (34,35). Avidins are functionally defined by their ability to bind biotin with high affinity and specificity without recognizing or binding any other physiological compound with any strength. For practical purpose, their binding can be regarded as irreversible (36,37). The molecular properties of avidins are summarized in Table 1.

Avidins are small oligomeric proteins made up of four identical subunits, bearing a single binding site for biotin. Avidin is a 66-kDa glycosylated protein, commonly isolated from hen egg white and shows a strong positive net charge. Streptavidin, a non-glycosylated analog, isolated from *Streptomyces avidinii*, in contrast to avidin is nearly neutral at physiological pH, with an isoelectric point of approximately 6 (38). Biotin is a 244-Da molecule, and is commercially avail-

Table 1 Molecular Properties of Avidin and Streptavidin

	Avian avidin	Streptavidin
Molecular weight	66,000	65,000
Number of subunits	4	4
Subunit MW	16,000	16,000
Biotin binding sites/mole	4	4
K_d of biotin complex	10^{-15}	10^{-15}
Oligosaccharide/subunit	1	0
Mannose/subunit	4.5	—
Glucosamine/subunit	3	—
Isoelectric point	10.5	6

able with several linkers that facilitate reactions with proteins. These linkers also afford spacers to allow biotin to interact more effectively with avidin after conjugation. Biotinylation of MoAb has been shown to have minimal effects on the biodistribution of antibodies (25). Biotin is recognized by a functional "head" region, which binds avidin, and a functionally irrelevant carboxyl "tail" end, which can be chemically altered with little or no effect on the molecule.

A number of options have been explored to take advantage of the avidin-biotin interaction in increasing the tumor localization for clinical purpose of MoAb and their conjugates (39).

4. Radioisotope Labeling

Radioisotope labeling of biotin, avidin, or streptavidin is either done directly to the protein (radioiodination) or by covalently linking a chelating agent, which in turn can bind a suitable radionuclide (indirect method) (40). In the case of biotin, the conjugation of a chelating agent is obtained by reacting the activated carboxyl group of biotin with a variety of functional groups present on almost all classes of compounds. The most commonly used chelating agents for indirect labeling are the polyaminocarboxylic acids (EDTA) and (DTPA) and their chemically modified derivatives. The molecular integrity of biotin or avidin is not altered significantly by radiolabeling, and reactivity of these proteins is preserved in 90% to 100% of unlabeled corresponding molecules (41).

For therapeutic applications, the choice of a suitable isotope is quite limited. Yttrium-90 (^{90}Y), indicated as one of the four best therapeutic radionuclides for use in conjunction with tumor-associated antibodies (42), is certainly very appropriate. It can easily be obtained with a ^{90}Sr/^{90}Y generator (43), has a physical half-life of 2.7 days, and is a pure, high-energy beta emitter (E_{max} beta = 2.28 MeV; E_{ave} beta = 0.94 MeV) (44,45). Recent studies have shown that yttrium complexes with the macrocyclic chelating agents presented enhanced thermodynamic and kinetic stability relative to an open-chain analogue (46,47). In particular, the 12-membered ring 1,4,7,10-tetraazacyclododecane-N,N',N'',N'''-tetraacetic acid (DOTA) has been shown to form remarkably stable complexes with yttrium under physiological conditions, prompting the synthesis of several derivatives of DOTA for linkage to monoclonal antibodies (MoAbs) (48).

A recent biodistribution study in tumor-bearing mice according to a three-step pretargeting approach indicated that, despite the fast blood clearance of ^{90}Y-labeled-biotin ($T_{1/2}$ = 1.3 ± 0.6 h) (49), ^{90}Y-DOTA-biotin with a noncleavable spacer arm was superior to ^{90}Y-DTPA-biotin (50). A DOTA-biotin ligand (NeoRx Corporation, Seattle, WA) consisting of the DOTA chelating agent linked to biotin via an amino acid side chain modified by amide N-methylation in order to prevent the action of the biotinidase (51), is capable of binding ^{90}Y with high specific activity and is currently used in pretargeted radioimmunotherapy trials (52).

II. CLINICAL APPLICATIONS OF THE AVIDIN/BIOTIN SYSTEM

Several protocols have been devised to exploit the high affinity between avidin and biotin in the clinical settings (21,25). Two major methods are used with the aim to improve the delivery of radionuclides to tumors.

A. Two-Step Method

This approach has been initially proposed based on the in vitro conjugation of streptavidin to the antibody which is administered first, followed, 2 to 3 days later, by the injection of radiolabeled biotin (41). Optimization of this pretargeting system in murine and canine animal models has been reported (53,54). Basically, three components have been proposed: antibody-streptavidin conjugate, galactose-albumin-biotin clearing agent, and radiobiotin.

An imaging study on 10 patients with documented squamous cell carcinoma of the lung, pretargeted with 1.0 mg of MoAb (HMFG1) conjugated with streptavidin followed 2 to 3 days later by 74 MBq of ^{111}In-labeled biotin, showed decreased activity levels in all normal organs and in blood and clear images obtained as little as 2 h postinjection of radiobiotin (55). However, in this clinical trial a clearing agent "chase" was not used which probably would have benefited the quality of the images.

An alternative approach has also been used to target intraperitoneal tumors. Intraperitoneal injection has been proposed to increase the tumor-to-nontumor ratio in such cases and IP over IV advantages has been described in humans (56). In this system, intraperitoneal injection of biotinylated MoAbs (first step) is followed 1 to 2 days later by the administration of radiolabeled streptavidin, thus exploiting at best, the specific binding of the biotinylated antibody onto the tumor (57).

B. Three-Step Method

The locoregional approach is feasible when tumor is confined to the peritoneal cavity or in other locoregional approaches. In the presence of widespread disease, a systemic injection of the tracer is nonetheless required. A three-step approach has been designed for these cases, where conjugates need to be cleared not only from a well-defined body cavity, but from the entire blood pool. In this technique,

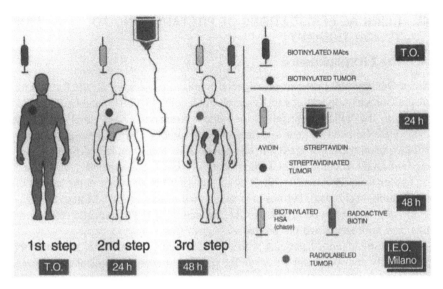

Figure 1 Three-step strategy. Biotinylated antibodies are injected (IV) and allowed to localize onto the target (step 1). One day later avidin/streptavidin are injected (IV) (step 2). After 24 h, when unbound streptavidin and circulating avidin-MoAb complexes have been cleared from circulation, radiolabeled biotin is injected (IV) (step 3). A second "chase" of biotinylated human serum albumin (HSA) is administered a few minutes prior to the radioactive biotin injection.

the excess of circulating biotinylated MoAbs are removed as cold complexes, which are taken up and metabolized by the liver. This is the major factor in background reduction and is obtained prior to label injection.

Schematically (Fig. 1), biotinylated MoAbs are first injected (step 1), followed by injection of avidin and streptavidin one day later (step 2). The second injection carries a twofold purpose: (a) the removal of excess circulating biotinylated antibodies in the form of cold complexes via avidin (fast clearance), and (b) the targeting of tumor cells with streptavidin (slower clearance). Thereafter radiolabeled biotin, which will selectively bind to streptavidin and thus to the tumor, is injected (step 3). The use of a second "chase" of biotinylated human serum albumin, with the purpose to decrease the radiation burden in circulation administered a few minutes prior to the radioactive biotin, has been also proposed (49).

A three-step protocol is currently used at the European Institute of Oncology in Milan for the treatment of high grade gliomas with encouraging results (52).

III. CLINICAL APPLICATIONS OF PRETARGETING TO TUMOR THERAPY

A. The EIO Experience

Since October 1994, as part of a special finalized project within the framework of the Clinical Applications of Research in Oncology (ACRO) and in collaboration with the Italian Association for Cancer Research, Phase I and II therapy trials were initiated to treat a variety of solid tumors. During these preliminary studies, several clinical grade MoAbs had become available, including antitenascin, antifolate receptor, anti-CD20, and anti-TAG-72. Subsequently, we focused on antitenascin MoAbs since their target (tenascin) is abundant in the stroma of brain tumors (gliomas), but not in normal cerebral tissues (58). Moreover, high-grade gliomas are good targets for the evaluation of the therapeutic efficacy of this new approach since the prognosis is grim (59).

The treatment of patients with ovarian carcinoma and other solid tumors is currently underway and we are in the process of accruing clinical data during follow-up.

B. Therapy of Gliomas

High-grade gliomas constitute more than 40% of malignant brain tumors and are characterized by an extremely poor prognosis (59). This fact has stimulated the search for new therapies, including gene therapy (60) and the use of monoclonal antibodies in association with cytotoxic agents (61).

Using a three-step technique, we have treated 45 eligible patients with histologically defined grade III and IV gliomas documented by CT or MRI scan prior to therapy. All patients were in progression after conventional treatments and they were initially evaluated with a three-step scintigraphic study using ^{99m}Tc-labeled biotin in order to assess the clinical application of the pretargeting approach.

The first step of the protocol consisted of biotinylated antitenascin monoclonal antibodies in 100 mL of physiological saline, injected IV over a period of 20 min at a dose of 35 mg/m^2. Avidin and streptavidin were then administered IV 24 to 36 h after the antibody as follows: 20 to 30 mg avidin as a rapid bolus (first chase), and 50 mg streptavidin in 100 mL saline with 2% human albumin, 30 min after the avidin. Two milligrams of the noncleavable DOTA-biotin ligand (NeoRx Corporation, Seattle, WA) was labeled with ^{90}Y-chloride and administered 24 h after streptavidin infusion (third step) in a dose ranging from 2.22 to 2.97 GBq/m^2 (60 to 80 mCi/m^2) per cycle.

To permit scintigraphic monitoring of radiolabel localization, the therapeutic dose was mixed with 74-111 MBq of indium-111 (^{111}In) (a gamma source) bound to 0.05 mg DOTA-biotin. Ten minutes before the injection of radioactive

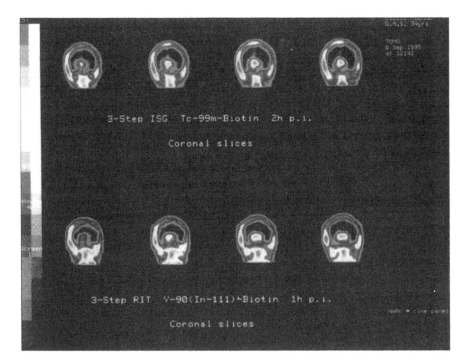

Figure 2   Tomographic images in a patient with frontal glioblastoma. Above images: immunoscintigraphic evaluation obtained 2 h postinjection of ^{99m}Tc-biotin; high uptake of radioactive biotin is present in the frontal lobes. Below images: the same pattern of uptake was observed in the scintigraphic evaluation 1 h after the injection of ^{90}Y-biotin (spiked with ^{111}In).

biotin, 20 mg biotinylated human serum albumin was administered IV to reduce circulating levels of streptavidin (second chase). The similar distribution pattern of radioactive biotin in a patient with frontal glioblastoma, prior to therapy (3-step ISG) and 1 hour after treatment, is documented in the tomographic images shown in Figure 2.

The patients were followed as inpatients for 72 h after the administration of the therapeutic dose.

In order to determine the biological *half-life* of the radiopharmaceuticals, blood samples were withdrawn from 10 patients at time 5 min, 10 min, 15 min, 20 min, 30 min, 1 h, 3 h, 15 h, and 24 h after therapy, and thereafter, for a total of 3 days. In the same patients, complete urinary collection was obtained over 3 days with samples at 2 h, 16 h, 24 h, 36 h, 48 h, and 72 h. The percentage of the injected dose excreted through the kidneys as a function of time was measured. The retention of the activity in the body, observed from the images, was compared with urine excretion at each time with good agreement.

Blood and urine samples were counted for In-111 to predict the biodistribution of Y-90 based on the assumption that In-111 and Y-90 have the same in vivo behavior. One hour, 16, 24, 48 and whenever possible 72 h after injection of radioactive biotin, whole-body biodistribution studies were performed using a dual-head gamma camera equipped with medium energy collimators (Maxuus, General Electric). Planar views were acquired using 20% window centered in the energy of both 172 and 247 keV peaks.

The sequence of distribution images observed for In-111 was used to extrapolate the activity versus time of Y-90 in critical organs (liver, kidney, and brain) and in tumor. Residence times (τ) and half-lives ($T_{1/2}$ α and $T_{1/2}$ β) were obtained adapting a biexponential model to the experimental curve.

The objective therapeutic response was evaluated from CT of MRI images of the brain acquired 40 to 60 days after therapy and, whenever possible, repeated every 2 to 3 months thereafter; a clinical evaluation was also performed. The clinical evaluation of all patients began 2 months after treatment. At this stage, tumor mass reduction occurred in 9/45 (20%) patients (MR+PR+CR); 55% had a stabilization of the disease (SD) and 25% did not respond to therapy (Fig. 3).

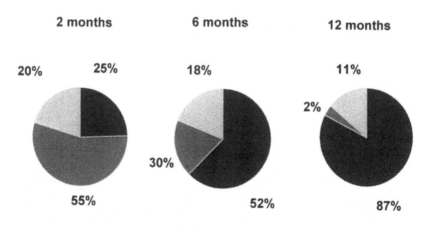

Figure 3 Summary of therapeutic responses at various follow-up times. CR, complete response; PR, partial response; MR, minor response; SD, stable disease; PD, progressive disease.

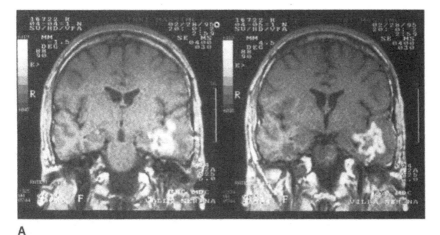

A

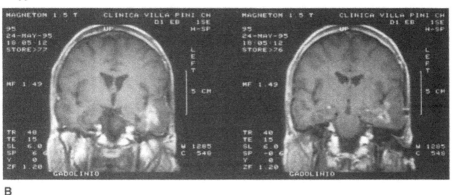

B

Figure 4 MRI study of a patient with glioblastoma. Panel A shows a mass (recurrence) in the left temporal lobe; he was in progression after surgery and radiotherapy. Panel B shows the same section of the brain 3 months after the first cycle of RIT with evidence of a partial regression of the tumor mass.

Of the nine patients with reduced tumor mass at 2 months, six had grade IV glioma and three had grade III glioma. The proportion of patients with a decrease of tumor mass remained stable at 2 and 6 months of follow-up (respectively 20% and 18%) while the percentage of those in progression increased from 25% to 52%. At 12 months' follow-up, all three patients with anaplastic glioma were still in good condition, while one glioblastoma patient had a minor response at 9 months and another is still in excellent condition more than 2 years after the first treatment (total of 11% MR+PR+CR). Two examples of tumor mass reduction at 3 and 7 months after therapy are documented in the MRI images shown in Figures 4 and 5, respectively.

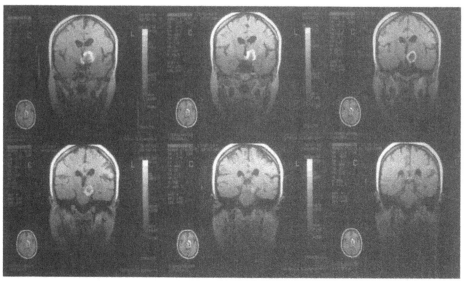

A

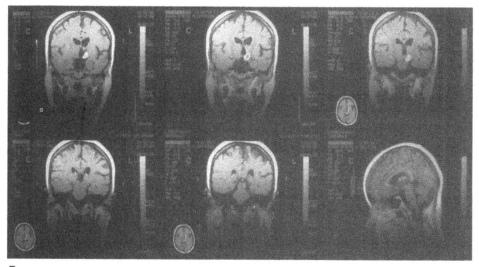

B

Figure 5 MRI study (coronal slices) of a 35-year-old patient. Panel A shows anaplastic astrocytoma in the left talamic area; the tumor was in progression after radiotherapy (surgery was not indicated). Panel B is the same section of the brain 7 months after the first cycle of RIT, showing a considerable reduction of the tumor mass. The patient received another cycle of RIT, and she is alive and in good condition more than 2 years after treatment.

IV. TOXICITY AND IMMUNOGENICITY

The data accrued so far in the therapy trials have shown that the treatment was well tolerated by all patients. None developed renal or liver alterations during follow-up. Most patients had bone marrow toxicity (82%, grade 0–II); 2/5 patients treated with the highest dose of ^{90}Y developed grade III–IV toxicity.

Even if these patients received granulocyte-macrophage colony-stimulating factors, transfusions, and antibiotics, full recovery occurred in all patients after 4 to 6 weeks. A small number of patients (6%), who had previously received streptavidin for diagnostic purposes, developed a mild allergic reaction during therapeutic streptavidin administration. Another group (18%) presented with allergic reactions (generally grade I) to streptavidin when the treatment was repeated a second time. Only 4% of the patients developed grade I allergic reactions either to MoAb or to avidin.

Some data on hematological toxicity are reported in Figure 6. Most patients (82%) had low toxicity (grades 0–II) consisting of thrombocytopenia or thrombocytopenia and neutropenia. The relation between administered dose/m^2 and toxicity grade, assessed with Spearman's rank-correlation and chi-square test, indicated a slight but not statistically significant correlation between dose and toxicity. However, after the second cycle, 2/5 patients treated with the highest dose developed grade III–IV toxicity, versus 0/13 of those treated with lower doses.

The probability that the components of the pretargeting systems (murine MoAbs, avidin, and streptavidin) may cause specific immune responses is well documented in the literature (25,55). Previous data, obtained in a group of 49 patients submitted to a pretargeted (three-step) ISG, have shown that less than 5% of the patients developed an immune response to the biotinylated mouse antibodies (HAMA) and less than 30% developed an antiavidin response (HAVA). Severe immune responses to streptavidin (HASA) have been observed in about 65% of the patients injected with 2 mg biotinylated MoAbs, 5 mg avidin, and 5 mg streptavidin (62). These data are in agreement with previous results where HAMA and HAVA responses were reported (28).

Immunogenicity data obtained in 34 patients treated with pretargeted RIT confirmed the trend reported in ISG studies. HAMA response was observed in 15% of patients, HAVA in 38%, and HASA in 85% of treated patients.

The unexpected and interesting finding that the HAMA response is reduced when biotinylated MoAbs are injected according to the three-step protocols, has been confirmed in all of these pretargeted trials. Whether this is due to biotinylation of the antibody or to the modified pharmacokinetics of the pretargeting strategy is still under evaluation (23). Some low-titer avidin responses were found in untreated patients, so the high frequency of avidin antibodies after treatment could represent a secondary response. No patients had streptavidin antibodies

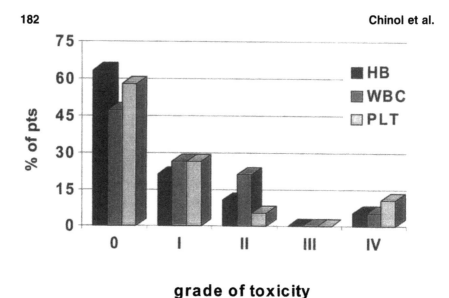

grade of toxicity

Figure 6   Hematological toxicity after one cycle of three-step pretargeted RIT.

before exposure, but all responded after a single exposure. Conversely, 47% of patients developed antibody against murine IgG after a second cycle and 60% after a third cycle.

V.   PHARMACOKINETICS AND DOSIMETRY

The serum clearance of Y-90-labeled biotin through the DOTA macrocycle ligand also reveals two components. All patients submitted to the three-step therapy trials had closely similar ^{90}Y-DOTA-biotin activity profiles in blood (Fig. 7) with mean $T_{1/2}\alpha$ of 1.2 ± 0.8 h, $T_{1/2}$ β of 14.8 ± 13.6 h, resulting in an absorbed dose to the bone marrow of 0.8 ± 0.5 cGy (range 0.3 to 1.1)/37 MBq. Thus the total dose for bone marrow was less than 2 Gy per cycle.

The rate of urinary excretion showed instead a large variability among patients especially for the first day after therapy, with a cumulative $70\% \pm 28\%$ of the injected dose excreted within the first 24 h and less than $5\% \pm 2\%$ in the next 24 to 40 h (Fig. 8).

Absorbed doses were calculated according to the MIRD formalism (63) using the residence times (τ) obtained from the experimental curves for each tissue and the S values relating the cumulative activity in the source organs to the absorbed dose in the target organs. A homogeneous distribution of the activity

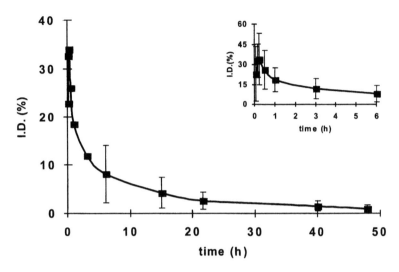

Figure 7 Representative ^{90}Y-DOTA-biotin blood clearance curve. The percent of the injected dose measured in patient blood is plotted versus the time postinjection of radiolabeled biotin. The small graph shows the standard deviations of the first part of the curve (until 6 h).

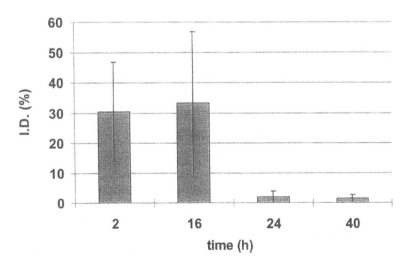

Figure 8 Histogram showing the rate of urinary excretion. The percent of the injected dose measured in patient urine is plotted versus the time postinjection of radiolabeled biotin.

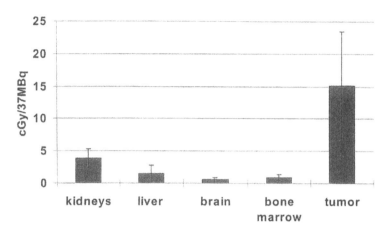

Figure 9 Mean absorbed doses (cGy/37 MBq) in tumor (gliomas) and in critical organs. Note the higher uptake in tumor compared to nontarget organs.

in the organs and tumor was assumed. The dose absorbed by the tumor was calculated using the tumor mass obtained from MRI or CT images.

The dose delivered to the bone marrow, which is the organ most affected by therapy with Y-90, was calculated from the activity of blood samples with the assumption of nonspecific uptake and homogeneous distribution. The contribution of the free Y-90 deposition in bone was not considered based on the extremely high in vivo stability of the binding between Y-90 and DOTA (47). The absorbed doses, obtained in the group of patients with gliomas treated according to a systemic three-step protocol, were as follows: 2.7 ± 1.6 cGy/37 MBq in kidneys, 1.5 ± 1.0 cGy/37 MBq in liver, and 0.6 ± 0.3 cGy/37 MBq in brain; the dose delivered to the tumor was 15.2 ± 8.7 cGy/37 MBq (Fig. 9).

VI. THERAPY OF OTHER SOLID TUMORS

Pretargeting protocols have been also applied to the treatment of other solid tumors. In a pilot study, we have treated 15 patients with recurrent ovarian carcinoma after surgery and chemotherapy. The radioimmunotherapy (RIT) was performed according to a three-step pretargeting approach, injecting IP a mixture of biotinylated MoAbs raised against ovarian carcinoma MoV18 and B72.3 (20 + 20 mg) followed by 150 mg streptavidin diluted in 1.5 liters saline by slow infusion. As the third step, ^{90}Y-labeled-biotin (1665 to 1850 MBq) was administered by IV injection. Preliminary results seem to indicate the absence of toxicity

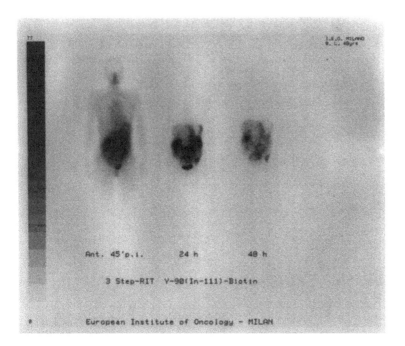

Figure 10 Whole-body images of a patient, with ovarian carcinoma and documented diffused tumor mass in the peritoneal cavity, acquired 45 min, 24 and 48 h after IV injection of ^{90}Y-biotin spiked with ^{111}In. The three-step pretargeting was performed by injecting intraperitoneally biotinylated MoAbs and streptavidin (steps 1 and 2) while the radioactive biotin was administered IV (step 3). The double routes of administration allowed to target high levels of MoAbs and streptavidin onto the tumor by IP injection and to deliver the radioactive biotin through systemic circulation. This approach overcomes the drawbacks of adhesion of radioactivity in the peritoneal cavity typical of a locoregional RIT.

and a good response in the peritoneal cavity but longer follow up is needed before definite conclusions can be made. Figure 10 shows an example of a scintigraphic study, according to this new pretargeting protocol, in a patient affected by ovarian carcinoma after the IV injection of a therapeutic dose of ^{90}Y-biotin spiked with ^{111}In.

We have also treated a patient with oropharyngeal carcinoma in local relapse after surgery, chemotherapy, and radiotherapy. The persistent disease was documented by CT/MRI and three-step ISG (Fig. 11) 10 weeks after the end of chemoradiotherapy. He received a cocktail of biotinylated MoAbs (anti-CEA, B72.3) in order to target the largest number of tumor cells (first step) and 2.59

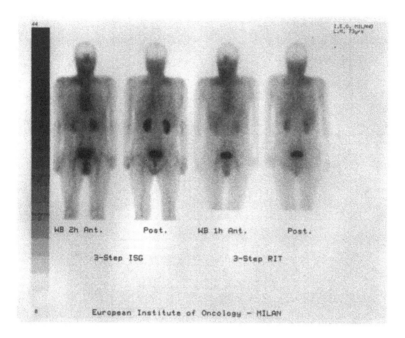

Figure 11 Scintigraphic studies on a patient with oropharyngeal carcinoma. Left: Whole-body scan (anterior and posterior projections) obtained 2 h after a three-step ISG with ^{111}In-biotin demonstrating high uptake at the level of the right laterocervical/submandibular and supraclavicular regions, corresponding well with radiological examinations. Right: Whole-body scan (anterior and posterior projections) acquired 1 h after the injection of the therapeutic dose of ^{90}Y-biotin, spiked with ^{111}In. It confirms the same pattern of uptake obtained in the three-step ISG before therapy.

GBq of ^{90}Y-DOTA-biotin as third step. He has shown an objective benefit, documented by CT/MRI, with a complete response lasting for more than 1 year (Fig. 12). He is still in excellent condition with no evidence of disease. This case appears to be the first example of clinical complete remission after combined modality treatments including ^{90}Y-biotin three-step RIT for head and neck carcinoma (64).

VII. CONCLUSIONS

The potential advantage in cancer therapy of pretargeting protocols, especially the three-step approach, with respect to the use of directly labeled antibodies,

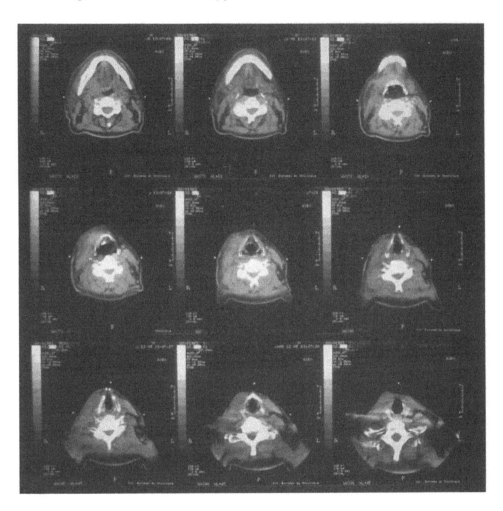

Figure 12   Panel A: CT scan of the neck of the same patient of Figure 11 performed before RIT, showing residual tumor mass in the right submandibular region. Panel B: MRI scan of the neck performed 7 months after RIT (2.59 GBq of ^{90}Y-DOTA-biotin), showing no evidence of tumor.

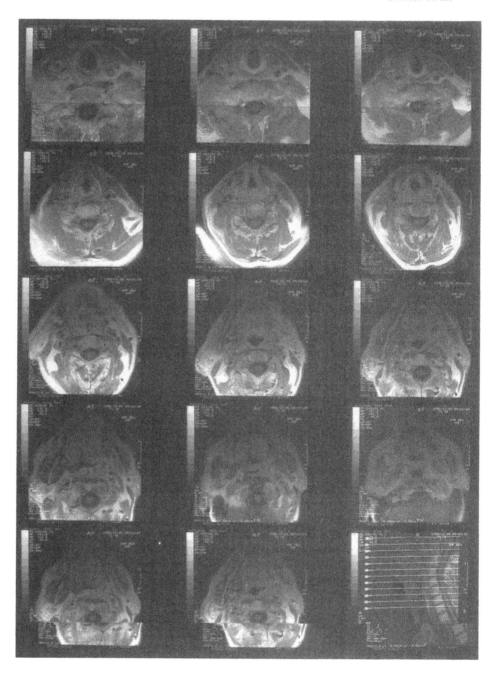

Figure 12 Continued

lies in the lower toxicity observed which has allowed administration of high doses of therapeutic radionuclides, such as Y-90, without bone marrow toxicity. Pilot studies, applied to the treatment of advanced stage tumors, have shown that this approach interferes with the progression of tumors and produces tumor regression in patients no longer responsive to other conventional therapeutic modalities. The potentiality of pretargeting based on the avidin/biotin system may be exploited in the near future to convey a variety of cytotoxic substances, other than radioactivity, onto cancer cells.

In a recent study a three-step antibody/avidin targeting approach was applied to increase the local concentration and the persistence of biotinylated human tumor necrosis factor α (bio-TNF) on a mouse tumor. Moreover, the same study showed that cell-bound TNF was still able to induce cytolytic effects in vitro, as well as decrease the tumorigenicity of a mouse lymphoma in vivo (65).

REFERENCES

1. Wawrzynczak EJ. Systemic immunotoxin therapy of cancer: advances and prospects. Br J Cancer 1991; 64:624.
2. Mach JP, Buchegger F, Forni M. Use of radiolabelled monoclonal anti-CEA antibodies for the detection of human carcinoma by external photoscanning and tomoscintigraphy. Immunol Today 1981; 2:239.
3. Epenetos AA, Britton KE, Mather S. Targeting of iodine-123-labelled tumor associated monoclonal antibodies to ovarian, breast, and gastrointestinal tumors. Lancet 1982; 2:999.
4. Larson SM. Radiolabelled monoclonal anti-tumor antibodies and therapy. J Nucl Med 1985; 26:538.
5. Buraggi GL, Callegaro L, Mariani G, Turrin A, Cascinelli N, Attili A, Bombardieri E, Terno G, Plassio G, Dovis M. Imaging with ^{131}I-labeled monoclonal antibodies to a high-molecular-weight melanoma-associated antigen in patients with melanoma: efficacy of whole immunoglobulin and its F(ab')$_2$ fragments. Cancer Res 1985; 45: 3378.
6. Fazio F, Paganelli G. Antibody-guided scintigraphy: targeting of the "magic bullet." Eur J Nucl Med 1993; 20:1138.
7. Kim JA, Triozzi PL, Martin EW. Radioimmuguided surgery for colorectal cancer. Oncology 1993; 7:55.
8. Leichner PK, Koral KF, Jaszczak RJ, Green AJ, Chen GTY, Roeske JC. An overview of imaging techniques and physical aspects of treatment planning in radioimmunotherapy. Med Physics 1993; 30:569.
9. Chetanneau A, Barbet J, Peltier P, Le Doussal JM, Gruaz-Guyon A, Bernard AM, Resche I, Rouvier E, Bourguet P, Delaage M. Pretargetted imaging of colorectal cancer recurrences using an In-111-labelled bivalent hapten and a biospecific antibody conjugate. Nucl Med Commun 1994; 15:972.
10. Schlom J. Basic principles and application of monoclonal antibodies in the manage

ment of carcinomas: the Richard and Hinda Rosenthal Foundation Award Lecture. Cancer Res 1986; 46:3225.

11. Hirai H. Use of tumor receptors for diagnostic imaging. Acta Radiol 1990; 374:57.

12. Kuhn JA, Corbisiero RM, Buras RR, Carroll RG, Wagman LD, Wilson LA, Yamauchi D, Smith MM, Kondo R, Beatty D. Intraoperative gamma detection probe with presurgical antibody imaging in colon cancer. Arch Surg 1991; 126:1398.

13. Strand SE, Zanzonico P, Johnson TK. Pharmacokinetic modeling. Med Physics 1993; 20:515.

14. Hazra DK, Britton KE, Lahiri VL, Gupta AK, Khanna P, Saran S. Immunotechnological trend in radioimmuno-targeting: from 'magic bullet' to 'smart bomb.' Nucl Med Commun 1995; 16:66.

15. Mann BD, Cohen MB, Saxton RE, Morton DL, Benedict WF, Korn EL, Spolter L, Graham LS, Chang CC, Burk MW. Imaging of human tumor xenografts in nude mice with radiolabeled monoclonal antibodies. Limitations of specificity due to non-specific uptake of antibody. Cancer 1984; 54:1318.

16. Johnson DA, Baker AL, Laguzza BC, Fix DV, Gutowski MC. Antitumor activity of L/1C2-4-desacetylvinblastine-3-carboxhydrazide immunoconjugate in xenografts. Cancer Res 1990; 50:1790.

17. Jain RK. Haemadynamic and transport barriers to the treatment of solid tumors. Int J Radiat Biol 1991; 60:85.

18. Goodwin DA, Meares CF, McCall MJ, McTigue M, Chaovapong W. Targeted immunoscintigraphy of murine tumors with indium-111-labeled bifunctional haptens. J Nucl Med 1988; 29:226.

19. Paganelli G, Riva P, Deleide G, Clivio A, Chiolerio F, Scasselati GA, Malcovati M, Siccardi AG. In vivo labelling of biotinylated monoclonal antibodies by radioactive avidin: a strategy to increase tumor radiolocalization. Int J Cancer 1988; 2:121.

20. LeDoussal JM, Martin M, Gautherot E, Delaage M, Barbet J. In vitro and in vivo targeting of radiolabeled monovalent and divalent haptens with dual specificity monoclonal antibody conjugates: enhanced divalent hapten affinity for cell-bound antibody conjugate. J Nucl Med 1989; 30:1358.

21. Paganelli G, Malcovati M, Fazio F. Monoclonal antibody pretargetting techniques for tumour localization: the avidin-biotin system. Nucl Med Commun 1991; 12:211.

22. Bos ES, Kuijpers WHA, Meesters-Winters M, Pham DT, de Haan AS, van Doornmalen AM, Kaspersen FM, van Boeckel CAA, Gougeoun-Bertrand F. In vitro evaluation of DNA-DNA hybridization as a two step approach in radioimmunotherapy of cancer. Cancer Res 1994; 54:3479.

23. Sung C, van Osdol WW. Pharmacokinetic comparison of direct antibody targeting with pretargeting protocols based on streptavidin-biotin binding. J Nucl Med 1995; 36:867.

24. Magnani P, Paganelli G, Modorati G, Zito F, Songini C, Sudati F, Koch P, Maecke HR, Brancato R, Siccardi AG, Fazio F. Quantitative comparison of direct antibody labeling and tumor pretargeting in uveal melanoma. J Nucl Med 1996; 37:967.

25. Paganelli G, Magnani P, Zito F, Villa E, Sudati F, Lopalco L, Rossetti C, Malcovati M, Chiolerio F, Seccamani E, Siccardi AG, Fazio F. Three-step monoclonal antibody tumor targeting in carcinoembryonic antigen-positive patients. Cancer Res 1991; 51: 5960.

26. LeDoussal JM, Barbet J, Delaage M. Bispecific-antibody-mediated targeting of radiolabeled bivalent haptens: theoretical, experimental and clinical results. Int J Cancer 1992; 7:58.
27. Kobayashi H, Sakahara H, Hosono M, Yao Z-S, Toyama S, Endo K, Konishi J. Improved clearance of radiolabeled biotinylated monoclonal antibody following the infusion of avidin as a "chase" without decreased accumulation in the target tumor. J Nucl Med 1994; 35:1677.
28. Paganelli G, Magnani P, Siccardi AG, Fazio F. In: Goldenberg DM, ed. Cancer Therapy with Radiolabeled Antibodies. Boca Raton, FL: CRC Press, 1995:239.
29. Rosebrough SF. Pharmacokinetics and biodistribution of radiolabeled avidin, streptavidin and biotin. Nucl Med Biol 1993; 20:663.
30. Brennan M, Davison PF, Paulus H. Preparation of bispecif antibodies by chemical recombination of monoclonal immunoglobulin G1 fragments. Science 1985; 229:81.
31. Suresh MR, Cuello AC, Milstein C. Bispecific monoclonal antibodies from hybrid hybridomas. Methods Enzymol 1986; 121:210.
32. Wickstrom E. Oligodeoxynucleotide stability in subcellular extracts and culture media. J Biochem Biophys Methods 1986; 13:97.
33. Stella M, DeNardi P, Paganelli G, Magnani P, Mangili F, Sassi I, Baratti D, Gini P, Zito F, Cristallo M. Avidin-biotin system in radioimmunoguided surgery for colorectal cancer. Dis Colon Rectum 1994; 37:335.
34. Wilchek M, Bayer EA. The avidin biotin complex in bioanalytical applications. Anal Biochem 1988; 171:1.
35. Wilchek M, Bayer EA. The avidin biotin complex in immunology. Immunol Today 1984; 5:39.
36. Green NM. Avidin-1. The use of [^{14}C] biotin for kinetic studies and for assay. Biochem J 1963; 89:585.
37. Green NM. Avidin. Adv Prot Chem 1975; 29:85.
38. Hamilton TC, Ozols RF, Longo DL. Biologic therapy for the treatment of malignant common epithelial tumors of the ovary. Cancer 1994; 60:2054.
39. Oehr P, Westermann J, Biersack HJ. Streptavidin and biotin as potential tumor imaging agents. J Nucl Med 1988; 29:728.
40. Hnatowich DJ. Recent developments in the radiolabeling of antibodies with iodine, indium, and technetium. Semin Nucl Med 1990; 20(1):80.
41. Hnatowich DJ, Virzi F, Rusckowski M. Investigations of avidin and biotin for imaging applications. J Nucl Med 1987; 28:1294.
42. Wessels BW, Rogus RD. Radionuclide selection and model absorbed dose calculations for radiolabeled tumor associated antibodies. Med Phys 1984; 11(5):638.
43. Chinol M, Hnatowich DJ. Generator-produced yttrium-90 for radioimmunotherapy. J Nucl Med 1987; 28:1465.
44. Montravadi VP, Spigos DG, Tan WS, Felix EL. Intraarterial yttrium-90 in the treatment of hepatic malignancy. Radiology 1982; 142:783.
45. Stewart JSW, Hird V, Snook D, Dhokia B, Sivolapenko G, Hooker G, Taylor-Papadimitriou J, Rowlinson G, Sullivan M, Lambert HE, Coulter C, Mason WP, Soutter WP, Epenetos AA. Intraperitoneal yttrium-90 labelled monoclonal antibody in ovarian cancer. J Clin Oncol 1990; 8(12):1941.

46. Riesen A, Zehnder M, Kaden TA. Synthesis, properties, and structures of mononuclear complexes with 12- and 14-membered tetraazamacrocycle-N,N′,N″,N‴-tetraacetic acids. Helv Chim Acta 1986; 69:2067.

47. Moi MK, Meares CF. The peptide way to macrocyclic bifunctional chelating agents: synthesis of 2-(p-nitrobenzyl)-1,4,7,10-tetraazacyclododecane-N,N′,N″,N‴-tetraacetic acid and study of its yttrium (III) complex. J Am Chem Soc 1988; 110: 6266.

48. Cox JPL, Craig AS, Helps IM. Synthesis of C- and N functionalised derivatives of 1,4,7-triazacyclonon-ane-1,4,7-triyltriacetic acid (NOTA), 1,4,7,10-tetra-azacyclo-dodecane-1,4,7,10-tetrayltetra-acetic acid (DOTA), and diethylenetriaminepenta-acetic acid (DTPA): bifunctional complexing agents for the derivatisation of antibodies. J Chem Soc Perkin Trans 1990; 1:2567.

49. Paganelli G, Chinol M, Grana C, DeCicco C, Cremonesi M, Meares C, Franceschini R, Tarditi L, Siccardi AG. Optimization of the three-step pretargeting approach for diagnosis and therapy in cancer patients. J Nucl Med 1995; 36(suppl 5):225P.

50. Chinol M, Paganelli G, Sudati F, Meares C, Fazio F. Biodistribution in tumour-bearing mice of two ^{90}Y-labelled biotins using three-step tumour targeting. Nucl Med Commun 1997; 18:176.

51. Su F-M, Gustavson LM, Axworthy DB, Lyen LJ, Theodore LJ, Fritzberg AR, Reno JM. Characterization of a new Y-90 labeled DOTA-biotin for pretargeting. J Nucl Med 1995; 36(suppl 5):154P.

52. Paganelli G, Grana C, Chinol M, Cremonesi M, DeCicco C, DeBraud F, Robertson C, Zurrida S, Casadio C, Zoboli S, Siccardi AG, Veronesi V. Antibody guided three-step therapy for high grade glioma with yttrium-90 biotin. Eur J Nucl Med 1999; 26:348.

53. Axworthy DB, Fritzberg AR, Hylarides MD, Mallett RW, Theodore LJ, Gustavson LM, Su FM, Beaumier PL, Reno JM. Preclinical evaluation of an anti-tumor monoclonal antibody/streptavidin conjugate for pretargeted ^{90}Y radioimmunotherapy in a mouse xenograft model. J Immunother 1995; 16:138.

54. Beaumier PL, Axworthy DB, Fritzberg AR, Hylarides MD, Mallett RW, Theodore LJ, Gustavson LM, Su FM, Reno JM. The pharmacology of pretargeting components: optimizing therapeutic targeting. Q J Nucl Med 1995; 39:20.

55. Kalofonos HP, Rusckowski M, Siebecker DA, Sivolapenko GB, Snook D, Lavender JP, Epenetos AA, Hnatowich DJ. Imaging of tumor in patients with indium-111-labeled biotin and streptavidin-conjugated antibodies: preliminary communication. J Nucl Med 1990; 31:1791.

56. Epenetos AA, Munro AJ, Stewart JSW, Rampling R, Lambert HE, McKenzie CG, Soutter WP, Rahemtulla A, Hooker G, Sivolapenko G, Snook D, Courtenay-Luck N, Dhokia B, Krausz T, Taylor-Papadimitriou J, Durbin H, Bodmer WF. Antibody-guided irradiation of advanced ovarian cancer with intraperitoneally administered radiolabelled monoclonal antibodies. J Clin Oncol 1987; 5:1890.

57. Paganelli G, Belloni C, Magnani P, Zito F, Pasini A, Sassi I, Meroni M, Mariani M, Vignali M, Siccardi AG, Fazio F. Two-step tumour targetting in ovarian cancer patients using biotinylated monoclonal antibodies and radioactive streptavidin. Eur J Nucl Med 1992; 19:322.

58. Natali PG, Nicotra MR, Bigotti A, Borri C, Castellani P, Risso AM, Zardi L. Com-

parative analysis of the expression of the extracellular-matrix protein tenascin in normal and human fetal, adult and tumor tissues. Int J Cancer 1991; 47:811.

59. Black PM. Brain tumors. N Engl J Med 1991; 324:1555.
60. Culver KW, Ram Z, Wallbridge S, Ishii H, Oldfield EH, Blaese RM. In vivo gene transfer with retroviral vector-producer cells for treatment of experimental brain tumors. Science 1992; 256:1550.
61. Zalutsky MR, Moseley RP, Coakham HB, Coleman RE, Bigner DD. Pharmacokinetics and tumour localisation of ^{131}I-labeled anti-tenescin monoclonal antibody 81C6 in patients with gliomas and other intracranial malignancies. Cancer Res 1989; 49: 2807.
62. Paganelli G, Chinol M, Maggiolo M, Sidoli A, Corti A, Baroni S, Siccardi AG. The three-step pretargeting approach reduces the human anti-mouse antibody response in patients submitted to radioimmunoscintigraphy and radioimmunotherapy. Eur J Nucl Med 1997; 24:350.
63. Weber DA, Eckerman KF, Dillman LT, Ryman JC. Radionuclide Data and Decay Schemes. MIRD Pamphlet. New York: Society of Nuclear Medicine, 1989:72.
64. Paganelli G, Orecchia R, Jereczek-Fossa B, Grana C, Cremonesi M, De Braud F, Tradati N, Chinol M. Combined treatment of advanced oropharyngeal cancer with external radiotherapy and three-step radioimmunotherapy. Eur J Nucl Med 1998; 25:1336.
65. Moro M, Pelagi M, Fulci G, Paganelli G, Dellabona P, Casorati G, Siccardi AG, Corti A. Tumor cell targeting with antibody-avidin complexes and biotinylated tumor necrosis factor α^1. Cancer Res 1997; 57:1922.

8

Evolution of a Pretarget Radioimmunotherapeutic Regimen

Louis J. Theodore, Alan R. Fritzberg, Jody E. Schultz, and Donald B. Axworthy
NeoRx Corporation, Seattle, Washington

I. INTRODUCTION

The potential of using antibodies directed to tumor-associated antigens has been the basis of a great deal of work for the selective delivery of radiation to tumors, giving rise to the field of radioimmunotherapy (RIT). Despite its theoretical appeal, this approach has been only modestly successful to date for the treatment of carcinomas including lung, colon, breast, prostate, and pancreatic cancers. Conventional RIT, a modality involving direct covalent coupling of a radionuclide or radiometal chelate to immunoglobulins, has unfortunately exhibited suboptimal therapeutic efficacy due to inadequate delivery of radiation to tumors.

Major limitations of this approach have been a result of a mismatch among the properties of the radioactive therapeutic agent, the physical constraints associated with tumor targeting, and the pharmacokinetic properties of antibody proteins. Antibodies accrete slowly at tumors and are eliminated slowly from the circulation (1). Use of radiolabeled antibodies, therefore, results in prolonged exposure of radiosensitive tissues, particularly marrow, due to the extended time within the circulation. Additionally, the extended time required for tumor localization of the antibody results in loss of tumoricidal potency of the radionuclide due to ongoing isotopic decay. As a result, the therapeutic utility of conventional RIT has been generally limited by unacceptable bone marrow toxicity (2). Bone marrow support can be given to bypass that toxicity, but adds significantly to complexity and cost of the treatment. Press et al. (3) have provided marrow support for RIT of lymphoma and reached doses which resulted in more durable responses. Amelioration of marrow toxicity by this method subsequently served to determine the lung as a second organ of toxicity, the result of circulating antibody radionuclide, and thereby define an extramedullary maximum tolerated dose (MTD).

Pretargeted radioimmunotherapy regimens using a number of protocols or methodologies have been proposed as an alternative approach designed to address the limitations associated with conventional RIT (4–7). In these systems, antibodies, which have been modified or derivatized to carry a high-affinity secondary receptor, are used in an initial localization step. Following tumor localization and either passive or facilitated clearance of the majority of residual antibody from the vascular space and normal tissues, radiation is delivered to the tumor in a final step by administration of a cytotoxic radionuclide covalently attached or chelated to a second binding component or ligand. Ideally, unlike whole antibodies, the radiotherapeutic second component should have biodistribution and pharmacokinetic characteristics consistent with rapid and efficient tumor localization resulting in minimal toxicity to red marrow and normal organs.

II. BIOTIN/STREPTAVIDIN-BASED PRETARGETING

Over the years, a number of pretargeting approaches have been reported to maximize radioisotope delivery to tumor based on the biotin/avidin-type binding interaction (4,5,7,8). The pretarget system and reagents that we have developed and employed also make use of this system, and specifically make use of biotin- and streptavidin-binding interactions as the high-affinity secondary receptor system delivered to the tumor by the antibody-targeting construct. A feature of the avidin/streptavidin system is the tetrameric valency of biotin binding. Thus, the binding of four biotins for each streptavidin localized results in the potential for increasing tumor uptake by, in effect, amplifying the antigen/cell number.

The pretargeting system we have developed is made up of three components: a primary tumor-targeting component, a clearing-agent component, and an effector component. These components will be discussed in terms of their design, preparation, and in vivo properties.

A. First-Generation Pretargeting Reagents

The majority of our preclinical and clinical studies utilized first-generation reagents. These agents consisted of an antibody chemically conjugated to streptavidin, a clearing agent produced through derivatization of human serum albumin (HSA), and a radionuclide delivered as a DOTA chelate.

1. Antibody/Streptavidin Chemical Conjugates

Our first tumor-targeting chemical conjugate consisted of the antibody NR-LU-10 chemically coupled to streptavidin (SA) through the use of a heterobifunctional linker. NR-LU-10 is a murine antibody that recognizes a 40-kD glycoprotein antigen expressed on several epithelial tumors such as carcinomas of lung, colon, breast, prostate, and ovary. It is an antibody that has been extensively evaluated for conventional radioimmunotherapy using [186]Re in animal models (9) and patients (10). Succinimidyl 4-(N-maleimido-methyl)cyclohexane-1-carboxylate (SMCC) was used as the coupling agent to effect antibody coupling to streptavidin to form the NR-LU-10/SA chemical conjugate. The product conjugate was a heterogenous mixture consisting of about 80% SA:antibody in a 1:1 ratio and the remainder primarily in a 2:1 ratio (11).

The antibody/SA conjugate is administered in tumor antigen saturating doses, which results in homogeneous targeting of the tumor (12). In order to overcome slow tumor penetration kinetics, the conjugate is allowed to accumulate over a period of 24 to 48 hours (13). The role of the targeting vehicle is thus not to immediately render therapy itself, but rather to target the SA receptor to the tumor.

As assessed by dual-label studies in normal Balb/C and nude mice bearing human xenograft tumors, the pharmacokinetic properties of the NR-LU-10/SA conjugate paralleled that of the parent antibody. As shown in Figures 1 and 2, blood disappearance, tumor uptake and retention, and comparative organ and tumor biodistribution of the conjugate were essentially the same as with antibody

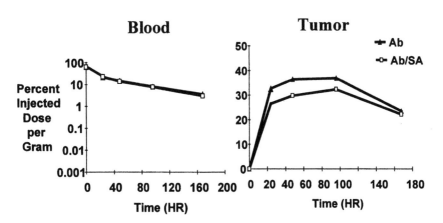

Figure 1 Comparative blood disappearance and tumor uptake and retention for ^{131}I-NR-LU-10 and ^{125}I-NR-LU-10/SA. *Note*: Blood curves for antibody and conjugate superimpose.

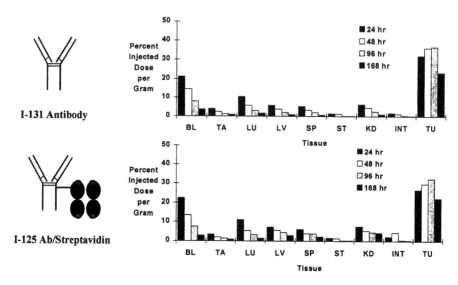

Figure 2 Comparative organ biodistribution study is shown at 24 hours postinjection of ^{131}I-NR-LU-10 and ^{125}I-NR-LU-10/SA in a dual-label, coinject study.

alone. This is remarkable for a tetrameric 66-kD SA bacterial protein conjugated to an antibody of 150 kD.

2.   Clearing Agent

Following localization of the antibody/SA component at the tumor site, a considerable mass of residual conjugate remains in the serum compartment. Administration of the radiotherapeutic effector at this point would result in substantial binding to the long-circulating antibody/SA conjugate, which would greatly reduce the advantage of pretargeting. To avoid this result, a clearing agent is given to remove the circulating conjugate and allow the effector to have relatively unimpeded access to the prelocalized antibody/SA at the tumor.

Initially proposed clearing agents were based on utilization of polyvalent macromolecular constructs which, by their nature and method of use, largely remained confined to the serum compartment (14). Agents of this type were designed to form crosslinks with antibody conjugate remaining in circulation. The resulting macromolecular aggregates formed were then removed by the liver through uptake by the reticuloendothelial system where the aggregates would subsequently be degraded.

Agents we have developed to facilitate clearance of the primary targeting component are based on an alternative mechanistic approach. This system proceeds via a binding protein or receptor on the surface of hepatocytes. This receptor, commonly referred to as the Ashwell receptor, is of a class II receptor type which appears to function solely to internalize bound ligands from extracellular fluids for the purpose of degradation (15). Following internalization, the receptor is recycled back to the cell surface. Interaction of the Ashwell receptor with most endogenous ligands is of high affinity with dissociation constants as low as the subnanomolar range (16). The receptor is specific for ligands containing terminal clustered galactosyl or N-galactosaminyl residues with three or more residues in close spatial proximity being requisite for maximal binding efficiency. Thus, ligands containing a sufficient plurality of galactosyl or N-galactosaminyl residues capable of adopting a complementary orientation may be expected to form high-affinity interactions with the triplex receptor.

The clearing agents synthesized for binding conjugate and clearing through the Ashwell receptor have been bispecific constructs which are derivatized with at least one biotin residue for rapid, noncovalent, high-affinity complexation with antibody SA conjugate and, secondly, are derivatized to a high level of galactosyl or N-acetyl galactosaminyl residues which allow for high-affinity interaction of any resultant complex that comes into contact with the hepatic Ashwell receptors.

HSA-Based Clearing Agent. The first-generation clearing agent utilizing the Ashwell receptor clearance mechanism was based on HSA, which served as a multireactive scaffold for derivatization with a low level of biotin residues (two on average) and a high loading of galactose residues (30 to 35). HSA was selected as the scaffold for preparation of the bispecific agent for a number of reasons. Firstly, literature precedent (17) indicated that serum albumins (BSA and HSA) could be effectively derivatized with galactosyl residues in a manner that rendered the resultant construct effective for binding to the hepatic lectin receptors with subsequent internalization. Secondly, such a clearing construct should have little difficulty in accessing and complexing with serum-associated conjugate while as a relatively large construct (MW 70 kD) with a relatively short serum half-life, it would have limited ability to diffuse out of the vascular compartment and access specifically tumor-targeted, extravascular conjugate. These properties were expected to minimally compromise the ability of subsequently administered radiotherapeutic biotin ligand to bind to tumor-associated conjugate.

Preclinical evaluation of the HSA-based clearing agent indicated that it was effective for removal of antibody/SA conjugate from circulation. Following IV administration of the Ab/SA chemical conjugate and subsequent administration of HSA clearing agent, 90% to 95% of residual circulating conjugate in either nude or Balb-C mouse animal models was removed (11). In nude mice bearing xenograft tumors, this level of clearance resulted in a sufficiently low background of circulating conjugate that an approximately 10-fold increase in tumor to blood ratios, versus conventional RIT, was achieved.

Facilitated clearance of conjugate using an optimized dose ratio of HSA-based clearing agent resulted in a reduction of serum conjugate concentration of >90% (Fig. 3) within 2 hours of administration. Apparent in the clearance curve is a small rebound of conjugate from the extravascular compartment back into the blood. The degree of rebound could be reduced with increased amounts of clearing agent. However, while immunohistochemical analysis showed no decrease of biotin-binding capacity in tumors pretargeted with the NR-LU-10/SA before or after administration of clearing agent at the optimized dose, a significant reduction of biotin-binding capacity was observed with administration of excess HSA-based clearing agent. This outcome was interpreted as being the result of hepatic uptake and catabolic degradation of the HSA clearing agent with resultant free biotin or low-molecular-weight biotin adducts being released back into circulation where they could then be carried to and bind tumor associated conjugate.

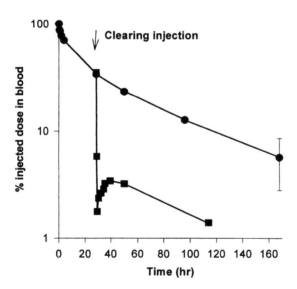

Figure 3 Effect of HSA clearing agent on blood disappearance in vivo. Balb/c mice (n = 3/group) were injected at t = 0 with 400 μg ^{125}I-NR-LU-10/SA conjugate. Blood samples (10 μL, n = 2/timepoint) were serially removed from the retro-orbital plexus and assayed for radioactivity. At 28.5 hours, mice were injected with either saline (●) or 200 μg of clearing agent (■). For the clearing-agent mice, blood was sampled at 28.5 (preinjection), 29, 29.5, 30.5, 32.5, 34.5, 35.5, 39.5, 50, and 114 hours. Control animals were sampled at 0.17, 0.5, 1.0, 2.0, 4.0, 28.5, 50.0, 72.0, 96.0, and 168 hours. Data are presented as the mean % ID in total blood ± SD of each group.

3. Radioactive Effector

A large number of therapeutic radionuclides are available for potential application. Yttrium-90 (^{90}Y) was selected for initial development. It is viewed as a superior choice for treatment of solid-tumor carcinomas due to its pure, high-energy β emission (2.27 MeV max beta) and commercial availability in high specific activity and purity. The agent used to carry the radionuclide to prelocalized tumor-bound streptavidin is illustrated in Figure 4. It is designated DOTA-biotin and is a bifunctional chelating agent which comprises an aminobenzyl-DOTA macrocycle, an N-methyl glycyl linker, and a biotinamide moiety (18). The DOTA macrocycle provides stable chelation of metals in the +3 oxidation state, the N-methyl glycyl linker was designed to provide maximal stability to enzymatic cleavage of the biotin amide bond by biotinidase, and the biotinamide moiety provides the very high affinity binding to SA. The hydrophilic properties of the radiometal-DOTA-linker moiety result in high specificity for renal excretion without significant organ retention (11).

The biodistribution properties of ^{90}Y chelated to DOTA-biotin is shown in Figure 5. The ligand chelate diffuse rapidly from the serum compartment throughout the total extracellular fluids with no localization in organs. Rapid renal excretion is observed ($t_{1/2}$ <15 min) in normal mice with no normal organ exhibiting >2% retention for all radiometals examined. These in vivo properties achieve nearly ideal expectations.

4. Preclinical Efficacy Data

The objectives of pretargeting include maintaining high absolute tumor uptake, rapid delivery of radiation to tumor, and sparing of bone marrow by rapid disappearance of radioactivity from the circulation and whole body. Preclinical biodistribution studies demonstrating these properties were initially done in a nude

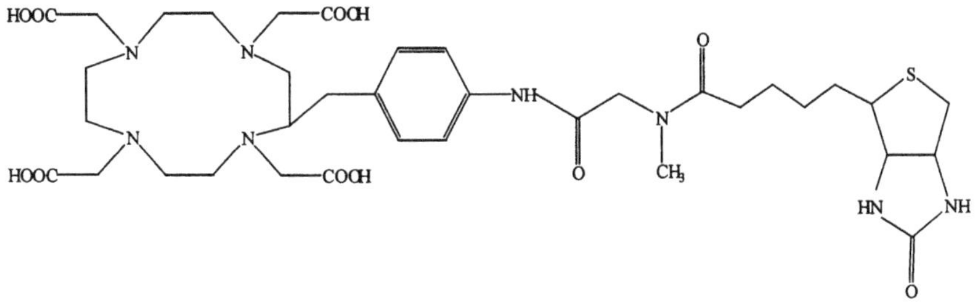

Figure 4 Structural formula of DOTA-biotin.

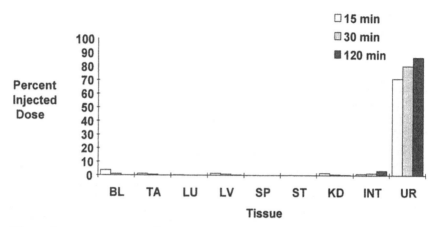

Figure 5 Biodistribution of ^{90}Y-DOTA-biotin chelate in normal mice, 15, 30, and 120 min postinjection. Data highlight rapid renal excretion with minimal normal organ retention.

mouse tumor xenograft model using the colon tumor cell line SW-1222. Figure 6 illustrates concentration of ^{90}Y-DOTA-biotin in tumor and in blood over time after initial pretargeting with NR-LU-10/SA at time zero, followed 26 hours later with a clearing agent, then followed 2 hours later with the ^{90}Y-DOTA-biotin. Comparison of the tumor-to-blood values of the pretargeted ^{90}Y to that for ^{125}I delivered by conventional ^{125}I-radiolabeled antibody shows an approximately 20-fold increase in specificity of radiation delivery and retention using the pretargeting approach. Importantly, absolute uptake (% ID/g) of radioactivity was maintained while gaining the advantages of rapid targeting and excretion of non-targeted radioactivity.

Preclinical therapy studies using a single dose of ^{90}Y has been shown to be effective in treating relatively large (200 mg) established tumors without toxicity. Figure 7 illustrates results from treatment of the small-cell lung cancer xenograft SHT-1 in which complete regressions occurred at doses as low as 200 μCi in the pretargeting format (11). A dose response relationship was evident in that a higher percentage of long-term cures (no tumor regrowth at >180 days) were observed at increased dose levels with 2/10 animals cured at doses of 200 μCi, 7/10 cured at 400 μCi, and 10/10 animals cured at 600 μCi. Similar efficacy using the pretarget approach was seen in other solid-tumor xenograft models including the MDA-MB-484 breast and SW-1222 colon tumor model systems (11). Treatment of MDA-MB-484 breast tumors with 800 μCi of pretargeted ^{90}Y-DOTA-biotin resulted in 8/10 cures. Analogously, treatment of SW-1222 colon tumors with 800 μCi of pretargeted ^{90}Y-DOTA-biotin resulted in 10/10 cures.

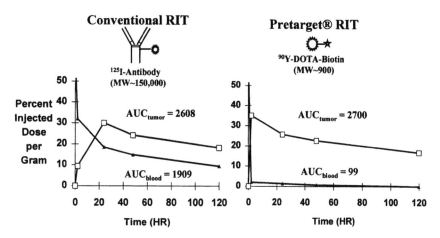

Figure 6 Concentration of ^{90}Y-DOTA-biotin in tumor and blood of SW-1222 tumor nude mice as final component of pretargeting protocol along with tumor and blood concentrations of ^{125}I-NR-LU-10 in SW-1222 tumor-bearing nude mice delivered in the conventional sense. Rapid tumor uptake and rapid disappearance from blood are notable for pretargeted ^{90}Y-DOTA-biotin.

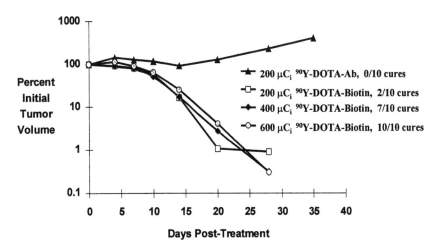

Figure 7 Radiotherapy of SHT-1 xenografts comparing conventional RIT with pretarget approach. Using conventional RIT, the MTD dose of 200 µCi of ^{90}Y only effected a delay in tumor growth. Pretargeting 200 µCi of ^{90}Y resulted in complete regressions and 2/10 cures. Higher doses resulted in greater cure rate, with 100% cure rate observed at 600 µCi.

B. Second-Generation Pretargeting Reagents

While the DOTA-biotin ligand has proven to be a stalwart of the pretarget regimen, refinements to the clearing agent and antibody/SA conjugate components improved the product's characteristics.

1. Synthetic Clearing Agent

A second-generation agent, designed to improve upon the HSA-based agent, is shown in Figure 8. This completely synthetic clearing agent, designated biotin-LC-NM-(Gal-NAc)$_{16}$, is also a bifunctional moiety consisting of biotin, joined through a modified aminocaproyl spacer, to the core of a four-generation dendrimeric backbone formed using repetitive bifunctional units (19). The outer dendrimeric shell is functionalized with 16 modified N-acetyl-galactosamine residues through aminopentyl linkages. The agent is administered in dose excess to antibody/SA conjugate. It has a relatively high volume of distribution, allowing it to access and bind to both vascular and extravascular conjugate. Vascular conjugate complexed with this agent is rapidly cleared. Through competitive in vitro binding assays, it was determined that while the affinity of this clearing agent for streptavidin is quite high, it is nonetheless significantly lower than that of natural biotin or of the subsequently administered radionuclide biotin-chelate ligand. Thus, although the clearing agent may also bind to significant amounts of extravascular conjugate under conditions of high doses, and thus in excess of tumor-associated conjugate, it does not compromise binding of subsequently administered biotin-chelate ligand. Numerous studies have been performed documenting that the ligand can effectively and completely compete off the clearing agent under in vivo conditions and time frames.

The significance of being able to utilize excess clearing agent is illustrated in the conjugate clearance curve illustrated in Figure 9. Use of stoichiometric ratios of clearing agent to conjugate in excess of what may be implemented with the HSA-based agent largely results in elimination of the rebound phenomenon associated with the HSA-based agent. Conjugate clearance is >95%, and binding

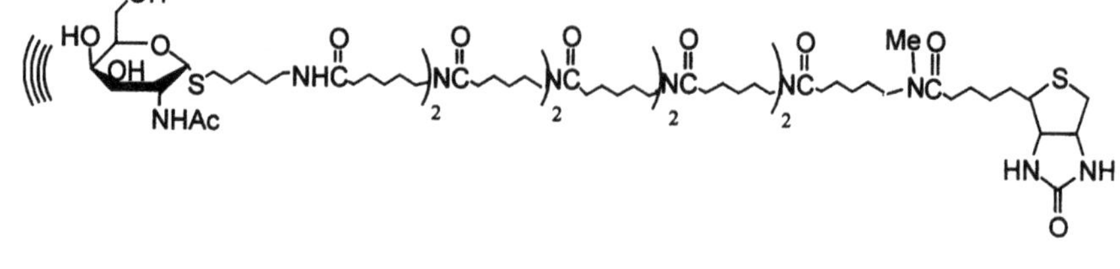

Figure 8 Structural formula of designated biotin-LC-NM-(Gal-NAc)$_{16}$.

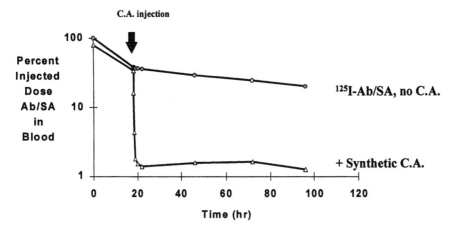

Figure 9 Effect of synthetic clearing agent on serum concentration of NR-LU-10/SA. Streptavidin conjugate is rapidly removed from serum compartment with minimal associated rebound.

capacity of tumor-associated conjugate to DOTA-biotin ligand is not compromised.

2. Antibody scFv-Streptavidin Fusion (scFv$_4$/SA) Proteins

As an alternative to the use of antibody/streptavidin chemical conjugates as the first component within our pretargeting system, we have developed fusion proteins consisting of antibody Fv fragments and genomic streptavidin (SA). The initial rationale for developing a fusion protein included providing a well-defined, homogeneous composition, a simplified manufacturing process, and a significantly lower cost in comparison to the chemical conjugate.

NR-LU-10 fusion protein (scFv$_4$/SA) was expressed from a genetic fusion of the single chain Fv of humanized NR-LU-10 fused to the genomic streptavidin of *Streptomyces avidinii*. The scFv$_4$/SA gene was fused in-frame with the streptavidin leader sequence and placed under control of the IPTG-inducible lac promoter. The mature scFv$_4$/SA fusion protein was produced in the periplasmic space of *E. coli* and formed a soluble tetramer of 172 kD (Fig. 10).

3. Pretargeting Using Antibody scFv$_4$-Streptavidin Fusion (scFv$_4$/SA) Protein Constructs

ELISA-based assessment of the NR-LU-10 fusion protein (scFv$_4$/SA) indicated that it bound to antigen approximately twice as effectively as the corresponding

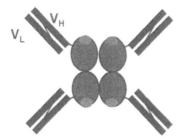

Figure 10   Humanized NR-LU-10 scFv₄/SA fusion protein.

antibody/SA chemical conjugate. The serum half-life of the fusion protein was approximately 40% that of the chemical conjugate in mice, and injection of synthetic clearing agent resulted in rapid clearance of the fusion protein (Fig. 11). Assessment of tumor-targeting and biodistribution properties of scFv₄/SA in nude mice bearing SW-1222 human colon carcinoma xenografts utilizing the full pretarget protocol, i.e., clearance with the synthetic clearing construct followed by injection of ^{111}In-DOTA-biotin, resulted in ^{111}In-DOTA-biotin biodistribution data consistent with that using chemical conjugate, as shown in Figure 12. However, the more rapid inherent disappearance of the fusion protein from blood and

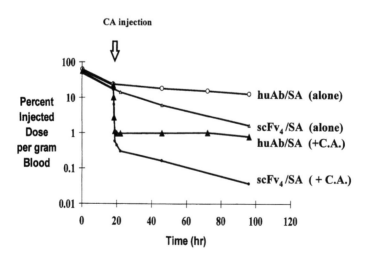

Figure 11   Natural clearance of the NR-LU-10 fusion protein and NR-LU-10 Ab/SA chemical conjugate and clearance facilitated with synthetic clearing agent.

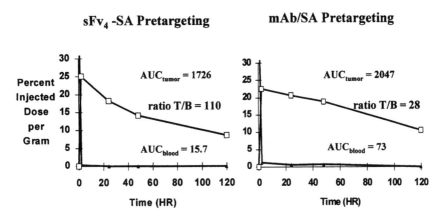

Figure 12 Comparative biodistribution of fusion protein and NR-LU-10/SA.

nonxenograft soft tissues, compared to that of the chemical conjugate, conferred a roughly threefold improvement in tumor-to-blood ratios of the ^{111}In-DOTA-biotin, reaching a value of approximately 100:1 at 2 hours after injection of the ^{111}In-DOTA-biotin.

Therapy studies using the fusion protein were performed in the nude mouse xenograft model using either the small-cell lung cancer cell line SHT-1, or the colon cancer cell line SW-1222. Animals were treated with 800 μCi ^{90}Y-DOTA-biotin and responses compared favorably to those carried out using the NR-LU-10/SA chemical conjugate. The data, along with comparative conventional therapy data for treatment in the SHT-1 xenograft model with nonpretargeted ^{90}Y-DOTA-biotin (albeit at a lower dose due to toxicity), are shown in Figure 13. All fusion-protein-treated animals exhibited dramatic tumor regressions with 9 of 10 animals all tolerating the treatment well and all going on to have complete, durable tumor regressions (>120 days without recurrence). Therapy studies with SW-1222 xenografts also showed dramatic tumor regressions with all mice (N = 10) tolerating the treatment well and 8/10 going on to have complete regressions, which is comparable to the analogous therapy study conducted using the chemical conjugate.

Production via fermentation in *E. coli* should result in significantly lower costs of production that are comparable to the costs for production of streptavidin alone. In addition, production of fusion proteins should result in a consistent, uniform formulation. For these reasons, fusion constructs of this type appear in general to be superior to antibody/SA chemical conjugates in our pretargeting format from clinical, commercial, and regulatory perspectives.

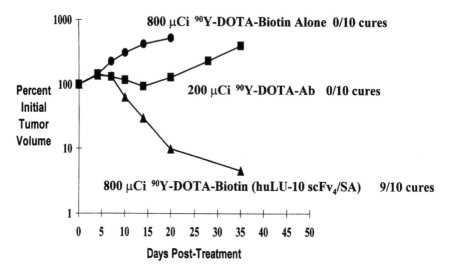

Figure 13   Human xenograft therapy of NR-LU-10 fusion protein in nude mice (SHT-1).

III. CLINICAL EVALUATION OF PRETARGET RIT AGAINST CARCINOMAS

A number of clinical studies have been conducted to evaluate many of the described components for use in pretarget protocols to treat carcinomas and lymphomas (20–23).

Phase I dose optimization and subsequent dose escalation trials have been performed for evaluation of the pretarget system incorporating NR-LU-10/SA chemical conjugate, HSA-based clearing agent, and DOTA-biotin ligand in the treatment of carcinomas. A subsequent Phase II trial using these reagents in the treatment of metastatic colon cancer has been reported (24).

We conducted a second, not yet reported, Phase I dose optimization study in which the HSA-based clearing agent was substituted with the synthetic clearing agent. The optimized protocol served as the basis for a Phase I/II study for the treatment of non-Hodgkin's lymphoma using a C2B8/SA chemical conjugate to pretarget to the CD-20 antigen expressed on mature B lymphocytes (25).

A. Phase I Optimization and Dose Escalation Studies Using HSA Clearing Agent

A Phase I optimization study (20) was carried out for initial clinical investigation into use of the pretargeting system. The pretargeting components consisted of murine NR-LU-10/SA chemical conjugate, HSA clearing agent, and ^{90}Y-DOTA-biotin. Forty-three patients with advanced cancers reactive to NR-LU-10 murine monoclonal antibody including colorectal, lung, gastroesophageal, bladder, breast, ovarian, and pancreatic cancer were studied. An optimized schema was determined by varying the doses of the three components as well as the timing of clearing agent and ^{90}Y-DOTA-biotin. Some patients received NR-LU-10/SA conjugate that was radiolabeled with ^{186}Re as an imaging tracer to assess biodistribution of the conjugate and the effectiveness of the clearing agent. ^{111}In-DOTA-biotin was coinjected with ^{90}Y-DOTA-biotin for quantitative imaging. Safety, biodistribution, pharmacokinetics, dosimetry, and antiglobulin formation were assessed.

Following the determination of an optimized reagent dosing and timing protocol, a 50-patient study was carried out to determine the maximum tolerated dose of pretargeted ^{90}Y-DOTA-biotin (21). As in the optimization trial all patients had refractory adenocarcinomas of a histological type known to react with the NR-LU-10 antibody.

B. Reagent Dose and Timing Optimization

1. NR-LU-10/SA Conjugate

NR-LU-10/SA conjugate doses were varied in order to achieve the highest intravascular concentrations that could still be effectively cleared from the body. This was done in an attempt to saturate available tumor antigen sites with conjugate and achieve uniform distribution of streptavidin throughout the tumor, though the latter was not directly evaluated. Doses of conjugate administered (IV in saline) ranged from 170 to 600 mg. Tumor uptake was assessed in conjunction with uptake in antigen-positive normal organs such as the kidney and gastrointestinal tract. As no obvious advantage to higher doses in regard to saturation of tumor and normal antigen-positive tissues was seen, 400 mg conjugate was initially chosen as the dose for the first component. Eventually, to achieve greater patient-to-patient consistency, conjugate dosing was based on estimated plasma volume. On this basis, a dose of 125 µg conjugate/mL plasma volume was adopted and instituted.

The mean serum clearance of conjugate was determined using ^{186}Re-NR-LU-10/SA from five patients that received only the radiolabeled conjugate. The elimination half-life of NR-LU-10/SA was 27.2 hours compared with 21.6 hours for the antibody. This was in good agreement with the similarities seen in animal model comparison studies.

Assessment of timing interval between conjugate and clearing agent administrations was based on preclinical and clinical studies with ^{186}Re-NR-LU-10 which suggested peak uptake at tumor to occur 24 to 48 hours after infusion. Given the pharmacokinetic similarities between whole antibody and conjugate, intervals of 24, 44 to 48, and 72 hours were investigated. In addition to optimization based on tumor uptake, the impact of this parameter on the eventual degree of conjugate clearance was evaluated. Longer intervals of time allowed greater passive clearance of conjugate. An intermediate interval appeared to offer the best compromise between maximum conjugate clearance nadirs following clearing agent administration and targeting of the radiometal-DOTA-biotin ligand. The uptake of radiometal-DOTA-biotin could be impacted by saturation of tumor-associated conjugate with endogenous biotin over time; thus, lower tumor uptake could result from waiting too long. Based on these considerations, a 48-hour interval was used in subsequent optimization studies.

2. Clearing Agent

Clearing agent dosage and time of administration postconjugate were varied with the intent of maximizing clearance of conjugate remaining in the circulation. The clearing agent was given IV over a period of 15 min, as a continuous infusion over a 24-hour period, or as discrete doses given at various times over 24 hours. Doses administered ranged from 110 to 600 mg with various ratios of clearing agent to conjugate remaining in the blood being examined. Imaging and blood clearance kinetics indicated that the best-performance consistency appeared to be achieved when the clearing agent to conjugate molar ratio was 10:1, correlating to a dose of 350 to 400 mg. Higher doses of clearing agent resulted in compromised uptake of administered ligand at the tumor in the final step. Clearing agent administration resulted in a rapid and significant reduction (>90%) of circulating conjugate. The additional dosing methods examined—IV bolus, continuous infusion over a 24 hour period, and discrete dosing given in two equal portions at various times over 24 hours—resulted in no obvious difference in methods. A bolus injection was thus implemented in subsequent studies for reasons of simplicity.

3. Radiometal DOTA-Biotin

Administration of radiochelate DOTA-biotin was initially carried out 4 hours after clearing agent. Use of this interval resulted in relatively high liver uptake of the radiometal chelate, approximately 12% of the injected dose. This observation was considered to be due to an insufficient interval of time for the conjugate to be maximally cleared from the serum compartment. Thus, a relatively significant fraction of conjugate was considered to still be available to bind ligand and subsequently undergo hepatic uptake. Increasing the interval to 10 hours or more resulted in significantly less liver uptake of the radiometal chelate. A convenient interval of 24 hours resulted in approximately 3% of the injected dose being taken up by the liver.

The dosage of DOTA-biotin was assessed at two levels—0.5 mg (n = 34), or 2 mg (n = 10). In patients who received the 2-mg dose, lower radiation absorbed doses were estimated in tumor compared to patients given the 0.5-mg dose. This was, of course, presumed to be due to lower ligand specific activity. A bolus administration of 0.5 mg was found to be as effective as a 15-min infusion and was therefore adopted.

Assessment in two patients of ^{111}In-DOTA-biotin distribution and elimination indicated the ligand to be excreted primarily into the urine. Images showed no retention in normal organs, no nonspecific tumor localization, and minimal hepatobiliary excretion. Because of the rapid extravasation of the radiometal DOTA-biotin from the vasculature, at 10 min postadministration only 19% of the injected dose remained in the serum, and by 8 hours <1% remained. The first-order serum half-life was 1.2 hours. Urinary excretion of the radiometal was as the intact ligand chelate. No free radioisotope was detected in the urine. Dosimetry estimates of interest for ^{90}Y-DOTA-biotin by itself were whole body, 0.13 rad/mCi; bone marrow, 0.047 rad/mCi; kidneys, 1.3 rad/mCi; and liver, 0.11 rad/mCi.

The serum disappearance of 0.5 mg ^{111}In-DOTA-biotin administered in the pretargeting format and calculated from 22 patients was biexponential with a mean alpha half-life of 0.4 hour and a beta half-life of 33 hours. The first-order plasma elimination constant was 10.3 hours. At 2 hours, 10% of the injected dose remained in circulation. Chromatographic analysis indicated that by 6 hours, all of the radiometal-DOTA-biotin remaining in serum was conjugate bound. Rapid urinary excretion of free radiometal ligand resulted in decreased blood pool background at early time points. Estimates made by whole-body counting indicated that 36% of the injected radioactivity had been excreted by 2.5 hours and 65% had been excreted by 21 hours. Analysis of urine confirmed that the excreted radioactivity was intact radiometal-DOTA-biotin.

Localization of radiometal-DOTA-biotin to the tumor occurred within minutes of administration and remained in tumor through the last imaging time point at 115 hours. Abdominal images at 3 hours post-^{111}In-DOTA-biotin showed prominent activity in the kidneys and the gastrointestinal tract. That the kidney and intestine were prominent early and persisted indicated that the localization was due to expression of antigen in the collecting tubules of the kidney and in the mucosa of the intestinal tract. This was consistent with known expression of the NR-LU-10 or EpCAM antigen.

Several aspects of the clinical pretargeting optimization studies are noteworthy. The optimal schema was determined to include an NR-LU-10/SA conjugate dose of 125 μg/mL plasma volume, followed by clearing agent dosed at a 10:1 molar ratio of remaining serum conjugate at 48 hours postconjugate administration, followed 24 hours later with 0.5 mg radiometal-DOTA-biotin. Preliminary observations were: (a) administration of the individual components in a combined protocol was safe; (b) conjugate was effectively removed from circulation by the clearing agent to the liver, as indicated through tracer imaging using [186]Re radiolabel; and (c) the radiometal-DOTA-biotin rapidly localized to pretargeted conjugate or was excreted unchanged.

4. Normal Organ and Tumor Dosimetry

Absorbed dose estimates, from quantitative imaging data, were reported for 34 patients receiving 0.5 mg DOTA-biotin (22). The kidneys and the gastrointestinal (GI) tract received the highest radiation dose of the normal organs at 13.3 and 9.9 rad/mCi, respectively. GI doses, however, were reported to be likely underestimated since the standard medical internal radiation dose (MIRD) model assumes all activity to be in the luminal contents. As noted above, the GI localization of radioactivity is thought to be antigen mediated. The mean red marrow projected dose of ^{90}Y in 29 patients, based on ^{111}In, was 0.33 rad/mCi. This value was in accordance with that derived from direct counting of ^{90}Y in the serum (0.27 rad/mCi). Of the marrow doses calculated, <7% was contributed by free radiometal-DOTA-biotin, and 93% by the residual labeled conjugate. The average ^{90}Y tumor dose estimate was 20 rad/mCi in the nine patients who received the optimized protocol, and 12.7 rad/mCi from all patients receiving 0.5 mg DOTA-biotin ligand. Tumor dose estimates ranged from 1 to 40 rad/mCi. In the optimized group, the mean tumor-to-marrow dose ratio was 63:1.

5. Toxicity, Efficacy, and Human Antibody Response

No gradable hematological toxicities were reported for any patient on the optimization protocols, and nonhematological toxicities were minor. No tumor responses were observed at the doses used (10 mCi/m^2 ^{90}Y). Patients generally developed HAMA (antimurine antibody), HASA (antistreptavidin), and HACA (anticlearing agent) by the second week following therapy. Levels of immune response were sufficient to preclude the likelihood of giving additional courses of therapy.

C. Dose Escalation

A subsequent Phase I dose escalation trial was designed to evaluate the therapeutic potential of the pretargeting regimen in a variety of carcinomas and to determine the maximum tolerated dose of ^{90}Y-DOTA-biotin (21). Component doses and the administration schedule were as determined in the prior optimization study with the exception of the method for determining dose of clearing agent. The clearing agent dosage was calculated to be 1.04 times (mass basis) the dose of conjugate. This was determined to be approximately equivalent to dosing at a 10:1 molar ratio of remaining serum conjugate. As in previous groups of patients, the 50 patients entered were required to have malignant neoplasms of a type known to react with the NR-LU-10 antibody, such as colon, breast, ovary, lung, and prostate, that were refractory to standard therapy. The DOTA-biotin component was labeled with 3 to 5 mCi of ^{111}In and administered as a dose of ^{90}Y ranging from 25 to 140 mCi/m^2 (55 to 289 mCi). Escalation was in increments of 5 to 25 mCi/m^2 with two to three patients at each dose level. Dose-limiting toxicity was defined as grade III toxicity in all three patients, or grade IV toxicity in two of three patients at any level of ^{90}Y. Once dose-limiting toxicity was reached, additional patients were studied at lower dose levels to further confirm that an appropriate dose level of ^{90}Y was selected as the maximum tolerated dose for contemplated phase II studies.

1. Dosimetry

The biodistribution of ^{111}In-DOTA-biotin in organs and tumor was evaluated by quantitative planar gamma camera imaging. Tumors were considered to be evaluable for radiation dose estimation if they were large enough to be visualized with gamma camera imaging and if tumor volumetrics was available from CT scans. Marrow dosimetry was assessed from serum samples that were counted in a gamma counter.

Mean radiation absorbed dose estimate for tumor, from 14 patients with evaluable tumors, was 16.4 ± 13.4 SD rad/mCi (22). The dose to tumor was highly variable, with highest dose estimated at 46 rad/mCi ^{90}Y. In three of the patients that showed partial or minor responses, radiation absorbed dose to tumor was to be 1500, 5000, and 6000 rads.

Localization of radiation in the intestinal tract occurred immediately upon administration and was persistent, which indicated localization to antigen expressed on normal intestinal mucosa. Radiation absorbed dose to the intestinal tract, assuming deposition on the mucosa was determined in two ways. Using standard MIRD methods, which assume that the radioactivity is within the lumen of the intestinal tract, a radiation absorbed dose estimate of 10.3 ± 5.3 rad/mCi was calculated. To obtain more accurate estimates of dose from activity within the tissue wall, mathematical representations of folded intestinal tissue were utilized in the developed models to determine more relevant estimates (22). Using this method, the mean value of absorbed dose to the small intestine was calculated to be 49.2 ± 25.3 rad/mCi and for the large intestine 34.8 ± 17.9 rad/mCi.

The mean kidney absorbed dose estimate was 11.5 ± 5.3 rad/mCi. In the Phase I optimization study, dose estimate to the kidney from ^{90}Y-DOTA-biotin alone was determined to be 1.3 rad/mCi. Thus, excreted free radiometaled ligand was not considered to significantly contribute to this total. This relatively high value was interpreted to be a result of crossreactivity of the NR-LU-10 antibody with normal renal tissue and, thus, a result of specific localization. Total kidney dose values ranged from 518 rads (25 mCi/m^2 injected) to 4506 rads (128 mCi/m^2 injected).

Bone marrow activity was not detected on the images of any of the patients. Thus, marrow doses were calculated assuming all marrow dose was from exposure of circulating radioactivity. The mean calculated radiation dose was 0.34 ± 0.08 rad/mCi ^{90}Y. Mean tumor-to-marrow dose ratio estimate was thus 48:1.

2. Toxicity

At doses of ^{90}Y < 100 mCi/m^2, myelosuppression was generally mild, although grade IV platelet suppression did occur in one patient with ovarian cancer who had been heavily pretreated with myelosuppressive chemotherapy. At ^{90}Y doses ≥ 100 mCi/m^2, hematological toxicity was variable, but was not dose limiting. Even at 140 mCi/m^2, only one of three patients experienced grade IV neutropenia, and none experienced grade III or IV thrombocytopenia.

Grade I/II elevations of liver function tests (LFT) were commonly observed. While higher-grade LFT elevations were noted in four patients, these abnormalities were not believed to be related to the therapy, but rather were associated with progressive disease.

Significant GI toxicity was observed and proved to be dose limiting. Nausea/vomiting and/or diarrhea correlated, in frequency and severity, with ^{90}Y dose escalation. From 100 to 140 mCi/m^2 grade III and IV toxicities appeared. This included cases of diarrhea requiring intravenous fluid replacement, and hemorrhagic cases. Patients that had received prior external-beam radiation to the abdomen for prostate cancer appeared to be more prone to diarrhea.

Two patients, one treated at 120 mCi/m^2 and one at 140 mCi/m^2, developed renal toxicity. Toxicity was in the form of elevated serum creatinine. Estimated dose to the patients' kidneys were 2170 and 3072 rads, respectively. Their respective creatinine levels were to 3.1 mg/dL at 12 months after treatment and 2.6 mg/dL after 13 months.

3. Tumor Responses

Generally, patients were evaluated for tumor responses 6 weeks after therapy. Partial responses, i.e., >50% decrease in tumor volume, occurred in 3 of 49 patients. One of the partial responders was a patients with ovarian cancer who received 75 mCi/m^2. The other two partial responders were patients with prostate cancer who received doses of 100 mCi/m^2 and 110 mCi/m^2 respectively. Lesser responses, i.e., 25% to 49% decrease in tumor volume, were seen in four patients. These patients included one with prostate cancer who was treated at 50 mCi/m^2, two with ovarian cancer who were treated at 65 and 80 mCi/m^2, and one with colon cancer who was treated at 80 mCi/m^2. Eighteen patients showed stable disease on follow-up CT scan, and 24 showed progressive disease.

4. Summary of Dose Escalation Study

This Phase I dose escalation trial was designed to evaluate the therapeutic potential of the optimized pretarget regimen in a variety of carcinomas and to determine the MTD of ^{90}Y that could be administered in the form of a DOTA-biotin chelate. Gastrointestinal toxicity, manifest in the form of grade III or IV diarrhea, was observed at 140 mCi/m^2. While grade III/IV diarrhea was also observed in two of six patients dosed at 120 to 128 mCi/m^2, no commensurate toxicity was observed in the five patients dosed at 108 to 110 mCi/m^2. These observations resulted in the selection of 110 mCi/m^2 as the MTD of ^{90}Y DOTA-biotin in the optimized formulation.

Partial and minor responses were observed in patients with prostate, ovarian, and colon cancer at ^{90}Y doses ranging from 50 to 110 mCi/m^2. Of 13 patients with prostate cancer who received 80 mCi/m^2 or more, two (15%) exhibited partial responses and six (46%) had stable disease. These observations suggested a need for further evaluation in more formalized Phase II therapy trials. Moreover, the response of these advanced cancers to just a single dose of the product suggests that multiple dosing, and also combination therapy with other agents, could be beneficial even in these cases.

D. Phase II Colon Cancer Study

A Phase II study was undertaken to evaluate the safety and efficacy of the pretargeting protocol in patients with metastatic colon cancer (24). Additional objectives of the study included evaluation of the duration of tumor response, time to tumor progression, quality of life, and immunoglobulin response. Twenty-five patients were treated at the previously established MTD of 110 mCi/m^2 of ^{90}Y-DOTA-biotin.

Patients received a dose of NR-LU-10/SA conjugate calculated at 125 µg/mL plasma volume. Clearing agent was dosed 48 hours later at a mass of 1.04 times that of administered conjugate. This was followed 24 hours later with 0.5 mg of ^{90}Y-DOTA-biotin. Dosimetry studies were not required or routinely performed, as ^{111}In-DOTA-biotin was not included for imaging.

1. Clinical Responses

There were two partial remissions (8%) produced in the study, with freedom from progression (FFP) of 16 weeks in both cases. Four patients had stable disease (16%) with FFP of 10 to 20 weeks as determined by tumor measurements made at the study sites.

2. Toxicity

Several toxicities were noted in the Phase II study that were similar to those experienced in the Phase I study. Grade 3 or 4 hematological toxicities resulted in some patients, which reached a nadir at 5 to 6 weeks posttreatment with resolution in 6 to 8 weeks. All patients had positive immune responses in the form of HAMA, HASA, and HACA. Hepatic toxicities, as indicated by elevated LFTs, were common but were transient and reversible. Persistent hepatic abnormalities were associated with progressive disease. Most patients had mild nausea and vomiting; one patient experienced grade 3 toxicity. At 7 to 8 months posttreatment, two patients developed signs of renal toxicity with significant elevations in serum creatinine levels, 3.1 and 6.8, that appeared independent of disease progression.

The more serious toxicity experienced was diarrhea. Twenty-two of the 25 patients (88%) had gradable diarrhea, with eight patients having grade 3 or 4 toxicity. Included in the group experiencing grade 3 or 4 toxicities were those with prior radiation therapy, a history of diverticulitis, or underlying partial bowel obstruction. One patient experienced severe diarrhea, dehydration, and hypokalemia and died of a cardiac arrest after refusing hospitalization for 2 consecutive days prior to death. Although autopsy revealed severe underlying cardiac disease, the diarrhea and resulting hypokalemia could have contributed to the death.

3. Summary of Phase II Colon Cancer Study

While the response rate (8%) of patients enrolled in this Phase II study was comparable to that observed in Phase I (9%) at the higher dose levels of ^{90}Y-DOTA-biotin ($\geq$80 mCi/m^2), only 16% of Phase II patients had stable disease compared to 54% of Phase I patients. Additionally, the mean FFP for responders was shorter in the Phase II study than in the Phase I. These disparities may be attributable to study design, as colorectal cancer patients made up only 22% of the Phase I study group.

The incidence and severity of GI and hematological toxicity in the Phase II trial were greater than anticipated from the Phase I study. As the patients in the Phase II had no evidence of either myelosuppression or a greater number of risk factors for GI toxicity, the reason for this increased toxicity was less clear.

IV. SUMMARY AND FUTURE DIRECTIONS

Preclinical results using the pretargeting components and methods described have resulted in a dramatic demonstration of the therapeutic potential of this radionuclide delivery strategy. Single application of the pretarget protocol using first-generation components resulted in high cure rates in mice implanted with a number of human xenograft lines. Second-generation components proved as therapeutically effective. Additional in vivo characterization of these second-generation constructs suggested the potential for an improvement in clinical performance over first-generation agents in the form of further enhancement in tumor-to-blood ratios.

In summarizing the Phase I and Phase II trials, although a degree of efficacy against bulky, radiation-insensitive carcinomas was displayed, three issues were evident:

1. Although only a single dose was administered to refractory patients, response rates were far less than had been hoped.
2. Antigen expression on normal organs, GI epithelium, and kidney collecting tubules appeared to be the reason for radiation localization to these organs and resultant dose-limiting toxicity prior to significant tumor response.
3. While not dose limiting, in the face of GI toxicity, levels of hematopoietic toxicity were still sufficient to limit significant further escalation in dose.

Much of the normal organ toxicity may be attributable to use of the NR-LU-10 antibody. This was unexpected since the same antibody labeled with up to 555 mCi of ^{186}Re produced no such toxicity (26). Additionally, tumor dosimetry suggests that levels of expression of the EpCAM antigen were not outstanding. Pretargeting of the CD-20 receptor in a related trial to treat non-Hodgkin's lymphoma resulted in much higher doses of absorbed radiation, approximately 30 rads/mCi versus 15 rads/mCi in the carcinoma trial (24). Thus, even if less ubiquitously expressed, suitable antigenic targets with higher, clinically documented levels of tumor expression would seem to be needed and possible.

Numerous conventional RIT clinical trials have been undertaken targeting a variety of carcinoma tumor antigens, and indications of clinical utility have been reported. Targeting of mucin antigenic epitopes using the antibodies L6 (27) or BrE3 (28) have resulted in some encouraging responses in breast cancer trials. Additionally, carcinoembryonic antigen (CEA) (29–31) and tumor-associated glycoprotein-72 (TAG-72) (32–34) also appear to be good tumor specific targets, based on dosimetry data accrued from breast and colon cancer trials.

Targeting to one of the alternative tumor antigens discussed, using a streptavidin fusion protein cleared with the synthetic clearing agent, should result in lowered normal organ uptake or targeting of radionuclide, enhanced tumor targeting, and lowered marrow exposure due to enhanced clearance. Additional enhancement may be obtained through simultaneous targeting of multiple tumor antigens using a cocktail of targeting fusion proteins. Cocktail targeting would appear to be particularly applicable to the described pretarget regimen, which calls for using antigen-saturating amounts of fusion protein to effectively replace each of a variety of different tumor antigens by a single streptavidin-like protein. This is in contrast to cocktail targeting in the conventional sense, which is constrained by the total amount of radiation that may be administered and subsequent use of subsaturating quantities of antibody (35).

Pretargeted radiotherapy also lends itself to the use of alternative radionuclides. DOTA forms highly stable chelates with many +3 metals and, as mentioned earlier in this chapter, ^{90}Y, ^{111}In, and ^{177}Lu have been shown to have equivalent radiometal chelate biodistribution properties with the DOTA-biotin reagent. ^{90}Y, with its 2.27 MeV beta maximum energy, has good penetration and maximizes potential for treating larger tumors (36). Lutetium (^{177}Lu) emits beta particles of lower energy in the same range as ^{131}I and thus may be more effective for small metastases (see O'Donoghue, Chap. 1). DOTA also forms stable complexes with lead and bismuth, which provides potential for delivering alpha radiotherapy via pretargeting. ^{212}Pb decays with a 10.6-hour half-life into the alpha emitter, while ^{212}Bi has a 1-hour half-life. Preliminary xenograft model studies demonstrated good selective tumor targeting of the ^{212}Pb-DOTA-biotin and decay product ^{212}Bi in the pretargeting format (37). Thus, a wide range of radionuclide properties can be used in the pretargeting system with potential advantages in the treatment of disease ranging from palpable tumors to micrometastases.

ACKNOWLEDGMENT

Supported in part by NIH grant CA71221 (Alpha Radiotherapy via Pretargeted Lead-212).

REFERENCES

1. Fritzberg AR. Biorecognition of antibodies in vivo: potential in drug targeting. J Mol Recognit 1996; 9:309–315.
2. Langmuir VK. Radioimmunotherapy: clinical results and dosimetric considerations. Nucl Med Biol 1992; 19:213–225.
3. Press OW, Eary JF, Appelbaum FR, Martin PJ, Badger CC, Nelp WB, Glenn S, Butchko G, Fisher D, Porter B. Radiolabeled-antibody therapy of B-cell lymphoma with autologous bone marrow support. N Engl J Med 1993; 329:1219–1224.
4. Goodwin DA, Meares CF. Pretargeting. General principles. Cancer 1997; 80:2675–2680.
5. Paganelli GM, Fazio F. Monoclonal antibody pretargeting techniques for tumor localization: the avidin/biotin system. Nucl Med Commun 1991; 12:211–234.
6. Le Doussal J-M, Martin M, Gautherot E, Delaage M, Barbet J. In vitro and in vivo targeting of radiolabeled monovalent and divalent haptens with dual specificity monoclonal antibody conjugates: enhanced divalent hapten affinity for cell-bound antibody conjugate. J Nucl Med 1989; 30:1358–1366.

7. Hnatowich DJ, Virzi F, Rusckowski M. Investigations of avidin and biotin for imaging applications. J Nucl Med 1987; 28:1294–1302.
8. Wilchek M, Bayer EA. The avidin/biotin complex in immunology. Immunol Today 1984; 184:39–43.
9. Beaumier PL, Venkatesan P, Vanderheyden J-L, Burqua WD, Kunz LL, Fritzberg AR, Abrams PG, Morgan AC Jr. Re-186 radioimmunotherapy of small cell lung carcinoma xenografts in nude mice. Cancer Res 1991; 51:676–681.
10. Breitz HB, Weiden PL, Vanderheyden J-L, Appelbaum JW, Bjorn MJ, Fer MF, Wolf SB, Ratliff BA, Seiler CA, Foisie DC, Fisher DR, Schroff RW, Fritzberg AR, Abrams PG. Clinical experience with Re-186-labeled monoclonal antibodies for radioimmunotherapy: results of Phase I trials. J Nucl Med 1992; 33:1099–1112.
11. Axworthy DB, Reno JM, Hylarides MD, Mallett RW, Theodore LJ, Gustavson LM, Su F-M, Hobson LJ, Beaumier PL, Fritzberg AR. Cure of human carcinoma xenografts by a single dose of pretargeted yttrium-90 with negligible toxicity. Proc Natl Acad Sci USA 2000; 97:1802–1807.
12. Sung S, Van Osdol WW. Pharmacokinetic comparison of direct antibody targeting with pretargeting protocols based on streptavidin-biotin binding. J Nucl Med 1995; 36:867–876.
13. Breitz HB, Fisher DR, Weiden PL, Durham JS, Ratliff BA, Bjorn MJ, Beaumier PL, Abrams PG. Dosimetry of rhenium-186-labeled monoclonal antibodies: methods, prediction from technetium-99m-labeled antibodies and results of Phase I trials. J Nucl Med 1993; 34:908–917.
14. Goodwin DA, Meares CF, McCall MJ, McTigue M, Chaovapong W. Pretargeted immunoscintigraphy of murine tumors with indium-111 labeled bifunctional haptens. J Nucl Med 1988; 29:226–234.
15. Ashwell G, Harford J. Carbohydrate-specific receptors of the liver. Annu Rev Biochem 1982; 72:3–20.
16. Hardy MR, Townsend RR, Parkhurst SM, Lee YC. Different modes of ligand binding to the hepatic galactose/N-acetylgalactosamine lectin on the surface of rabbit hepatocytes. Biochemistry 1985; 24:22–28.
17. Vera DR, Krohn KA, Stadalnik RC, Scheibe PO. Tc-99m galactosylneoglycolalbumin: in vitro characterization of receptor-mediated binding. J Nucl Med 1984; 25:779–787.
18. Axworthy DA, Theodore LJ, Gustavson LM, Reno JM. U.S. Patent 5,608,060 (1997).
19. Theodore LJ, Axworthy DB. Cluster Clearing Agents. PCT Application International. Publication No. WO97/46098 (1997).
20. Breitz HB, Weiden PL, Beaumier PL, Axworthy DB, Seiler C, Su F-M, Graves S, Bryan B, Reno JM. Clinical optimization of pretargeted radioimmunotherapy (PRIT™) with antibody-streptavidin conjugate and ^{90}Y-DOTA-biotin. J Nucl Med 2000; 41:131–140.
21. Breitz H, Knox S, Weiden P, Goris M, Murtha A, Bryan J, Axworthy D, Seiler S, Su F-M, Beaumier P, Reno J. Pretargeted radioimmunotherapy with antibody streptavidin and Y-90 DOTA-biotin (Avicidin). Results of a dose escalation study. J Nucl Med 1998; 39:71P. Abstract.
22. Breitz JB, Fisher DR, Goris ML, Knox S, Ratliff B, Murtha AD, Weiden PL. Radia-

tion absorbed dose estimation for ^{90}Y-DOTA-biotin with pretargeted NR-LU-10/ streptavidin. Cancer Biother Radiopharm 1999; 14:381–395.

23. Breitz HB, Weiden PL, Appelbaum JW, Stone DM, Axworthy DB, Fisher DR, Press O, Abrams PG. Pretargeted radioimmunotherapy (PRIT™) for treatment of non-Hodgkin's lymphoma (NHL). Cancer Biother Radiopharm 2000; 15:15–29.

24. Knox SJ, Goris ML, Tempero M, Weiden PL, Gentner L, Breitz H, Adams GP, Axworthy D, Gaffigan S, Bryan K, Fisher DR, Colcher D, Horak ID, Weiner LM. Phase II trial of yttrium-90-DOTA-biotin pretargeted by NR-LU-10 antibody-strep-tavidin in patients with metastatic colon cancer. Clin Cancer Res 2000; 6:406–414.

25. Tedder TF, Engel P. CD20: a regulator of cell-cycle progression of B lymphocytes. Immunol Today 1994; 15:450–454.

26. Su F-M, Lyen L, Breitz HB, Weiden PL, Fritzberg AR. [186]Rhenium MAG2GABA antibody radiolabeling for high dose radioimmunotherapy studies. Proceedings of the Fourth International Symposium of Technitium in Chemistry and Nuclear Medicine, Seminario Maggiore, Bressnanone, Italy, 12–14 Sept 1994.

27. DeNardo SJ, O'Grady LF, Richman CM, Goldstein D, O'Donnel RT, DeNardo DA, Kroger LA, Lamborn KR, Hellstrom KE, Hellstrom I, DeNardo GL. Radioimmuno-therapy of advanced breast cancer using I-131-chL6 antibody. Anticancer Res 1997; 17:1745–1752.

28. Schrier DM, Stemmer SM, Johnson T, Kasliwal R, Lear J, Matthes S, Taffs S, Duf-ton C, Glenn SD, Butchko G, Ceriani RL, Rovira D, Bunn P, Shall EJ, Bearman SI, Purdy M, Cagnoni P, Jones RB. High-dose [90]Y Mx-diethylenetriaminepenta-acetic acid (DTPA)-BrE-3 and autologous hematopoietic stem cell support (AHSCS) for the treatment of advanced breast cancer: a Phase I trial. Cancer Res Suppl 1995; 55:5921s.

29. Yu B, Carrasquillo J, Milenic D, Chung Y, Perentesis P, Feuerstein I, Eggensperger D, Qi C-F, Paik C, Reynolds J, Grem GC, Siler K, Schlom J, Allegra C. Phase I trial of iodine-131-labeled COL-1 in patients with gastrointestinal malignancies: influence of serum carcinoembryonic antigen and tumor bulk on pharmacokinetics. J Clin Oncol 1996; 6:1798–1809.

30. Wong JYC, Williams LE, Yamauchi DM, Odom-Maryon T, Esteban JM, Neumaier M, Wu AM, Johnson DK, Primus FJ, Shively JE, Raubitschek AA. Initial experience evaluating [90]yttrium radiolabeled anti-carcinoembryonic antigen chimeric T84.66 in a Phase I radioimmunotherapy trial. Cancer Res 1995; 55:5929–5934s.

31. Behr TM, Sharkey RM, Juweid ME, Dunn RM, Vagg RC, Ying Z, Zhang CH, Swayne LC, Vardi Y, Siegel JA, Goldenberg DM. Phase I/II clinical radioimmuno-therapy with an iodine-131-labeled anti-carcinoembryonic antigen murine mono-clonal antibody IgG. J Nucl Med 1997; 38:858–870.

32. Murray JL, Macey JD, Kasi LP, Rieger P, Cunningham J, Bhadkamkar V, Zhang H-Z, Schlom J, Rosenblum MG, Podoloff DA. Phase II trial of ^{131}I-CC49 Mab with alpha interferon in colorectal cancer. Cancer Suppl 1994; 73(3):1057–1066.

33. Murray JL, Macey DJ, Grant EJ, et al. Phase II ^{131}I-CC49 Mab plus alpha interferon (rIFNa) in breast cancer. J Immunother 1994; 16:162. Abstract.

34. Leichner PK, Akabani G, Colcher D, Harrison KA, Hawkins WG, Eckblade M, Baranowska Kortylewicz J, Augustine SC, Wisecarver J, Tempero MA. Patient-

specific dosimetry of indium-111 and yttrium-90-labeled monocloncal antibody CC49. J Nucl Med 1997; 38(4):512–516.

35. Meredith RF, Khazaeli MB, Plott WE, Grizzle WE, Liu T, Schlom J, Russel CD, Wheeler RH, LoBuglio AF. Phase II study of dual ^{131}I-labeled monoclonal antibody therapy with interferon in patients with metastatic colorectal cancer. Clin Cancer Res 1996; 2:1811–1818.

36. Fritzberg AR, Wessels BW. Therapeutic radionuclides. In: Wagner HN, ed. Principles of Nuclear Medicine, 2nd ed. Philadelphia: Saunders, 1995:229–234.

37. Su F-M, Beaumier P, Axworthy D, Reno J, Fisher D, Fritzberg A. Pretargeted radioimmunotherapy in tumored mice using an in vivo Pb-212/Bi-212 generator. J Nucl Med 1998; 39:91P. Abstract.

9
Extracorporeal Techniques in Radioimmunotherapy

Sven-Erik Strand, Hans-Olov Sjögren, JianQing Chen,* and Cecilia Hindorf
Lund University, Lund, Sweden

Jan G. Tennvall and Michael Garkavij
Lund University Hospital, Lund, Sweden

Rune Nilsson and Bengt E. B. Sandberg
Mitra Medical Technology AB, Lund, Sweden

I. INTRODUCTION

A major problem in achieving effective immunotargeting is the poor tumor-to-blood activity ratio which rarely reaches values sufficiently high to give effective radioimmunotherapy (RIT) or permit accurate diagnostic radioimmunoimaging (RII). This is of particular importance in RIT, where the toxic effect of conjugates on critical organs (marrow) is normally a limiting factor due to high absorbed doses from the relatively long circulation time of intact monoclonal antibodies (MAbs). Although MAb fragments such as Fab or $F(ab')_2$ are cleared more rapidly from the blood and penetrate more easily into solid tumors than the intact antibodies, most MAb fragments do not accumulate sufficiently in tumors to achieve the desired therapeutic effect (1).

There are currently a number of methods described which aim to increase the tumor-to-blood activity ratio by artificially decreasing the amount of the radioimmunoconjugate (RIC) in the blood while retaining the level of the conjugate in the tumor. The various strategies to enhance the tumor-to-normal tissue ab-

---

* *Current affiliation:* University of Missouri, Columbia, Missouri.

sorbed dose ratios (including extracorporeal technique) have been reviewed (1). This chapter will focus on extracorporeal techniques.

In view of this, it is not surprising that the use of various extracorporeal techniques for the removal of circulating RIC has been contemplated (2–4). Our group has proposed the extracorporeal immunoadsorption (ECIA) technique (5). Extracorporeal techniques are generally employed for the removal of pathogenic or otherwise undesirable agents from the bloodstream of patients with various severe diseases. In numerous cases it has been proven efficient and sometimes life saving. Most notable is the success of dialysis in the treatment of renal failure (>700,000 patients on chronic treatment worldwide).

II. PRINCIPAL WAYS FOR EXTRACORPOREAL DEPLETION

There are two principal ways to control levels of systemically administered immunoconjugate by extracorporeal means; either the patient's plasma is continuously or stepwise removed and replaced by donated plasma or by albumin solutions, or the patient's plasma or whole blood is cleared by the use of specific adsorption devices. Both these methods have been explored clinically. Any technique where blood is exchanged by continuous or discontinuous withdrawal follows an exponential curve with respect to clearance efficiency (Fig. 1).

Removing exogenous or endogenous toxic agents from the circulation by plasma exchange in an online setting is standard procedure for a number of diseases and syndromes. However, such treatments are not without serious drawbacks. If a patient's plasma is replaced by albumin solution, rarely more than one plasma volume can be processed due to the fact that essential components in plasma, such as coagulation factors, must not be decreased by more than that. Hence, it is inconceivable that more than 60% to 65% of nonbound immunoconjugate could be removed from the patient's plasma through such means. If on the other hand the patient's plasma is exchanged for donated human plasma, hypersensitivity may occur. There is also a risk of contamination.

A more attractive method is the selective removal of undesirable agents from blood circulation, with a simultaneous return of the purified blood to the patient, thus avoiding loss of essential blood components and eliminating the need for replacement solutions. These methods are typically based on the principle of affinity adsorption, although size and physical properties could also be utilized. In extracorporeal affinity treatment, a substance selective for the component to be removed is covalently bound to a matrix through which the blood or plasma is passed (Fig. 2).

Clinical extracorporeal adsorption systems for processing human plasma are available for the removal of immunoglobulin by the use of Protein-A in the

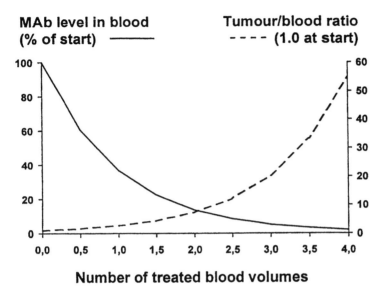

Figure 1 A theoretically calculated curve illustrating the improvement of the tumor-to-blood ratio as a function of number of blood volumes processed. The concentration of immunoconjugate at start of the affinity adsorption is set to 100%, and the tumor-to-blood ratio is assumed to be 1.0. After three blood volumes have been processed, about 95% has been removed and the ratio has increased to 20.

treatment of autoimmune diseases (6) or to avoid early rejection of transplanted organs (7), and for the removal of low-density lipoprotein (LDL), in the treatment of hypercholesterolemia by the use of immobilized anti-LDL antibodies (8).

Any device used with the purpose to specifically remove RIC must rely on the presence of structural entities on the immunoconjugate accessible for binding to the device. These structural entities can either be an integral part of the immunoconjugate or be artificially conjugated to the immunoconjugate prior to administration to the patient. An example of the former is the use of immobilized antibodies directed against specific and accessible epitopes present on the immunoconjugate. An extracorporeal system utilizing immobilized anti-isotypic (anti-species) antibodies directed against immunoconjugate based on mouse MAbs has been developed and clinically evaluated (9).

Over the past 5 or 6 years most pharmaceutical companies in the field have focused their efforts on alternatives to mouse monoclonal antibodies for various types of immunotargeting. It is generally acknowledged that xenotypic monoclonal antibodies give rise to production of human antibody directed against the administered monoclonal antibodies (10). To minimize these effects attempts

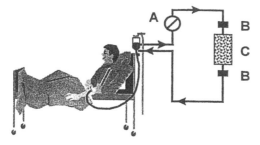

Adsorption system for whole blood

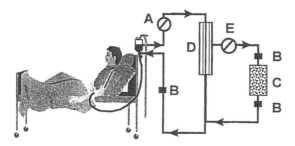

Adsorption system for plasma

Figure 2   Principal outline of the affinity-adsorption systems for the treatment of whole blood and plasma, respectively. (A) Blood pump. (B) Air detector with pressure monitor. (C) Adsorption device. (D) Plasma separation device (plasma filter or online centrifuge). (E) Plasma pump.

have been made to humanize part of the mouse monoclonal antibodies by replacing mouse structures for the corresponding human structures (11). In the long term there is little doubt that new generations of immunoconjugates will be based on monoclonal antibodies with structures closely related to that of human IgG. Consequently, such exogenous humanized antibodies (foreign) might differ from the endogenous human antibodies (own) only with respect to the specific antigen-binding region.

Any general affinity adsorption device has to be based on artificially introduced characteristics of the exogenous antibodies in order to differentiate between own and foreign IgG. This can be achieved by the labeling of the exogenous antibody with affinity ligands (12,13). Such affinity ligands should exhibit a high affinity as well as high specificity toward a given receptor immobilized to the adsorbent. Another prerequisite is that the affinity labeling of the immuno-conjugate must not significantly alter the tumor-binding properties of the mono-clonal antibodies, or affect the biodistribution or enhance the immunogenicity of the conjugate. The stability of the conjugate is also important since successful extracorporeal removal of non-target-bound conjugates will be dependent on the presence of accessible affinity ligand moieties on the conjugate. Furthermore, if the affinity ligand is an endogenous substance, the content in human blood must be low so as not to interfere with the adsorption of the conjugate to the device. Furthermore, the immobilized receptor utilized must not interfere with the blood through activation or inhibition of vital physiological processes. The use of biotin (vitamin H) as affinity ligand in conjunction with immobilized avidin/streptavidin fulfill most of the above described criteria.

III. RADIOLABELING AND BIOTINYLATION OF IMMUNOCONJUGATES

A successful combination of procedures for biotinylation and radiolabeling of immunoconjugates is a prerequisite for the use of ECAT based on the biotin-avidin concept.

Many papers regarding the optimal radionuclide for radioimmunotherapy have been published (14–17). Due to its familiarity, relatively simple labeling, appropriate physical half-life, ready availability, and low cost, ^{131}I has been used in many experiments and clinical RIT studies. In our experience, the appropriate means of combining radiolabeling and biotinylation varies for different types of MAbs. Direct iodination has been successfully used for MAb L6 radiolabeling in conjunction of biotinylation (12,18) and for other MAbs by the Paganelli group (19), whereas it is less straightforward to apply these techniques for BR96 (20). Instead, the use of N-succinimidyl-3-(tri-n-butylstannyl)benzoate (NSTBB) for BR96 iodination, followed by subsequent biotinylation with N-hydroxysuccini-mido-biotin, has proven more successful (20,21). Chelates such as SCN-Bz-CHX-A-DTPA and TFP MAG_2-GABA (tetrafluorophenyl mercaptoacetylglycylglycyl-gamma-aminobutyrate) have been found appropriate for indium and rhenium labeling of biotinylated BR96 (22,23). The maintenance of tumor cell binding properties was confirmed on tumor cell lines in vitro. The in vivo stability of the radiolabeled and biotinylated BR96 was examined by determining free radioactivity and the binding to avidin-agarose in plasma. The biodistribution of the radiolabeled BR96 with or without biotin was further compared in the colon car-cinoma isografted Brown Norwegian (BN) rat model. In Table 1, a comparison of biodistribution of the biotin-coupled and non-biotin-coupled radiolabeled BR96 (with ^{125}I, [188]Re, or ^{111}In) at 48 h postinjection in the colon carcinoma isografted BN rats is given. As seen in the table, there is a close resemblance in activity uptake in tumors and normal tissues for nonbiotinylated and biotinylated MAb.

Table 1 Biodistribution of the Biotin-Coupled and Non-Biotin-Coupled Radiolabeled-BR96 (with ^{125}I, ^{188}Re, or ^{111}In) at 48 h Postinjection in Colon Carcinoma Isografted BN Rats (% injected activity per gram tissue)

	^{125}I-BR96	^{125}I-BR96-biotin	^{188}Re-BR96	^{188}Re-BR96-biotin	^{111}In-BR96	^{111}In-BR96-biotin
Tumor (im)	2.19 ± 0.40	1.79 ± 0.74	2.07 ± 0.62	1.78 ± 0.37	2.57 ± 0.32	2.68 ± 0.38
Tumor (sr)	2.91 ± 0.17	2.51 ± 0.69	2.76 ± 0.66	2.41 ± 0.76	6.54 ± 1.36	5.61 ± 0.79
Testicle	0.17 ± 0.01	0.15 ± 0.00	0.16 ± 0.02	0.14 ± 0.02	0.41 ± 0.09	0.43 ± 0.05
Liver	0.52 ± 0.03	0.49 ± 0.04	0.27 ± 0.11	0.29 ± 0.09	1.14 ± 0.18	1.13 ± 0.23
Spleen	0.31 ± 0.02	0.28 ± 0.03	0.18 ± 0.04	0.19 ± 0.02	0.32 ± 0.04	0.31 ± 0.02
Kidney	0.28 ± 0.03	0.28 ± 0.05	0.48 ± 0.04	0.49 ± 0.05	0.54 ± 0.06	0.49 ± 0.05
Colon	0.24 ± 0.05	0.22 ± 0.02	0.32 ± 0.08	0.32 ± 0.08	0.42 ± 0.18	0.52 ± 0.08
Lung	0.31 ± 0.02	0.30 ± 0.00	0.37 ± 0.09	0.34 ± 0.04	0.63 ± 0.09	0.60 ± 0.04
Bone marrow	0.24 ± 0.02	0.16 ± 0.11	0.21 ± 0.03	0.20 ± 0.05	0.35 ± 0.16	0.40 ± 0.12
Blood	0.64 ± 0.09	0.58 ± 0.05	0.82 ± 0.13	0.82 ± 0.09	1.12 ± 0.15	1.08 ± 0.09

Biotinylation of proteins such as immunoglobulins can be achieved through various means. The amino groups in proteins can be conjugated by the use of biotinyl-p-nitrophenyl esters or biotinyl-N-succinimide esters. The coupling can also be achieved by the use of carbodiimide and equivalent coupling reagents. In all these cases the biotinyl group will be linked to the ε-amino groups of lysine residues forming a biocytin derivative, although a limited number of α-amino groups may also be conjugated. The combined radioiodination and biotinylation of immunoconjugates have been extensively investigated (19). However, exploiting primary amino groups for biotinylation purposes may cause some problem in the cases where the same amino groups are needed for the radionuclide labeling. This may not severely hamper the use of these agents, provided that biotinylation is accomplished prior to the radiolabeling. It is probably of minor importance whether the radionuclide is buried inside the IgG molecule or exposed on the surface. The biotin groups, however, must at least to some extent be available on the surface of the immunoglobulin in order to be captured by the immobilized avidin. Although natural biotin carries a short spacer of four carbon atoms, which together with the four carbon atoms of the lysine residue side chain should distance the biotin double ring from the backbone structure of the immunoglobulin, there might still in some cases be an advantage to introduce spacers of various length.

Alternative ways of preparing biotin derivatives reacting with groups other than amino groups are also commonly used. Among these are biotinyl hydrazide which reacts with sugar residues and biotinyl-bromoacetyl hydrazide or biotin maleimide, which reacts with sulfhydryls and other strong nucleophiles. Biotinyl-diazoanilide can be used to conjugate biotin to phenol or imidazole functions. To achieve sufficiently high avidin binding capacity without significant alteration of the antigen-binding properties of the immunoconjugate, the number of conjugated biotin moieties should be limited but high enough to ensure that nearly all individual MAbs carry at least one biotin residue. The optimal number will most likely vary from MAb to MAb and depend on the conditions for extracorporeal removal, but something in the range of three to five biotin residues per MAb will probably be appropriate.

Although there is some controversy regarding the physical states of biotin in human blood, in a recent study of 10 healthy persons of both sexes, the average total amount of biotin was found to be 483 pmol/L (276 to 785 pmol/L) (24). Thus, on average a patient having 6 L blood will carry about 15 μg of extracellular biotin. This amount of extracellular biotin should be capable of blocking about 1 mg of immobilized avidin, assuming that all four binding sites for biotin are available on the immobilized avidin. Hence, the presence of naturally occurring extracellular biotin is unlikely to interfere with the efficiency of the extracorporeal depletion. Due to the short duration of biotin depletion it is very unlikely that the patients will show any manifestations of biotin deficiency.

The stability of the biotinyl linkage is of utmost importance, since this concept of extracorporeal removal will rely on the presence of biotin residues on the MAb. Naturally occurring biotin is recycled from biocytin by the cleavage into lysine and biotin, through the activity of a group of enzymes called biotinidase (25). However, these enzymes are sensitive to steric hindrance near the biotin carboxyl function, making it unlikely that biotin groups directly linked to the protein would be removed from the MAb molecule prior to the extracorporeal depletion (26). The relatively short time interval of the immunoconjugate circulating in blood prior to the extracorporeal removal should also be considered.

IV. DOSIMETRIC CONSIDERATIONS AND THERAPEUTIC RATIO

DeNardo et al. (27) emphasize that the imaging efficacy is dependent on amount of radionuclide in target and normal tissues; i.e., the tumor-to-normal-tissue activity ratio at the time point of imaging has to be as large as possible, while the therapy efficacy is dependent on cumulative activity in target and normal tissues; i.e., the tumor-to-normal-tissue residence time- or absorbed dose ratio has to be as large as possible.

The absorbed dose to different organs/tissues in radionuclide therapy is usually calculated using the MIRD S-formalism (28). Mean absorbed dose in the target region, $\overline{D}$, is calculated as the product of the cumulated activity in the source region, $\tilde{A}$, and the S-value. Here are the simplified equations describing the MIRD formalism presented (summation for type of radiation and summation of contribution from more than one source region are omitted).

$$\overline{D} = \tilde{A} \cdot S \tag{1}$$

The cumulated activity, $\tilde{A}$, is determined from the biological parameters (the source region's uptake and clearence) and is calculated as the time integral of the time-activity curve for an organ or tissue (the source organ):

$$\tilde{A} = \int_0^\infty A(t)dt \tag{2}$$

The physical parameters is gathered in the S-value:

$$S = \Delta \cdot \frac{\phi}{m} \tag{3}$$

where Δ is emitted energy per decay of the radionuclide, ϕ is absorbed fraction, and m is the mass of the target region. (See Chapter 2 in this volume for a more extensive review of the MIRD S-formalism.)

When radionuclide therapy is combined with ECAT the calculation of mean absorbed dose has to be done in a slightly modified way. The S-value for a given region remains the same whether ECAT is performed or not, but the cumulated activity is changed (Fig. 3). Mean absorbed dose in an organ/tissue after extracorporeal immunoadsorption, $\overline{D}_{ECAT}$ is then calculated as:

$$\overline{D}_{ECAT} = \tilde{A}_{ECAT} \cdot S \tag{4}$$

The cumulative activity when extracorporeal immunoadsorption is performed, $\tilde{A}_{ECAT}$, is calculated as the time integral of the time-activity curve as before, but the integration should be divided into three different time periods—the first period describing biokinetics from injection point to start of ECAT, the second describ-

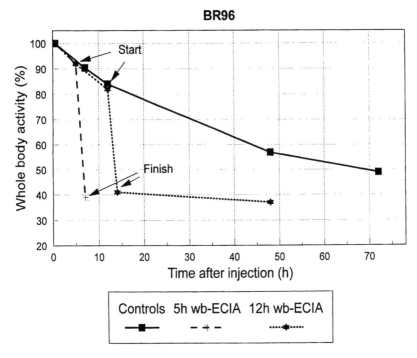

Figure 3 Whole-body activity curves after injection of ^{125}I-chiBR96-biotin in either controls or rats subjected to wb-ECAT.

ing clearance during ECAT, and a third period for the biokinetics from stop of
ECAT to infinity (29).

$$\tilde{A}_{\text{ECAT}} = \int_0^{\text{ECAT start}} A_{\text{before ECAT}}(t)dt + \int_{\text{ECAT start}}^{\text{ECAT stop}} A_{\text{ECAT}}(t)dt$$
$$+ \int_{\text{ECAT stop}}^{\infty} A_{\text{after ECAT}}(t)dt \tag{5}$$

The curve describing the removal of activity during ECAT, $A_{\text{ECAT}}(t)$, should be
determined experimentally, with a scintillation camera as described in an experimental model (13) or by blood samples measured with a gamma counter as described for patients (30). If this is not possible during ECAT, a monoexponential
decrease of activity could be assumed if the activity is known immediately before
and after performance of ECAT (31). This assumption, of course, introduces an
uncertainty in the cumulated activity, but since the time to perform ECAT is
short compared to the whole integration time, this error would be small and could
probably be neglected.

An often reported quantity is the therapeutic index, i.e., the ratio of absorbed doses to tumor and to critical organs. Therapeutic index is reported to
compare the efficency of radioimmunotherapy with and without ECAT. The reason for performing ECAT is to maintain a high absorbed dose to the tumor while
decreasing absorbed dose to critical organs, so the therapeutic index should be
higher when combining radioimmunotherapy with ECAT than radioimmunotherapy alone. Values of therapeutic index obtained both from theoretical estimations
and from experiments reported in the literature are given in Table 2.

Reported values on therapeutic characteristics for radioimmunotherapy
with and without ECAT vary considerably, as seen in Table 2. This variation is
due to several factors, but the main reasons are different ECAT systems and
different theoretical models employed. The interval between injection of radioimmunoconjugate and start of ECAT, the choice of critical organ for evaluating
therapeutic index, and the choice of radionuclide for therapy, all will influence
the therapeutic index, as is elucidated in the theoretical models.

A compartmental model describing experimental data on the pharmacokinetics of an antibody labeled to ^{111}In and the removal of activity during ECAT
was developed by Hartman et al. (34). Their simulation of starting time of ECAT
postinjection shows a decrease of percent removed activity with an increased
onset time of ECAT postinjection and the simulation of duration of ECAT shows
increase in percent removed activity with an increase in duration time of ECAT.

Norrgren et al. (33) have constructed a compartmental model from bioki-
netic data to theoretically evaluate the efficacy of ECAT. The model involves
13 compartments and for each compartment the influence of ECAT on the time-
activity curve for an organ is simulated. A simulation of treatment efficiency for

Table 2 Theoretically and Experimentally Obtained Therapeutic Characteristics

Experimental model	Radio-nuclide	Therapeutic characterisitics	Reference
Patients, anti-immunoglobulin system	^{111}In	$\tilde{A}_{blood}$ mean decrease is 21% and 43% (two calculation models)	(29)
Theoretical simulation Extravascular tumor	^{123}I ^{125}I ^{131}I	^{a}T/BM = 8; T/BM$_{ECAT}$ = 7 T/BM = 0; T/BM$_{ECAT}$ = 2 T/BM = 23; T/BM$_{ECAT}$ = 44	(32)
Compartment model Theoretical model	^{211}At ^{90}Y ^{125}I	^{a}T/WB$_{ECAT}$ = 0.8; T/BM$_{ECAT}$ = 0.15 T/WB$_{ECAT}$ = 1.75; T/BM$_{ECAT}$ = 1.25 T/WB$_{ECAT}$ = 0.75; T/BM$_{ECAT}$ = 0.4	(33)
Patients, anti-immunoglobulin system	^{111}In	D$_{BM}$ decreased 29–56% while D$_T$ remained the same with ECAT	(30)

^{a} T/WB: Ratio of absorbed dose to tumor and whole body; T/BM: ratio of absorbed dose to tumor and bone marrow.

different starting times of ECAT shows that the highest ratio of tumor and blood activity is obtained if the starting time for ECAT corresponds to the time for the highest activity uptake in the tumor. Norrgren et al. (33) pointed out that the therapeutic ratio varies depending on which critical organ is chosen, tumor-to-whole-body ratio is, for example, higher than tumor-to-bone-marrow ratio.

DeNardo et al. (27) have done a simulation to optimize adsorption onset time regarding ratio of tumor to blood absorbed dose. From their simulation it is confirmed that blood clearance rate, tumor uptake and clearance rate, and radio-nuclide decay influence the optimal starting time of the adsorption procedure.

Some models show an increase in plasma activity after termination of adsorption (33,34). This increase is probably a redistribution of activity from the extravascular compartment, due to the rapid decline in plasma activity during ECAT. If the duration time of the adsorption is increased, the simulation shows a larger redistribution of activity after end of ECAT procedure (34).

Sgouros (32) has calculated absorbed dose to the tumor as a function of tumor radii, showing that different radionuclides give different homogeneity of absorbed dose. The simulations by Sgouros of radioimmunotherapy in combination with plasmapheresis show for example a very high therapeutic index when ^{125}I is used in a model with a hematologic tumor; however, the absorbed dose in the tumor is highly nonuniform. As almost no absorbed dose is delivered to the central part of the tumor, the efficacy of the therapy will be low.

This understanding indicates the need for microdosimetric considerations rather than using mean absorbed dose. By varying the amount of MAb administered in the simulation, Sgouros shows that a larger amount MAb results in a more uniform absorbed dose profile in the tumor. The latter should be followed by ECAT to decrease the absorbed dose to normal tissues and increase the therapeutic ratio.

V. STUDIES OF EXTRACORPOREAL AFFINITY SYSTEMS ON ANIMALS

Experimental studies with ECAT in animals have been reported by our group. Athymic rats as well as euthymic Brown Norwegian (BN) rats were used in these studies. The athymic rats were inoculated with human melanoma tumor (UMT10) subcutaneously and intramuscularly, or with human lung carcinoma (H2981) intramuscularly and beneath the left kidney capsule. The BN rats were injected intramuscularly and beneath the left kidney capsule with colon carcinoma chemically induced in the same strain. Details of these experiments are published elsewhere (12,35,36).

Three radioiodinated and biotinylated MAbs, murine 96.5, murine L6 or chimeric (chi) BR96, and ^{188}Re or ^{111}In and biotinylated BR96, were employed (12,35–37). Quality control of radiolabeled and biotinylated MAbs included cell binding capacity, the presence of free isotopes in the preparations as well as binding to avidin gel prior to injection (12).

Before ECAT was performed, the animals underwent arterial (a. carotis communis) and venous (v. jugularis) catheterization. In studies of ^{125}I-96.5-biotin and ^{125}I-L6-biotin, the catheters were connected to the ECAT system 24 or 48 h postinjection, and the blood was then pumped through a hollow fiber plasma filter. The separated plasma was passed through the adsorption column, which contained 1 to 1.5 mL of avidin agarose at a flow rate of 0.2 mL/min, and the processed plasma was then mixed with the blood cells and returned via the venous catheter. During a 3-hour treatment three plasma volumes were passed through the column.

There are some appearent disadvantages in using a p-ECAT system in rats—hemolysis during plasma separation, hypervolemic effects, the complexity of tubing connections, and the long time required for preparation. An alternative avenue using ECAT was therefore explored (Fig. 2). This system enables direct adsorption of biotinylated MAb from unseparated blood, and includes only a peristaltic blood pump, an adsorption column, and connecting tubings with a drop chamber. The adsorption column (1.5 mL) contained avidin covalently linked to larger-size agarose beads. Blood was pumped from the arterial catheter through the adsorption column at a flow rate of 1.0 to 1.5 mL/min. The adsorption treatment lasted 2 h.

The rats were divided into a control group (to be given radiolabeled MAb only) and an ECAT group. The p-ECAT was performed 24 h after the injection of ^{125}I-96.5-biotin or ^{125}I-L6-biotin. Wb-ECAT was accomplished 12 h postinjection of ^{125}I-chiBR96-biotin. The difference in timing was dependent on the MAb kinetics and not the selected adsorption technique.

Blood sampling and whole-body imaging were performed immediately after the injection of MAb, just before start of ECAT, immediately after termination of adsorption, and at 48 and 72 h after the injection of MAb. The animals were killed either after termination of the adsorption or 24 h (L6) or 33 h (chiBR96) after completion of the procedure.

At dissection, the tumors as well as several organs (bone marrow, liver, lungs, right kidney, thigh muscles, pancreas, bowel, spleen, stomach, lymph nodes, and thyroid) were removed, weighed, and measured for activity. The activity uptake was expressed in percent of the injected activity per gram tissue (%IA/g), corrected for decay. T/N uptake ratios were based on the %IA/g of tumor and %IA/g of normal tissue.

Immediately after p-ECAT, whole-body activity for ^{125}I-L6-biotin was reduced by 38%. Scintigraphic visualization of implanted tumors in the region of the kidney was greatly improved and was in several cases only possible after ECAT. Approximately 80% to 95% of the circulating plasma activity was removed. The plasma activity was found to increase only slightly during the 24 h following the completion of ECAT. The ECAT procedure improved T/N ratios by a factor of 2.5 to 8.4 (median 3.15) for lungs, and 6.3 to 35.7 (median 12.6) for bone marrow. The reduction of activity in liver, lung, bone marrow, and kidney 24 h after ECAT was more pronounced than that in tumors, so the T/N ratios were still elevated compared with untreated rats at the same time postinjection.

Similar results for BR96 were found for both iodinated and rhenium-labeled and biotinylated BR96. By using wb-ECAT, radioactivity of whole body was reduced by about 50% (Fig. 3) and plasma activity by about 85%. Both directly after completion of wb-ECAT and 33 h later, the displayed activity uptake in tumors was not significantly different from that of control animals ($P > .05$), and had approximately similar time-activity curves. The activity in bone marrow, liver, kidney, lung, pancreas, and bowel directly after completion of wb-ECAT was reduced by 40%. The activity removed by ECAT from normal organs correlated very well with blood content in respective organ (12). Activity uptake ratios after completion of ECAT are shown in Figure 4.

The present studies showed that ECAT was applicable to different MAbs labeled by different isotopes, and resulted in substantially improved tumor-to-normal-tissue ratios.

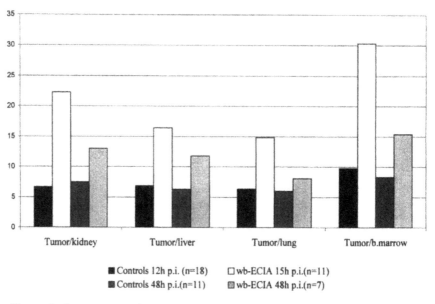

Figure 4 Improvement of tumor-to-normal-organ activity ratios after wb-ECAT in comparison with corresponding controls.

VI. CLINICAL CONSIDERATIONS OF EXTRACORPOREAL TREATMENTS

Extracorporeal systems utilizing immobilized antispecies antibodies has been evaluated for antibody tumor imaging. In 21 patients treated with a device comprising goat antimouse MAbs, there was substantially improved image contrast (9,29,30).

The same technique has been exploited in RIT, albeit to a limited number of patients. By using the goat antimouse antibody adsorption device to remove non-tumor-bound ^{131}I-labeled L6 in the treatment of breast cancer and ^{131}I-labeled Lym-1a monoclonal antibody directed to B-cell lymphoma, De Nardo et al. reported a depletion of 65% to 85% of the activity in total body, whereas tumor radioactivity was not significantly altered (27,38,39).

Hence, the clinical feasibility of the above described procedure has been demonstrated and the predicted reduction in plasma activity and bone marrow absorbed dose has been verified. However, the specificity of this goat antimouse antibody clearly dictates the need for a more general technique which is not limited to the adsorption of antibodies of mouse origin. Principally such adsorbents could be based on immobilized anti-idiotypic antibodies. However, if the concept is going to gain widespread use it is not feasible to develop an affinity adsorption system specific for only a particular type of antibody. This can be circumvented by the labeling of the immunoconjugate with affinity ligands such as biotin.

After administration, the immunoconjugate will gradually begin to metabolize. Any adsorption technique based on immobilized antibodies directed against specific epitopes of the immunoconjugate will depend on the intact structure of the epitope, whereas in the case of removing affinity-labeled antibodies it is sufficient that the cytotoxic moiety is adjacent to at least one of the artificially introduced affinity groups (biotinyl residues). Hence, the cytotoxic moiety can be removed from the blood circulation even if the immunoconjugate is partly metabolized.

This general concept of catching the immunoconjugates independent of their properties could in principle facilitate the use of a cocktail of different monoclonal antibodies directed against different cell surface antigens. These could later be simultaneously removed from the blood circulation with the one and same adsorption device, provided they are all labeled with the very same affinity group.

One major advantage with the use of the combination of biotin/avidin compared to other extracorporeal concepts is its applicability to the processing of whole blood.

A treatment system based on the processing of plasma is quite cumbersome and requires much more advanced equipment than the simpler processing of whole blood. Furthermore, separation of plasma from blood cells through plasma filtration sometimes leads to activation of complement and hemolysis. This is well known in all extracorporeal treatments where plasma separation is used. Hence, all extracorporeal systems based on the processing of plasma require a careful monitoring of infusion of rather large amounts of citrate to the extracorporeal circuit in order to diminish complement activation.

Compatibility with whole-blood processing requires that the immobilized protein does not interact with or activate blood cells and that the binding strength and binding rate constant are sufficiently high. Immobilized antimonoclonal IgG could interact with the F_c receptor of passing immune cells, and the limited binding strength could severely restrict its use in the processing of whole blood, at least when performed at reasonable flow rates. On the contrary, in recent publications (36,40), we have shown that our biotin/avidin concept is also applicable to the processing of whole blood.

Two vascular accesses are mainly needed for an extracorporeal affinity treatment—one for the channeling of blood from the patient to the extracorporeal circuit, and the other for the return of processed blood to the patient. Central vein catheterization is a well-established and widely used procedure to obtain vascular access for extracorporeal treatment. The femoral vein, the subclavian vein, and the external and internal jugular veins have all been utilized for tempo-rary or permanent vascular access. These catheterizations can allow blood flow rates up to 400 mL/min. Citrate and/or heparin are used for anticoagulation of the circuit.

The blood clearance rate is defined as the volume of blood quantitatively depleted of the immunoconjugate per minute, and is expressed as mL/min. In a male patient with a body weight of 75 kg, the blood volume is about 6 L. At a hematocrit of 0.50 the patient has about 3 L of plasma. During a whole-blood adsorption, blood is assumed to be drawn from the patient and passed through the adsorbent at 100 mL/min. At a hematocrit of 0.50, the amount of plasma passing through the adsorbent is 50 mL/min. As the adsorption efficacy is 100%, the blood clearance will be 100 mL/min. In order to process three plasma volumes (9 L), three blood volumes (18 L) has to be processed. The process will require 3 hours of adsorption.

During a plasma adsorption, blood is assumed to be drawn from the patient and passed through the plasma separator at 100 mL/min. As the hematocrit during extracorporeal treatment may not exceed 0.70 in the blood circuit, the maximal tolerable plasma flow rate is 25 mL/min. At this flow rate of blood, the amount of plasma passing through the adsorbent is then 25 mL/min. As the adsorption efficacy is 100%, the blood clearance is 50 mL/min. To process three plasma volumes (9 L), six blood volumes (36 L) has to be processed. The process will require 6 hours of adsorption. Therefore, plasma adsorption will require the dou-ble treatment time, and the processed volume of blood will be two times greater.

VII. SUMMARY AND FUTURE

Extracorporeal immunoadsorption, above all whole-blood ECAT, seems to be a both promising and probably clinically feasible tool for improving absorbed dose ratio for tumor to normal tissues. By using biotinylated MAbs and avidin col-umns, there is no need to develop a new adsorbent for each antibody system used in contrast to the use of antiantibody columns. The time for implementation of ECAT is crucial to its success and can be tailored to each antibody employed as to tumor growth kinetics.

Nonmyeloablative (anti-CD20) RIT is well tolerated and appears to be es-pecially effective at inducing durable remissions in a high proportion of patients with low-grade and transformed non-Hodgkin's lymphoma in whom multiple chemotherapy regimens have failed (41). In the more radioresistant de novo inter-mediate and high-grade non-Hodgkin's lymphoma nonmyeloablative therapy seems not equally successful.

Bone marrow reconstitution, transplantation, or peripheral blood stem cell harvest has made it possible to increase the activity of radiolabeled antibody administered. Signs of radiotoxicity in other organs sensitive to radiation (lungs, kidney, and liver) might then appear. Press et al. (42) have used this approach in treating non-Hodgkin's lymphoma with success, but noted lung toxicity when the lung absorbed dose exceeded 25 Gy. DeNardo et al. have demonstrated that patients tolerated higher activities of ^{131}I Lym-1 with less evidence for myelosupression after immunoadsorption than did patients not having immunoadsorption (43).

As ECAT offers the opportunity of administering higher radioactivity by circumventing toxicity in organs sensitive to radiation, future clinical applications of this procedure might be treatment of the less radiosensitive de novo intermediate and high-grade non-Hodgkin's lymphoma.

Only a small percentage of patients with disseminated solid tumors can be cured with current cytostatic regimens. Because solid tumors are far less sensitive to radiation and show more heterogeneous growth than lymphoma, RIT might only be considered when tumor burden is small. Riethmüller et al. (44) have proven in a randomized study that adjuvant treatment with nonradiolabled MAb 17-1A to patients with colorectal cancer of stage C Dukes' significantly reduced the overall death rate and especially the recurrence rate of distant metastases. The study has now been continued on colorectal carcinoma with proven minimal residual disease in bone marrow.

In light of preceding discussions, RIT might only be considered when the distant cancer metastases show a limited tumor burden, intrinsic radiosensitivity, and feasible antigenic characteristics. In patients with metastases disclosing a fast cell proliferation, repeated RIT and subsequent ECAT with short time intervals (in conjunction with a MAb with fast tumor uptake) should be considered to maintain a high absorbed dose rate in the tumor for a longer time.

The effect of ECAT might be further improved in conjunction with other immunological approaches, e.g., together with cytokines. By combining ECAT with preload (i.e., idiotypic MAb prior to the radiolabeled one), a synergistic improvement of T/N ratios for MAb L6 has been achieved in our experimental model (18).

Buchsbaum et al. (45) have demonstrated that by fractionated RIT a higher concentration of radiolabled MAb was maintained in the tumor periphery for a longer period of time than would have occurred with a single administration. Thus, both absorbed dose and the dose rate were increased in the proliferating portion of the tumor. It might be possible that a prior treatment of radiolabled MAb results, for a later treatment with the same radiolabled MAb, with an accumulation of cells in G2-M phases of the cell cycle (46). By using genetically engineered antibody fragments [preferably (Fab′)$_2$] and thereby achieving rapid tumor targeting, repeated ECAT and MAb injections might be employed to further increase tumor activity as well as tumor dose rates. Even when low immunogenic antibodies in a repeated ECAT strategy are used, there is always a risk of evoking antiantibodies in the host. ECAT might however also offer an opportunity to remove human antimouse, human antichimeric, or human antihuman antibodies by passing the patient's blood through the adsorbent column previously saturated with biotinylated antibody.

ACKNOWLEDGMENTS

This work has been supported by grants from the Swedish Cancer Foundation grants 2353-B95-09XAB, 3635-B96-02XAB; the Gunnar, Arvid and Elisabeth Nilsson Foundation; the Mrs Berta Kamprad Foundation; and the John and Augusta Persson Foundation. The authors would like to express their gratitude to Professor Ingegerd Hellström and Professor Karl Erik Hellström for the gift of MAbs BR96 and L6.

REFERENCES

1. Schreiber GJ, Kerr DE. Strategies to enhance the localization of anticancer immunoconjugates. Curr Med Chem 1995; 2:616–629.
2. Wahl RL, Piko CR, Beers BA, Geatti O, Johnson J, Sherman P. Systemic perfusion: a method of enhancing relative tumor uptake of radiolabeled monoclonal antibodies. J Nucl Med 1987; 28:715.
3. Wahl RL, Piko CR, Beers BA, Geatti O, Johnson J, Sherman P. Systemic perfusion: a method of enhancing reative tumor uptake of radiolabeled monoclonal antibodies. Nucl Med Biol 1988; 15:611–616.
4. Maddock SW, Maddock EN, Quittner SF, Hamstra A, Pastusiak H. Immunoadsorption of circulating monoclonal antibody. In: 7th International Congress of Immunology. New York: Gustav Fisher Verlag, 1989:771.
5. Strand S, Norrgren K, Ingvar C, Erlandsson K, Persson EC. Plasmapheresis as a tool for enhancing contrast in radioimmunoimaging and modifying absorbed doses in radioimmunotherapy. Med Phys 1989; 16:465. Abstract.
6. Bygren P, Freiburghaus C, Lindholm T, Simonsen O, Thysell H, Wieslander J. Goodpasture's syndrome treated with staphylococcal protein-A immunoadsorption. Lancet 1985:1295–1296.
7. Palmer A, Taube DH, Welsh K, Bewick M, Gjorstrup P, Thick M. Removal of anti-HLA antibodies by extracorporeal immunoadsorption to enable renal transplantation. Lancet 1989:10–12.
8. du Moulin A. LDL immunoapheresis technique. In: Gotto AM, Mancini M, Richter WO, Schwandt P, eds. Treatment of Severe Hypercholeserolemia in the Prevention of Coronary Heart Disease. Basel: Karger, 1990:170–174.
9. Lear JL, Kasliwal RK, Feyerabend AJ, Pratt JP, Bunn PA, Dienhart DG, Gonzales R, Johnson TK, Bloedow DC, Maddock SW, Glenn SD. Improved tumor imaging

with radiolabeled monoclonal antibodies by plasma clearance of unbound antibody with anti-antibody column. Radiology 1991; 179:509–512.

10. Dillman RO. Human antimouse and antiglobulin responses to monoclonal antibodies. Antibody Immunoconj Radiopharm 1990; 3:1–9.

11. Riechmann L, Clark M, Waldmann H. Reshaping human antibody for therapy. Nature 1988; 332:323–327.

12. Norrgren K, Strand S, Nilsson R, Lindgren L, Sjögren H. A general extracorporeal immunoadsorption method to increase tumor-to-normal tissue ratio in radioimmunoimaging and radioimmunotherapy. J Nucl Med 1993; 34:448–454.

13. Norrgren K, Strand S, Nilsson R, Lindgren L, Lilliehorn P. Evaluation of extracorporeal immunoadsorption for reduction of the blood background in diagnostic and therapeutic applications of radiolabeled monoclonal antibodies. Antibody Immunoconj Radiopharm 1991; 4:907–914.

14. Breitz HB, Weiden PL, Vanderheyden J, Appelbaum JW, Bjorn MJ, Fer MF, Wolf SB, Ratliff BA, Seiler CA, Foisie DC, Fisher DR, Schroff RW, Fritzberg AR, Abrams PG. Clinical experience with rhenium-186-labeled monoclonal antibodies for radioimmunotherapy: results of phase I trials. J Nucl Med 1992; 33:1099–1112.

15. Camera L, Kinuya S, Garmestani K, Brechbiel MW, Wu C, Pai LH, McCurry TJ, Gansow OA, Pastan I, Paik CH, Carrasquillo JA. Comparative biodistribution of indium and yttrium-labeled B3 monoclonal antibody conjugated to either 1B4M-DTPA or 2B-DOTA. Eur J Nucl Med 1994; 21:640–646.

16. Schuster JM, Garg PK, Bigner DD, Zalutsky MR. Improved therapeutic efficacy of a monoclonal antibody radioiodinated using N-succinimidyl 3-(tri-n-butylstannyl) benzoate. Cancer Res 1991; 51:4164–4169.

17. Srivastava SC. Criteria for the selection of radionuclides for targeting nuclear antigens for cancer radioimmunotherapy. Cancer Biother Radiopharm 1996; 11:43–50.

18. Garkavij M, Tennvall J, Strand S, Norrgren K, Lindgren L, Nilsson R, Sjögren H. Enhanced radioimmunotargeting of 125I-L6-biotin monoclonal antibody (MAb) by combining preload of cold L6 MAb and subsequent immunoadsorption. Cancer Res 1995; 12:5874–5880.

19. Paganelli G, Stella M, Zito F, Magnani P, De Nardi P, Mangili F, Baratti D, Veglia F, Di Carlo V, Siccardi AG, Fazio F. Radioimmunoguided surgery using iodine-125-labeled biotinylated monoclonal antibodies and cold avidin. J Nucl Med 1994; 35:1970–1975.

20. Chen JQ, Strand S, Sjögren HO. Optimization of radioiodination and biotinylation of monoclonal antibody chimeric BR96: an indirect labeling using N-succinimidyl-3-(tri-n-butylstannyl)benzoate conjugate. Cancer Biother Radiopharm. 1996; 11: 217–226.

21. Chen JQ, Strand S, Isaksson M, Ljunggren K, Sjögreen K, Garkavij M, Tennvall J, Sjögren H. Biodistribution and pharmacokinetics of 125-I/131-I pair-labeled, biotinylated chimeric BR96 in colon carcinoma isografted rats. Tumor Targeting 1996; 2:204–214.

22. Chen JQ, Strand S, Brechbiel MW, Gansow OA, Sjögren HO. Combination of biotinylation and indium-111 labeling with chelate SCN-Bz-CHX-A-DTPA for chimeric BR96: biodistribution and pharmacokinetic studies in colon carcinoma isografted rats. Tumor Targeting 1996; 2:66–75.

23. Chen JQ, Strand S, Tennvall J, Hindorf C, Sjögren H. Biodistribution and pharmaco-kinetics of biotinylated 188Re-chiBR96 in colon carcinoma isografted rats. Tumor Targeting 1998; 3:87–95.

24. Mock DM, Malik MI. Distribution of biotin in human plasma: most of the biotin is not bound to protein. Am J Clin Nutr 1992; 56:427–432.

25. Heard GS, Grier RE, Weiner DL, Secor McVoy JR, Wolf B. Biotinidase—possible mechanism for the recycling of biotin. Ann NY Acad Sci 1985; 447:400.

26. Wolf SB, Hymes J, Heard GS. Biotinidase. Methods Enzymol 1990; 184:103–111.

27. DeNardo GL, Maddock SW, Sgouros G, Scheibe PO, DeNardo SJ. Immunoadsorption: an enhancement strategy for radioimmunotherapy. J Nucl Med 1993; 34:1020–1027.

28. Loevinger R, Budinger TF, Watson EE. In: MIRD Primer for Absorbed Dose Calculations. New York: Society of Nuclear Medicine, MIRD, 1991.

29. Johnson TK, Maddock SW, Kasliwal R, Bloedow DC, Hartmann C, Feyerabend A, Dienhart DG, Thickman D, Glenn S, Gonzales R, Lear J, Bunn PA. Radioimmunoadsorption of KC-4G3 antibody in peripheral blood: implications for radioimmunotherapy. Antibody Immunoconj Radiopharm 1991; 4:885–893.

30. Dienhart DG, Kasliwal R, Lear JL, Johnson TK, Bloedow DC, Hartmann C, Seligman PA, Miller GJ, Glenn SD, McAteer MJ, Thickman D, Feyerabend A, Maddock EN, Maddock SW, Bunn PA. Extracorporeal immunoadsorption of radiolabeled monoclonal antibody: a method for reduction of background radioactivity and its potential role during the radioimmunotherapy of cancer. Antibody Immunoconj Radiopharm 1994; 7:225–252.

31. Schindhelm K. Transport and kinetics in synthetic and immunospecific adsorption columns. Artif Organs 1989; 13:21–27.

32. Sgouros G. Plasmapheresis in radioimmunotherapy of micrometastases: a mathematical modeling and dosimetrical analysis. J Nucl Med 1992; 33:2167–2179.

33. Norrgren K, Strand S, Ingvar C. Contrast enhancement in RII and modification of the therapeutic ratio in RIT: a theoretical evaluation of simulated extracorporeal immunoadsorption. Antibody Immunoconj Radiopharm 1992; 5:61–73.

34. Hartmann C, Bloedow DC, Dienhart DG, Kasliwal R, Johnson TK, Gonzales R, Bunn PA. A pharmacokinetic model describing the removal of circulating radiolabeled antibody by extracorporeal immunoadsorption. J Pharm Biopharm 1997; 19: 385–403.

35. Garkavij M, Tennvall J, Norrgren K, Nilsson R, Strand S, Lindgren L, Sjögren H. Improving radioimmunotargeting of tumors: variation in the amounts of MAb L6 combined with an immunoadsorption system. Acta Oncol 1993; 32:853–859.

36. Garkavij M, Tennvall J, Strand S, Sjögren H, Chen JQ, Nilsson R, Isaksson M. Extracorporeal whole blood immunoadsorption enhances radioimmunotargeting of 125-I-labeled BR96-biotin monoclonal antibody in syngeneic rat tumor model. J Nucl Med 1997; 38:895–901.

37. Chen JQ, Strand S, Tennvall J, Lindgren L, Hindorf C, Sjögren HO. Extracorporeal immunoadsorption vs. avidin "chase" to enhance tumor-to-normal tissue ratio for biotinylated 188Re-chiBR96. J Nucl Med 1997; 38:1934–1939.

38. DeNardo GL, DeNardo SJ, Maddock SW, Zeiter PC, Maddock EN, Matthews KJ.

Efficacy of immunophoresis to reduce myelosuppression in radioimmunotherapy. J Nucl Med 1992; 33:863–864.

39. DeNardo SJ, O'Grady LF, Warhoe KA, Kroger LA, Hellstrom I, Hellstrom KE, Maddock SW, DeNardo GL. Radioimmunotherapy in patients with metastatic breast cancer. J Nucl Med 1992; 33:862–863.

40. Garkavij M, Tennvall J, Strand S, Nilsson R, Chen JQ, Lindgren L, Isaksson M, Eriksson H, Sjögren H. Extracorporeal immunoadsorption (ECIA) from whole-blood based on avidin-biotin concept: evaluation of a new method. Acta Oncol 1996; 53: 309–312.

41. Kaminski MS, Zasadny KR, Francis IR, Fenner MC, Ross CW, Milik AW, Estes J, Tuck M, Regan D, Fisher S, Glenn SD, Wahl RL. Iodine-131-anti-B1 radioimmunotherapy for B-cell lymphoma. J Clin Oncal 1996; 14:1974–1981.

42. Press OW, Eary JF, Appelbaum FR, Martin PJ, Nelp WB, Glenn S, Fisher DR, Porter B, Matthews DC, Gooley T, Bernstein ID. Phase II trial of 131-I-B1 (anti-CD20) antibody therapy with autologous stem cell transplantation for relapsed B cell lymphomas. Lancet 1995; 346:336–340.

43. DeNardo GL, DeNardo SJ. Treatment of B-lymphocyte malignancies with 131-I-Lym-1 and 67CU-2IT-BAT-Lym-1 and opportunities for improvement. In: Goldenberg DM, ed. Cancer Therapy with Radiolabeled Antibodies. Boca Raton, FL: CRC Press, 1995:217–227.

44. Rietmuller G, Schneider-Gedäcke E, Schlimok G, Schmiegel W, Raab R, Höffken K, Gruber R, Pichlmaier H, Hirche H, Pichlmayr R, Buggisch P, Witte J. Randomised trial of monoclonal antibody for adjuvant therapy of resected Dukes' C colorectal carcinoma. Lancet 1994; 343:1177–1183.

45. Buchsbaum DJ, Khazaeli MB, Liu T, Bright S, Richardson K, Jones M, Meredith RF. Fractionated radioimmunotherapy of human colon carcinoma xenografts with 131-I-labeled monoclonal antibody CC49. Cancer Res 1995; 55:5881–5887.

46. Meredith RF, Khazaeli MB, Liu T, Plott G, Wheeler RH, Russel C, Colcher D, Schlom J, Schochat D, LoBuglio AF. Dose fractionation of radiolabeled antiodies in patients with metastatic colon cancer. J Nucl Med 1992; 33:1648–1653.

10

Radioimmunotherapy in the Treatment of Non-Hodgkin's Lymphoma

Monica S. Krieger
Corixa Corporation, Seattle, Washington

Paul L. Weiden and Hazel B. Breitz
Virginia Mason Medical Center, Seattle, Washington

O. Press
University of Washington and Fred Hutchinson Cancer Research Center, Seattle, Washington

G. L. DeNardo
University of California, Davis, California

I. INTRODUCTION

Non-Hodgkin's lymphoma (NHL) is a worldwide health problem. In the United States, approximately 250,000 individuals are afflicted with 56,800 new cases diagnosed annually. Since the early 1970s the incidence of the disease has nearly doubled, although the rate of increase appears to be slowing (1).

Many types of non-Hodgkin's lymphomas have been defined based on the type of cancer cells. Over the years, different classification systems have been used. The commonly used systems group lymphoma by cell type and rate of growth into three categories: highly aggressive, aggressive, and indolent.

Prognosis and treatment options are directly related to aggressiveness of the disease. Combination chemotherapy is curative for 30% to 50% of patients with advanced-stage, aggressive non-Hodgkin's lymphoma. These patients, however, account for only 5% of the patient population. In contrast, few patients with low-grade lymphoma and less than half of those with intermediate-grade lymphomas are cured with combination chemotherapy. Despite some improvements in treatment, median survival is only 9 years.

Immunotherapy with monoclonal antibodies may be a useful alternative or adjunct to chemotherapy or radiation therapy in the management of NHL. Unconjugated, tumor-specific monoclonal antibodies, or tumor-specific antibodies conjugated to a radionuclide or other cytotoxic agent can be used to target tumor cells. This chapter will provide a history of the use of unconjugated monoclonal antibodies, but focus on the use of radioimmunoconjugates to treat patients with non-Hodgkin's lymphoma. Data published in abstract form, as well as in published papers, will be included to provide a current picture of this evolving field.

II. UNMODIFIED MONOCLONAL ANTIBODIES

In 1975, Kohler and Milstein published their report describing the production of monoclonal antibodies (MAbs) by hybridomas (2). Within a few years, monoclonal antibodies were developed that bound to the surface of malignant, hematopoietic cells. Clinical investigators hypothesized that these antibodies could be used to target and destroy malignant cells. The rationale for employing unconjugated monoclonal antibodies in cancer therapy depends on (a) lysis of tumor cells via complement-mediated cytotoxicity (CMC) or antibody-dependent, cell-mediated cytotoxicity (ADCC), or (b) induction of apoptosis.

Based on these hypotheses, a number of Phase I studies were conducted evaluating murine monoclonal antibodies for treatment of patients with hematologic malignancies. The majority of the patients enrolled on the studies were refractory to prior chemotherapeutic regimens. Despite this patient history, some patients achieved a response after treatment with a monoclonal antibody. However, as the summary of the results below and the data in Table 1 illustrate, clinical results were largely disappointing.

A. Clinical Results with Murine Monoclonal Antibodies

In 1979, the first patient was treated with a monoclonal antibody directed against a lymphoma-associated antigen (3). In vitro studies demonstrated that this antibody (Ab 89) could mediate complement-dependent lysis and macrophage adherence, but not ADCC. A transient decrease in the number of circulating tumor cells and the appearance of circulating dead cells after infusion were reported.

Over the next 12 years, articles were published that described the use of monoclonal antibodies directed again various antigens (4–7). These studies were small, Phase I/II studies investigating the safety and efficacy of single or multi-dose infusion of antibodies. The toxicities observed were minimal. Although a

Table 1 Clinical Results Using Murine Monoclonal Antibodies in Non-Hodgkin's Lymphoma

Author	No. patients treated	Antibody	HAMA reported	Outcome/ response	Median duration of response
Nadler (3)	1	AB89	NR	Decrease in tumor cells	N/A
Press (4)	4	IF5	25%	1 PR	6 weeks
Hekman (5)	6	LLB	0	1 PR, 1 MR	6 months[a]
Hu (6)	10	Lym-1	0	3 MR	N/A
Scheinberg (7)	18	OKB7	28%	No responses	N/A
Meeker (8,9)	11	Anti-idiotype	45%	1 CR, 4 PR,	4 months
Brown (9)	11	Anti-idiotype + interferon	0	2 CR, 7 PR	7 months

Note: NR = not reported; N/A = not applicable.
[a] One patient was treated twice. The first remission was 3 months in length and the second was 6 months.

decrease in the number of circulating tumor cells was observed in all the studies, clinical responses were generally minor, experienced by few of the patients, and brief in duration. The studies provided some useful information regarding pharmokinetics, antibody localization, and the percentage of patients in whom the antibody elicited a response to human antimouse antibody.

The most successful results with tumor-specific, anti-idiotypic antibodies were those obtained by Ronald Levy and his coworkers (8). In the initial study, they reported treating patients with B-lymphocytic malignancy with murine monoclonal anti-idiotype antibodies prepared against the patient's own tumor. A subsequent study added treatment with alpha interferon in combination with the anti-idiotype antibody based on its known independent activity in follicular NHL and its synergistic activity with anti-idiotype antibodies in a murine lymphoma model (9). Substantial tumor regressions occurred with minimal toxicity in both trials, even in patients refractory to conventional chemotherapy. These responses continued to occur months after treatment, suggesting to the authors that the antibodies altered the idiotype-anti-idiotype network involved in the regulation of B-cell clones.

Levy and his colleagues encountered two obstacles in the treatment of patients. First, the presence of serum idiotype prevented murine antibody from reaching the lymph nodes, despite plasmapharesis and large doses of antibody. Second, an immune response to mouse Ig occurred in five of the 11 patients in the first study. Once an immune response was detected, additional infusions of antibody did not result in tumor response.

Taken together, these studies provided preliminary evidence for the clinical utility and lack of significant toxicity associated with the use of monoclonal antibodies. These results also illuminated some of the problems encountered in using murine monoclonal antibodies as therapeutic agents. Conceptually the use of monoclonal antibodies to kill malignant hematopoietic cells seemed very simple. In fact, the execution of this treatment was difficult to implement and the results were disappointing. The obstacles encountered included the following.

1. Difficulty in delivering the monoclonal antibody to the tumor. These difficulties were related to the fact that monoclonal antibodies are substantially larger than drugs generally used as chemotherapeutic agents. Consequently, the antibodies may have difficulty penetrating to sites of bulky disease. In addition, circulating tumor cells often bound to the antibody leading to rapid clearance from circulation.

2. Inability to exert cytotoxic effects. Classes and subclasses of monoclonal antibodies differed in their ability to activate complement and human effector cells. Murine IgM monoclonal antibodies were most effective in mediating cytotoxicity with human complement (10). In contrast, murine antibodies of the IgG_{2a} and IgG_3 type were most effective in mediating antibody-dependent, cell-mediated cytotoxicity (11).

3. HAMA responses. HAMA responses occurred in some patients, despite the fact that patients were immunosuppressed because of their disease and extensive chemotherapy. Although the clinical sequelae of a HAMA response was usually minor, treatment with multiple doses was precluded because of enhanced clearance of the antibody from circulation.

4. Antigen-negative cells. Antigen-negative variant cells arose during treatment and became the dominant cell type in the tumor, effectively rendering the tumor refractory to further therapy.

An understanding of these problems has helped clinical investigators to develop rational approaches to using monoclonal antibodies, human chimeric antibodies, and radioimmunoconjugates.

B. Clinical Results with Chimeric or Humanized Monoclonal Antibodies

Early studies indicated that murine monoclonal antibodies interacted poorly with human effector cells and complement. Consequently, investigators tried to enhance the antibody-effector interactions using chimeric and humanized monoclonal antibodies. A number of studies have been performed in patients with of non-Hodgkin's lymphoma; these studies are summarized below and in Table 2.

One of the first studies to suggest that genetically engineered antibodies might have an important use in the treatment of lymphoproliferative disorders

Table 2 Clinical Results Using Chimeric Monoclonal Antibodies in Non-Hodgkin's Lymphoma

Author	No. patients treated	Antibody	HAMA or HACA reported	Outcome/ response	Median duration of response
Hale (12)	2	CAMPATH-1H	None	Depletion of B cells	N/A
Maloney (15)	15	C2B8	None	2 PR, 4 MR	8.5 months
Maloney (16)	18	C2B8	None	6 PR, 5 MR	6.4 months
Maloney (17)	34	C2B8	None	3 CR, 14 PR	8.6 months
McLaughlin (18)	165	C2B8	<1%	10 CR, 70 PR	13 months[a]
Czucman (19)	40	C2B8 + CHOP	None	22 CR, 16 PR	Not reached

N/A = not applicable.
[a] Projected median time to progression.

was reported using genetically reshaped, human IgG_1 monoclonal antibody (CAMPATH-1H) to treat two patients with non-Hodgkin's lymphoma (12). Results were similar to those obtained with murine monoclonal antibodies; lymphoma cells were cleared from the blood and bone marrow in both patients.

The most successful clinical trials to date with a chimeric antibody were those conducted with an antibody directed against the B-cell antigen CD20 (C2B8, Rituxan). The CD20 B-lymphocyte surface antigen is expressed on almost all-mature B lymphocytes and on 95% of B-cell malignancies. The antigen plays a role in B-cell differentiation, B-cell cycle progression, and transmembrane channeling of calcium (13). There is no shedding of the antigen into circulation, and the antigen is not internalized after binding of the antibody. Most importantly, the antigen is not expressed on stem cells.

In vitro studies showed the ability of C2B8 to bind human C1q, mediate complement-dependent cell lysis of human B-lymphoid cell lines, and lyse human target cells through ADCC (14). In addition, the chimeric C2B8 antibody was significantly less immunogenic than murine monoclonal antibody in primates and humans.

The safety and efficacy of the chimeric antibody were evaluated in three studies of patients with relapsed low-grade B-cell lymphoma. One study evaluated a single dose of C2B8 antibody (15) and the other two evaluated four weekly doses (16,17). In all studies there were some treatment-related symptoms during infusion; however, no serious toxicity was reported. CD20+ B cells were rapidly and specifically depleted in the peripheral blood and generally remained depleted for at least 2 to 3 months. Toxicities were reversible and responses were observed even in heavily pretreated patients and those with bulky disease.

One hundred sixty-six patients were enrolled and 165 were treated in a multi-institutional trial for patients with relapsed, low-grade, or follicular lymphoma (18). The overall response rate of the intent-to-treat group was 48%, of which 6% were complete responses; the remainder were partial responses. The median follow-up duration was 11.8 months at the time of publication with a projected median time to progression for responders of 13.0 months. These efficacy data are similar to results seen with chemotherapy.

Based on the safety and efficacy observed during these studies the FDA approved Rituxan for marketing. Thus, C2B8 became the first antibody to be marketed for treatment of cancer in the United States and Europe, as well as the first new, single-agent biologic product marketed for treatment of non-Hodgkin's lymphoma in a decade.

Additional studies were conducted to evaluate the benefits obtained by combining Rituxan with conventional chemotherapy or other biological agents. The rationale for these studies was that the combination might take advantage of the low toxicity and independent activity of Rituxan and provide a synergy to improve outcome. Forty patients with NHL were enrolled and given multiple cycles of Rituxan and CHOP (19). There was an overall response rate of 95% in the intent-to-treat population, with 22 (55%) of the patients achieving a complete response and a median time to progression of 21.1 months. These results suggest that the combination of Rituxan with chemotherapy may provide significantly improved rates of response.

Over 15,000 patients have been treated with Rituxan. Although no serious toxicities were reported during the clinical studies, there have subsequently been at least eight deaths. In seven of the eight fatalities, severe symptoms occurred during the first infusion of Rituxan (20). In most cases, death was preceded by severe bronchospasm, dyspnea, hypotension, and/or angioedema.

III. RADIOLABELED MONOCLONAL ANTIBODIES

The effectiveness of monoclonal antibodies in the treatment of cancer may be significantly improved by conjugating the monoclonal antibodies with radionuclides, drugs, or toxins. The use of radioimmunotherapy (RIT) has proven to be effective in the treatment of patients with NHL for three reasons: the sensitivity of lymphocytes to radiation; the large number of target antigens on the surface of lymphocytes; and the vascular accessibility of the malignancies.

Radioimmunoconjugates possess two advantages over unconjugated monoclonal antibodies. First, they do not rely on the immune system to kill tumor cells. This is important since patients with cancer often have suppressed or defective immune systems. Second, the beta particles emitted by decaying radioactivity have an effect over several cell diameters. This results in "crossfire" from the antigen-positive cells and killing of neighboring antigen-negative cells.

A number of clinical trials have been performed involving various radioimmunoconjugates. Generally, targeting radiation to pan B-cell differentiation antigens, such as CD19, CD20, and CD22, has proven the most effective in clinical trials. These target antigens are expressed in high density and with high reliability on target cells. Approximately 99% of B-cell lymphomas express CD19, 95% express CD20, and 70% express CD22.

The choice of the radionuclide has also varied. Most of the evaluations have used either ^{131}I-labeled or ^{90}Y-labeled antibody. In addition, there have been several studies conducted by DeNardo and colleagues evaluating ^{67}Cu-labeled antibody (21–23). There is currently no consensus on which of these radionuclides is optimal (see Table 3). Yttrium-90 may be the best option for the following reasons:

    1. ^{131}I-labeled conjugates are degraded after internalization into tumor cells, resulting in free ^{131}I and ^{131}I-tyrosine circulating in the blood stream.

    2. The gamma rays emitted by ^{131}I may require isolation of the patient to prevent possible risks to family members and health care personnel.

    3. ^{67}Cu is a novel radionuclide that is not yet routinely available in adequate quantities for RIT. Commercial production would require adequate clinical demand.

    4. An analysis of the emission properties and decay mode of ^{90}Y-labeled antibody implies that tumors will be exposed to a higher dose of radiation that is more homogeneous in distribution.

The disadvantages of ^{90}Y are that it cannot be used for radioimmunoscintigraphy due to the absence of gamma radiation and it is more expensive than ^{131}I. However, ^{111}In can be used as a surrogate for ^{90}Y for imaging purposes, based on the assumption that its biodistribution will mimic that of ^{90}Y. In addition, the cost differential may be offset since the hospitalization time required is significantly shorter for patients treated with ^{90}Y.

Table 3 Comparison of Radionuclide Candidates

	Iodine-131	Yttrium-90	Copper-67
E_{max} beta (MeV)	0.81	2.27	0.57
Half-life (hours)	193	64	62
Mean range of β particles (mm)	0.40	2.8	0.27
Path length over which 90% of energy is absorbed (mm)	0.8	5.3	0.6
Relative rads/mCi	1[a]	5	1
Imageability	Yes	No	Yes
Specific activity	High	High	High

[a] Based on beta particle emissions.
Source: Ref. 47.

Traditionally, antibodies are conjugated directly to the radionuclide to form a radioimmunoconjugate. The sections below summarize results obtained with radioimmunoconjugates and are divided based on whether or not hematopoietic stem cell support was required. Recently, an approach has been evaluated where the radioactivity is decoupled from the antibody (see Pretarget technology below). Preliminary data using this Pretarget technology for patients with B-cell lymphomas will also be presented.

A. Radioimmunotherapy Without Stem Cell Support: Directly Labeled Conjugates

Those radiolabeled antibodies that have progressed the furthest toward clinical use include two anti-CD20 antibodies and a ^{131}I-labeled Lym-1 antibody. Clinical results obtained with these antibodies are summarized in Tables 4, 5 and 6.

B. Anti-CD20 Antibodies

There are two products in the late stages of development; one uses the antibody named anti-B1, while the other uses Y2B8.

C. Use of Radiolabeled Antibody: Anti-B1

Kaminski and colleagues at the University of Michigan (24) conducted a Phase I dose escalation trial to assess the toxicity and efficacy of nonmyeloablative doses of an anti-CD20 monoclonal antibody (anti-B1) labeled with iodine-131 (Bexxar, Coulter Pharmaceutical). Patients were administered a diagnostic dose and then a radioimmunotherapeutic dose predicted by the diagnostic dose. Sequential groups of patients were treated with whole-body radiation doses escalating in 10-cGy increments from 25 to 85 cGy. In an attempt to reduce normal, antigen-specific binding each dose of radiolabeled antibody was preceded by an infusion of unlabeled anti-B1 antibody in most patients.

Treatment was well tolerated; however, hematologic toxicity was dose limiting with 75 cGy being the maximally tolerated whole-body radiation dose. Twenty-eight of the 34 patients completed treatment; 79% achieved a response and 50% achieved a complete response (CR). The median duration of response was 357 days for all patients and 471 days for those patients who reached a complete response. Sixteen of 17 patients who achieved a response of 6 months or more in duration remain alive 6 years after treatment (25).

Based on the low toxicity and the clinical results, a trial was designed to evaluate the ^{131}I-labeled anti-B1 antibody in NHL patients (26). The study included 60 NHL patients who were refractory to chemotherapy. The primary clinical end point was the comparison between the patient's duration of remission on

Table 4 Clinical Results Using Radiolabeled Monoclonal Antibodies in Non-Hodgkin's Lymphoma

Author	No. patients treated	Antibody isotope	HAMA reported	Responses	Median duration of response
Without stem cell transplant					
Kaminski (24,48)	28	B1 [131]I	34%	14 CR, 8 PR	12 months >16.5 months if CR > than with previous chemotherapy
Kaminski (26)	60	B1 [131]I	5%	10 CR 30 PR	7 months
Knox (27)	18	B1 and YB8 [90]Y	22%	6 CR 7 PR	11.7 + months (projected)
Wiseman (29)	49	Y2B8 [90]Y	Not reported	13 CR 23 PR	
DeNardo (35)	25[a]	LYM-1 [131]I	30%[b]	3 CR 11 PR	18 months
DeNardo (36)	20[c]	LYM-1 [131]I	35%	7 CR 4 PR	14 months
With stem cell transplant					
Press (39)	19	B1, 1F5, and MB-1 [131]I	16%	16 CR, 2 PR	18 months
Press (41)	21	B1 [131]I	33%	17 CR[d], 1 PR	38 months

[a] 25 with NHL; 5 patients with CLL; and 3 additional patients.
[b] After multiple doses of Lym-1.
[c] One of these patients was entered twice. On the second occasion, the patient had another complete remission of 18.5 months' duration.
[d] The publication reports 16 patients achieved a CR; one patient converted from a PR to a CR after publication (42).

Table 5 Comparison of the Radiation Dose Delivered (cGy/mCi): Direct Targeting vs Pretarget (mean ± SEM)

Target	Direct targeting			Pretarget lymphoma ^{90}Y-labeled (n = 9)
	^{131}I anti-CD20 (47) (n = 7)	^{90}Y anti-CD20 (27) (n = 18)	Lym-1 (23) (n = 20)	
Tumors	10.6 ± 2.8[a]	26.9 ± 46.3	3.9 ± 2.6	28.7 ± 32.4
Whole body	0.7 ± 0.5	1.5 ± 0.8	0.4 ± 0.1	0.7 ± 0.1
Blood	4.1 ± 0.5	9.2 ± 4.8	Not reported	Not reported
Marrow	Not reported	Not reported	0.4 ± 0.1	0.3 ± 0.3
Kidneys	5.2 ± 0.5	Not reported	2.3 ± 0.9	4.8 ± 0.3
Liver	2.5 ± 0.1	9.9 ± 6.0	1.4 ± 0.3	1.5 ± 0.1
Lung	2.5 ± 0.3	Not reported	2.0 ± 0.4	0.6 ± 0.1
Spleen	5.2 ± 0.9	31.7 ± 54.0	2.2 ± 1.0	4.3 ± 0.3

[a] Reported as best tumor.

Table 6 Response to Treatment of Patients Treated with Pretarget Lymphoma

Patient no.	Total dose ^{90}Y (dose in mCi/m^2)	Response
9802.003	101 mCi	Nodes decreased >50%
	50 mCi/m^2	Abdominal mass decreased 30%
9802.004	57 mCi	Nodes decreased >50%
	30 mCi/m^2	One nodal mass increased
9802.005	51 mCi	CR by CT at 12 weeks
	30 mCi/m^2	
9806.001	109 mCi	90% decrease in tumor at 8 weeks
	50 mCi/m^2	
9806.002	93 mCi	80% decrease in tumor at 6 weeks
	50 mCi/m^2	
9806.003	86 mCi	CR at 10 weeks
	50 mCi/m^2	
9806.004	86 mCi	Progressive disease
	50 mCi/m^2	

[131]I-labeled antibody and the duration of remission on the patient's last chemotherapy.

The duration of response after treatment was not equivalent (>30 days difference) for 41 of the 60 patients. Eighty-one percent of the patients experienced a longer duration of response to ^{131}I-labeled antibody compared to only 19% who experienced a longer duration of response to prior chemotherapy ($P <$ .001). In addition, a response was observed in only 28% of patients following their last chemotherapy regimen compared to 67% of patients responding following a regimen of ^{131}I-labeled antibody ($P <$ .001).

D. Use of Radiolabeled Antibody: Anti-2B8

Knox and colleagues performed a Phase I/II dose escalation study of ^{90}Y-labeled murine anti-CD20 monoclonal antibody (2B8, IDEC Pharmaceutical) in patients with recurrent B-cell lymphoma (27). The primary objectives of the study were to determine the effect of infusing unlabeled antibody prior to labeled antibody and the maximum-tolerated dose as well as evaluate the safety and efficacy. Eighteen patients were treated; of these, 13 were treated with ^{90}Y-labeled anti-2B8 antibody, and five were treated with ^{90}Y-labeled anti-B1 antibody. Prior to treatment, biodistribution studies were conducted with ^{111}In-labeled antibody.

Groups of three or four patients were treated at escalating dose levels increasing from 13.5 to 50 mCi ^{90}Y anti-CD20 monoclonal antibody. The only significant toxicity was myelosuppression. Two of the patients receiving the 50-mCi dose required infusion of previously collected stem cells. The overall response rate following a single dose of therapy was 72%, with six complete responses and seven partial responses. Time to progression ranged from 3 to 29 months after treatment. These investigators also evaluated the use of unlabeled antibody prior to administration of the labeled antibody. Known sites of disease were visualized more easily, and the projected dose of radiation to the spleen and spine was decreased with preadministration of unlabeled antibody.

A subsequent, Phase I/II study evaluated the safety and efficacy of treatment with IDEC-Y2B8 in 50 patients with low- or intermediate-grade and mantle cell NHL (28–30). The amount of ^{90}Y-labeled antibody was dose-escalated from 0.2 mCi/kg to 0.4 mCi/kg. Adverse events were primarily hematologic, transient, and reversible. The overall response rate was 67% and the median time to progression for patients who responded was 12.9 months.

E. Use of Radiolabeled Antibody Lym-1

Lym-1 is a novel murine monoclonal antibody that recognizes a 31- to 35-kD antigen initially characterized as an HLA-DR variant (31). Additional studies isolating the Lym-1 antigen from Raji cell lysate led to the conclusion that the epitope is in the β-chain of HLA-DR10 (32). This antigen is expressed on the surface of malignant B-cells, but less so on normal lymphocytes (31,32). Consequently, only small amounts of Lym-1 were required for optimal lymphoma targeting.

Although *in vitro* studies indicated significant antitumor activity of Lym-1 against lymphoma cell lines, the unmodified antibody had little therapeutic effectiveness *in vivo* (6). Lym-1 was actually the first monoclonal antibody to be used as a radioimmunoconjugate to treat NHL. A patient with Richter's syndrome was treated in a compassionate-use protocol (33). This patient received a series of injections of ^{131}I-labeled Lym-1 that resulted in a dramatic clinical response including reduction of tumor volume and progression of circulating cellular elements toward normality.

Based on the response of this patient, the investigators proceeded to investigate the safety and efficacy of radiolabeled Lym-1 in other patients with advanced disease. Most of the other investigators evaluating radiolabeled antibodies have administered a single dose of radiolabeled antibody. DeNardo and colleagues decided to take the alternative approach of dividing the dose into multiple fractions (34). Their rationale for this approach was based on evidence that fractionated RIT increased the amount of radiation that could be safely administered.

Thirty patients, 25 with NHL and 5 with CLL, were treated using a series of low doses (35). Based on dosimetric studies, the investigators determined that a cumulative dose of 300 mCi (1200 rads) would be acceptable. Initially, the patients received doses of 30 mCi at 4-to-6-week intervals. Subsequently, the patients received 60-mCi doses at shorter intervals. Eleven of the 30 patients received the intended dose of 300 mCi. Nonhematologic toxicities were generally mild, with thrombocytopenia being the dose-limiting toxicity. The overall response rates were 57% for all eligible patients of all histologic grades and 94% for those patients who received >180 mCi.

A second study was designed to define the maximum-tolerated dose (MTD) and efficacy of at least the first two, of a maximum of four, doses of ^{131}I-Lym-1 given 4 weeks apart (36). Twenty patients with advanced NHL resistant to standard therapy, one of whom was treated twice, entered the study. Dose-limiting toxicity was thrombocytopenia at an MTD of 100 mCi/m^2 for each of the first two doses. Seven patients achieved a complete response with a mean duration of 14 months. All three patients treated at the MTD level had complete remissions.

DeNardo and colleagues have also used Lym-1 antibody radiolabeled with [67]Cu in 11 patients with advanced-stage lymphoma. (21) Patients were given unmodified Lym-1 followed by an imaging dose of 3.4 to 14.4 mCi [67]Cu-labeled Lym-1. In seven patients with superficial tumors that had been accurately measured, tumors regressed a mean of 48% within several days of infusion of the radiolabeled antibody. The mean ratio of the radiation dose was 32:1 for tumor to marrow, 24:1 for tumor to total body, and 1.5:1 for tumor to liver. The investigators concluded that high therapeutic ratios were achieved because of the long residence time of the radiolabeled antibody.

In a subsequent study, four patients received both ^{67}Cu- and ^{131}I-labeled Lym-1 to compare the two radiopharmaceuticals (22). The mean tumor concentration of ^{67}Cu-labeled Lym-1 was up to 2.8 times that of ^{131}I Lym-1. These results in combination with the longer half-life and lower radiation dose to the marrow of ^{67}Cu-labeled Lym-1 resulted in tumor-to-marrow therapeutic indices that were much higher for the ^{67}Cu-labeled Lym-1 than the ^{131}I Lym-1 (29 and 9.7, respectively). Thus, DeNardo and colleagues suggest that ^{67}Cu-labeled Lym-1 may be superior to ^{131}I-labeled Lym-1 for RIT.

Of particular interest is a retrospective analysis performed by these investigators evaluating dosimetric, pharmacokinetic, and other treatment-related parameters as predictors of patient outcome (37). Results were analyzed for 57 patients (52 with NHL and 5 with chronic lymphocytic leukemia, all heavily pretreated) treated with radiolabeled Lym-1 antibody. Logistic regression and proportional hazards models were used to evaluate treatment parameters for their ability to predict outcome. Two factors predicted improved survival: the occurrence of a complete or partial response, and the development of HAMA. Although the sample size is small, these results suggest that even patients who are heavily pretreated may benefit from treatment with radioimmunotherapy, and development of HAMA does not preclude treatment.

IV. HIGH-DOSE RIT AS A SINGLE AGENT WITH STEM CELL SUPPORT

A preliminary study by Press et al. (38) tested the effects of high-dose radiolabeled monoclonal antibody administered in conjunction with marrow transplantation for treatment of lymphoma. Four patients were treated with ^{131}I-labeled antibody (MB-1) estimated to deliver 380 to 1570 cGy to normal organs and 850 to 4260 cGy to tumor. Myelosuppression occurred in all patients. Complete tumor regressions were observed in all four patients.

A few years later, Press and colleagues (39) evaluated biodistribution, toxicity, and efficacy of two anti-CD20 antibodies (B1 and 1F5) and one anti-CD37 antibody (MB-1) labeled with ^{131}I in 43 patients with relapsed B-cell lymphoma. Sequential biodistribution studies were performed with escalating doses of trace-labeled antibody. Serial gamma camera imaging and tumor biopsies were used to estimate the doses of radiation absorbed by tumors and normal organs. Patients with a higher dose to tumor than to normal organs were eligible for therapeutic infusion. Twenty-four patients were eligible for therapeutic infusion, and 19 received therapeutic infusions of 234 to 777 mCi ^{131}I-labeled antibodies. Fifteen of the patients required autologous marrow reinfusion. Toxicities were moderate for patients who received <27 Gy to normal organs. Two of the four patients who received >27 Gy developed reversible cardiopulmonary toxicity. Of the 19 patients treated, complete remissions were in obtained in 16; eight of these patients were still in complete remission at 46 to 95 months after therapy (40).

Based on the results above, Press and colleagues (41) evaluated treatment with the maximum-tolerated dose (25 to 27 Gy) of radioactivity. Twenty-five patients with relapsed B-cell lymphomas were evaluated with trace-labeled doses and 22 patients achieved biodistributions considered adequate to receive a therapeutic infusion. Twenty-one patients were treated with therapeutic infusions of ^{131}I-B1 antibody calculated to deliver not more than 25 to 27 Gy to normal organs followed by autologous hematopoietic stem cell reinfusion. Of these 21 patients, 17 (81%) eventually achieved complete remission. The median duration of response in these patients was 38 months. At 6 years, the projected overall survival rates were 78% for patients with indolent lymphoma and 43% for patients with aggressive histologies (42).

These results, although encouraging, did not provide a cure for the majority of the patients. Consequently, Press (unpublished) initiated a study of the combination of ^{131}I-labeled B-1 antibody, high-dose chemotherapy, and autologous stem cell transplantation. This Phase I/II study is evaluating the maximum-tolerated dose of ^{131}I-labeled B-1 antibody with high-dose VP16 and cyclophosphamide and stem cell support. Preliminary results of the study indicated that the toxicities were significantly greater for the combination regimen than for single-agent therapy (40). Approximately 80% of the patients are disease free at 1 to 34 months posttransplant. Additional patients and studies will be required to determine if this approach provides sufficient benefits to outweigh the toxicities.

V. ALTERNATIVE APPROACHES: PRETARGET TECHNOLOGY

A. Introduction to Pretarget Technology

Pretarget technology was developed to decrease the amount of time that the radionuclide circulates in the blood irradiating the bone marrow, thereby allowing the administration of higher doses of radiactivity (43). In clinical studies evaluating Pretarget radioimmunotherapy in patients with various adenocarcinomas, bone marrow toxicity was not observed with doses as high as 140 mCi/m^2 ($\sim$266 mCi ^{90}Y) (44). This is more than five times the maximum-tolerated dose of ^{90}Y used in conventional studies of RIT for patients with non-Hodgkin's lymphoma. These results led to the expectation that Pretarget could be used to deliver more radiation to B cells in patients with non-Hodgkin's lymphoma and thereby increase the response rate without increasing the toxicity.

B.   Description of Pretarget Lymphoma

The Pretarget regimen uses three components: an antibody streptavidin conjugate, a clearing agent, and ^{90}Y-DOTA biotin. The antibody conjugate targets the strep-tavidin receptor to the tumor cells. After allowing sufficient time for the conjugate to reach the tumor, the clearing agent is administered to remove any conjugate that remains in circulation. The final component, ^{90}Y-DOTA biotin, binds to the streptavidin on the tumor via the avidin-biotin attraction.

C.   Pretarget Lymphoma: Clinical Results

The use of Pretarget is being evaluated for treatment of patients with relapsed or refractory NHL using a chimeric, anti-CD20 antibody (C2B8, Rituxan, Rituxi-mab) chemically conjugated to streptavidin (45,46). Ten patients have been eval-uated. Component dosing and schedule were based on previous clinical experi-ence with Pretarget technology.

Patients entered on the study were typical of those with relapsed, indolent NHL: six males and four females ranging in age from 31 to 64 (median 54.5 years). All patients had prior therapy: three had high-dose chemotherapy and peripheral stem cell transplant; one had ^{131}I-B1 antibody therapy; and six had prior Rituxan.

Gamma camera images were obtained to follow the biodistribution of the components and to estimate the radiation absorbed dose. The images demon-strated tumor targeting of the DOTA-biotin within 10 min after the injection and identified previously unknown disease in several patients. The dosimetry results for patients treated with Pretarget lymphoma are compared to those reported for patients treated with conventional RIT in Table 5.

Seven of the 10 patients were treated with doses of 30 to 50 mCi/m^2 ^{90}Y (51 to 109.2 mCi total dose). The regimen was safe and well tolerated. Three patients experienced grade 3 hematologic toxicity consisting of transient throm-bocytopenia and neutropenia; however, in all cases this resolved spontaneously. Other toxicities were minimal, consisting primarily of fatigue.

Preliminary response data are encouraging (see Table 6). Six of the seven patients who received doses of 30 to 50 mCi/m^2 showed evidence of antitumor activity. Two patients achieved a CR, two a PR, one a mixed response, and one stable disease. It is too early to assess the duration of the response.

Although these results are preliminary, they suggest that even heavily treated patients can tolerate high doses of radioimmunotherapy with Pretarget lymphoma. The possibility exists, therefore, that this technology can be used to deliver higher doses of radiation without requiring stem cell transplantation. If this hypothesis is true, patients may obtain high response rates and durable remis-sions without the toxicity and expense of stem cell transplantation.

VI. SUMMARY

Monoclonal antibodies and radioimmunoconjugates have been used by various investigators to treat patients with relapsed B-cell lymphomas. Objective remissions have been achieved in a high percentage of patients. However, most patients still relapse and ultimately die of lymphoma. Higher rates of response and longer durations of response have been obtained in patients treated with radioimmunoconjugates at doses requiring stem cell transplantation. Several alternative approaches are being investigated that may yield results equivalent to those obtained with high-dose chemotherapy including radioimmunoconjugates and chimeric antibodies in combination with other therapies and alternative delivery methods including the Pretarget approach.

REFERENCES

1. Cancer Facts & Figures—1999. Atlanta, GA: American Cancer Society, 1999.
2. Kohler G, Milstein C. Continuous cultures of fused cells secreting antibody of predefined specificity. Nature 1975; 256:495–497.
3. Nadler LM, Stashenko P, Hardy R, et al. Serotherapy of a patient with a monoclonal antibody directed against a human lymphoma-associated antigen. Cancer Res 1980; 40:3147–3154.
4. Press OW, Appelbaum F, Ledbetter JA, et al. Monoclonal antibody 1F5 (anti-CD20) serotherapy of human B cell lymphomas. Blood 1987; 69:584–591.
5. Hekman A, Honselaar A, Vuist WM, et al. Initial experience with treatment of human B cell lymphoma with anti-CD19 monoclonal antibody. Cancer Immunol Immunother 1991; 32:364–372.
6. Hu E, Epstein AL, Naeve GS, et al. A phase 1a clinical trial of LYM-1 monoclonal antibody serotherapy in patients with refractory B cell malignancies. Hematol Oncol 1989; 7:155–166.
7. Scheinberg DA, Straus DJ, Yeh SD, et al. A phase I toxicity, pharmacology, and dosimetry trial of monoclonal antibody OKB7 in patients with non-Hodgkin's lymphoma: effects of tumor burden and antigen expression. J Clin Oncol 1990; 8: 792–803.
8. Meeker TC, Lowder J, Maloney DG, et al. A clinical trial of anti-idiotype therapy for B cell malignancy. Blood 1985; 65:1349–1363.
9. Brown SL, Miller RA, Horning SJ, et al. Treatment of B-cell lymphomas with anti-idiotype antibodies alone and in combination with alpha interferon. Blood 1989; 73: 651–661.
10. Herlyn DM, Koprowski H. Monoclonal anticolon carcinoma antibodies in complement-dependent cytotoxicity. Int J Cancer 1981; 27:769–774.
11. Lubeck MD, Steplewski Z, Baglia F, Klein MH, Dorrington KJ, Koprowski H. The interaction of murine IgG subclass proteins with human monocyte Fc receptors. J Immunol 1985; 135:1299–1304.

12. Hale G, Dyer MJ, Clark MR, et al. Remission induction in non-Hodgkin's lymphoma with reshaped human monoclonal antibody CAMPATH-1H. Lancet 1988; 2:1394–1399.
13. Tedder TF, Engel P. CD20: a regulator of cell-cycle progression of B lymphocytes. Immunol Today 1994; 15:450–454.
14. Reff ME, Carner K, Chambers KS, et al. Depletion of B cells in vivo by a chimeric mouse human monoclonal antibody to CD20. Blood 1994; 83:435–445.
15. Maloney DG, Liles TM, Czerwinski DK, et al. Phase I clinical trial using escalating single-dose infusion of chimeric anti-CD20 monoclonal antibody (IDEC-C2B8) in patients with recurrent B-cell lymphoma. Blood 1994; 84:2457–2466.
16. Maloney DG, Grillo-Lopez AJ, Bodkin DJ, et al. IDEC-C2B8: results of a phase I multiple-dose trial in patients with relapsed non-Hodgkin's lymphoma [see comments]. J Clin Oncol 1997; 15:3266–3274.
17. Maloney DG, Grillo-Lopez AJ, White CA, et al. IDEC-C2B8 (Rituximab) anti-CD20 monoclonal antibody therapy in patients with relapsed low-grade non-Hodgkin's lymphoma. Blood 1997; 90:2188–2195.
18. McLaughlin P, Grillo-Lopez AJ, Link BK, et al. Rituximab chimeric anti-CD20 monoclonal antibody therapy for relapsed indolent lymphoma: half of patients respond to a four-dose treatment program. J Clin Oncol 1998; 16:2825–2833.
19. Czucman MS, Grillo-Lopez AJ, White CA, Saleh M, Gordon L. Treatment of patients with low-grade B-cell lymphoma with the combination of chimeric anti-CD20 monoclonal antibody and CHOP chemotherapy. J Clin Oncol 1999; 17:268.
20. Important Prescribing Information: Genentech and IDEC Pharmaceuticals, 1998.
21. DeNardo SJ, DeNardo GL, Kukis DL, et al. ^{67}Cu-2IT-BAT-Lym-1 pharmacokinetics, radiation dosimetry, toxicity and tumor regression in patients with lymphoma. J Nucl Med 1999; 40:302–310.
22. DeNardo GL, Kukis DL, Shen S, DeNardo DA, Meares CF, DeNardo SJ. ^{67}Cu-versus ^{131}I-labeled Lym-1 antibody: comparative pharmacokinetics and dosimetry in patients with non-Hodgkin's lymphoma. Clin Cancer Res 1999; 5:533–541.
23. Denardo GL, Denardo SJ, Kukis DL, et al. Maximum tolerated dose of ^{67}Cu-2IT-BAT-LYM-1 for fractionated radioimmunotherapy of non-Hodgkin's lymphoma: a pilot study. Anticancer Res 1998; 18:2779–2788.
24. Kaminski MS, Zasadny KR, Francis IR, et al. Iodine-131-anti-B1 radioimmunotherapy for B-cell lymphoma. J Clin Oncol 1996; 14:1974–1981.
25. Wahl RL, Zasadny KR, MacFarlane D, et al. Iodine-131 anti-B1 antibody for B-cell lymphoma: an update on the Michigan Phase I experience. J Nucl Med 1998; 39:21S–27S.
26. Kaminski M, Zelenetz A, Press O, et al. Multicenter phase III study of iodine-131 Tositumomab (anti-B1 antibody) for chemotherapy-refractory low-grade or transformed low-grade non-Hodgkin's lymphoma (NHL). ASH Meeting, Miami, FL, 1998.
27. Knox SJ, Goris ML, Trisler K, et al. Yttrium-90-labeled anti-CD20 monoclonal antibody therapy of recurrent B-cell lymphoma. Clin Cancer Res 1996; 2:457–470.
28. Wiseman G, White C, Witzig T, Gordon L. IDEC-Y2B8 radioimmunotherapy: baseline bone marrow involvement and platelet count are better predictors of hematologic toxicity than dosimetry (abstr 1721). Blood 1998; 92(suppl):417a.

29. Wiseman G, White C, Stabin M, Gordon L, Emmanouilides C. Therapeutic index of IDEC-Y2B8 radioimmunotherapy: up to 850 fold greater radiation dose to tumor than to normal organs (abstr 13). J Clin Oncol (Proc. ASCO) 1999; 18:4a.
30. Witzig L, White C, Wiseman G, Gordon C, Emmanoulides C. IDEC-Y2B8 radioimmunotherapy; responses in patients with splenomgaly (abstr 1721). Blood 1998; 92(suppl):417a.
31. Epstein AL, Marder RJ, Winter JN, et al. Two new monoclonal antibodies, Lym-1 and Lym-2, reactive with human B-lymphocytes and derived tumors, with immunodiagnostic and immunotherapeutic potential. Cancer Res 1987; 47:830–840.
32. Rose LM, Gunasekera AH, DeNardo SJ, DeNardo GL, Meares CF. Lymphoma-selective antibody Lym-1 recognizes a discontinuous epitope on the light chain of HLA-DR10. Cancer Immunol Immunother 1996; 43:26–30.
33. DeNardo SJ, DeNardo GL, O'Grady LF, et al. Treatment of a patient with B cell lymphoma by I-131 LYM-1 monoclonal antibodies. Int J Biol Markers 1987; 2:49–53.
34. Schlom J, Molinolo A, Simpson JF, et al. Advantage of dose fractionation in monoclonal antibody–targeted radioimmunotherapy. J Natl Cancer Inst 1990; 82:763–771.
35. DeNardo GL, DeNardo SJ, Lamborn KR, et al. Low-dose fractionated radioimmunotherapy for B-cell malignancies using I-131-LYM-1 antibody. Cancer Biother Radiopharm 1998; 13:239–254.
36. DeNardo GL, DeNardo SJ, Goldstein DS, et al. Maximum-tolerated dose, toxicity, and efficacy of (131)I-Lym-1 antibody for fractionated radioimmunotherapy of non-Hodgkin's lymphoma. J Clin Oncol 1998; 16:3246–3256.
37. Lamborn KR, DeNardo GL, DeNardo SJ, et al. Treatment-related parameters predicting efficacy of Lym-1 radioimmunotherapy in patients with B-lymphocytic malignancies. Clin Cancer Res 1997; 3:1253–1260.
38. Press OW, Eary JF, Badger CC, et al. Treatment of refractory non-Hodgkin's lymphoma with radiolabeled MB-1 (anti-CD37) antibody. J Clin Oncol 1989; 7:1027–1038.
39. Press OW, Eary JF, Appelbaum FR, et al. Radiolabeled-antibody therapy of B-cell lymphoma with autologous bone marrow support. N Engl J Med 1993; 329:1219–1224.
40. Press OW. Prospects for the management of non-Hodgkin's lymphomas with monoclonal antibodies and immunoconjugates. Cancer J Sci Am 1998; 4(suppl)2:S19–S26.
41. Press OW, Eary JF, Appelbaum FR, et al. Phase II trial of ^{131}I-B1 (anti-CD20) antibody therapy with autologous stem cell transplantation for relapsed B cell lymphomas. Lancet 1995; 346:336–340.
42. Press O. Radiolabeled antibody therapy of B cell lymphomas. In press 1999.
43. Breitz H, Weiden PL, PL B. Clinical optimization of pretargeted radioimmunotherapy (PRIT) with antibody-streptavidin conjugate and 90Y-DOTA Biotin. J Nucl Med 2000; 41:131–140.
44. Murtha A, Weiden P, Knox S, Breitz H, Goris M, Axworthy D. Phase I Dose Escalation Trial of Pretargeted Radioimmunotherapy (PRIT) with 90-Yttrium (abstr 1686). J Clin Oncol (Proc. ASCO) 1998; 17:438a.

45. Weiden P, Breitz H, Press O, et al. Radioimmunotherapy (RIT) in the Treatment of Non-Hodgkins Lymphoma (NHL): Advantage of Pretarget RIT (PRITR) (abstr 1709). Blood 1998; 92(suppl):414a.
46. Breitz H, Weiden P, Appelbaum J, Stone D, Axworthy D. Pretargeted radioimmunotherapy (PRIT) for treatment of non-Hodgkin's lymphoma (NHL): preliminary results (abstr 75). J Nucl Med 1999; 40:19p.
47. Grossbard ML, Press OW, Appelbaum FR, Bernstein ID, Nadler LM. Monoclonal antibody–based therapies of leukemia and lymphoma. Blood 1992; 80:863–878.
48. Kaminiski MS, Zasadny KR, Francis IR, et al. Radioimmunotherapy of B-cell lymphoma with [131I] anti-B1 (anti-CD20) antibody. N Engl J Med 1993; 329:459–465.

11
Radioimmunotherapy of Solid Tumors

Hazel B. Breitz and Paul L. Weiden
Virginia Mason Medical Center, Seattle, Washington

Paul L. Beaumier
Shin Nippon Biomedical Sciences USA, Everett, Washington

I. INTRODUCTION

It has been 45 years since the first indication that radioimmunotherapy (RIT) might be a feasible approach to therapy of cancer. Since then, especially during the past decade, many antibodies directed against tumor-associated antigens have been produced, successfully labeled with radionuclides, tested in xeno-graft models, and evaluated in Phase I clinical trials. Gamma-emitting radionuclides have been used to assess biodistribution and tumor targeting, and beta emitters have been used with therapeutic intent, but with limited success in solid tumors. To place RIT of solid tumors in context, this chapter will first briefly describe the historical aspects of radiolabeled antibodies, use of diagnostic radiolabeled monoclonal antibodies (radioimmunoscintigraphy), and the role of nonimmune, internally administered beta emission radiotherapy in the management of cancer patients. We shall then consider the choice of radionuclides and antibodies for RIT and preclinical RIT studies. Finally we will focus on clinical trials of RIT of those solid tumors not discussed in other chapters.

A. Historical Overview of Radiolabeled Antibodies

The first use of radiolabeled antibodies to detect a defined population of cells occurred in 1948 (1) when Pressman and Keighly demonstrated that ^{131}I-labeled antirat kidney antibodies selectively localized in rat kidneys following intravenous injection. Pressman also pioneered the use of radiolabeled antibodies for tumor localization (2) showing that ^{131}I-labeled specific antisera localized preferentially into rat sarcomas when compared to ^{125}I-labeled nonimmune serum.

In the 1960s and 1970s, Bale et al. (3) and Spar et al. (4) demonstrated that radiolabeled antifibrin antibodies localized in rat, dog, and human tumors (65% of 141 patients). McCardle et al. in 1974 reported tumor regression in one of two patients treated with ^{131}I-labeled antibodies to human fibrinogen (5).

A dramatic complete response in a patient with widely metastatic malignant melanoma treated with ^{131}I-labeled polyclonal antiserum raised against his own tumor was reported by Vial and Callahan in 1952 (6). Unfortunately 13 subsequent patients treated the same way did not respond. In 1974, Ghose et al. reported inhibition and complete suppression of the murine EL4 lymphoma with an ^{131}I-labeled anti-EL4 antibody (7). At this time it was realized that more specific antibodies were needed and that more deposition of radioactivity was required at the tumor for therapeutic effect.

Kohler and Milstein reported in 1975 that myeloma cells could incorporate DNA from programmed and stimulated B lymphocytes to produce an immortalized hybridoma that secreted monoclonal antibodies (8). This discovery made possible studies with highly purified, homogenous antibody reagents with consistent specificity.

Early studies of radiolocalization with monoclonal antibodies using ^{125}I or ^{131}I as the radionuclide established the feasibility of injecting radiolabeled monoclonal antibodies intravenously and achieving localization of the radioactivity at the site of tumor. The first reported study of a radiolabeled monoclonal antibody directed at a tumor antigen in vivo was carried out by Ballou et al. in 1979 who showed localization of an IgM antibody directed against the stage specific embryonic antigen (SSEA-1) expressed by human teratocarcinoma xenograft (9). Sufficient clinical-grade monoclonal antibodies to tumor-associated antigens became readily available for clinical trials in the 1980s.

B. Radioimmunoscintigraphy (RIS)

Gamma-emitting radionuclides linked to monoclonal antibodies directed against tumor-associated antigens have been shown to be of value in the staging and management of patients with cancer. Demonstration of the utility, efficacy, and clinical benefit of RIS has led to U.S. FDA approval of four murine, antibody-based radiopharmaceuticals for diagnostic purposes. In each case, an antibody with a limited spectrum of reactivity is labeled with a gamma-emitting radioisotope, injected into a patient, allowed to target tumor tissue. The patient is then imaged with a gamma camera. Each antibody/isotope combination differs in details of normal tissue reactivity, timing of the imaging procedure, and specificity and sensitivity in detecting tumor.

[99m]Tc-Nofetumomab merpentan, Verluma, is a ^{99m}Tc-labeled Fab fragment of the NR-LU-10 murine antibody, which is approved for staging small-cell lung cancer (10). It has a positive predictive value of 94% for diagnosis of extensive, as opposed to limited, disease. When used as a single test, a positive study obviates the need to perform a number of standard diagnostic staging tests. Satumomab pendetide, Oncoscint CR/OV, is an ^{111}In-labeled B72.3 intact murine monoclonal antibody approved for determining the extent and location of extrahepatic malignant disease in patients with colorectal and ovarian cancer (11,12). Arcitumomab, Cea-Scan, is a ^{99m}Tc-labeled anti-CEA Fab' fragment of a murine antibody approved for use in patients with colorectal cancer to determine location and extent of disease prior to surgical exploration in conjunction with CT scan (13). Prostascint, an ^{111}In-labeled intact murine antibody EC11, is approved to evaluate extent of disease prior to lymphadenectomy for patients with confirmed prostatic cancer and in patients with a high likelihood of recurrence of prostatic cancer, for example, patients with a rising PSA prior to exploratory surgery (14). The three last agents are all recommended for use in conjunction with standard diagnostic tests and are reported to influence patient management in approximately 25% of patients by defining extent of disease and detecting occult disease.

Nonimageable radiolabeled antibodies also are being utilized in the surgical management of colorectal cancer. Radioimmunoguided probes are being used intraoperatively to identify tumor deposits. The hand-held probe has a small scintillation crystal that detects gamma emissions which are then displayed audibly or visually according to the counts detected. Tumor deposits too small to be visible by the surgeon or with standard diagnostic tests can be detected. Tumor-free margins at the time of surgical resection can be more reliably attained, and regional nodal involvement can be detected. Arnold et al. reported that the use of the Neoprobe RIGScan device in conjunction with ^{125}I-labeled CC49 antibody enabled occult disease to be detected and that 14% of the patients studied were considered unresectable as determined by this technique (15). Probes that can detect imageable photons are also available, e.g., C-Trak, which detects ^{111}In-labeled antibodies.

C. Nonimmune Systemic Radiotherapy

Systemic radiotherapy has been utilized for decades in the management of patients with thyroid cancer. [131]I administered for ablation of residual thyroid tissue postthyroidectomy significantly reduces the likelihood of both local and distant recurrence. Treatment of metastatic thyroid cancer is of particular benefit in young patients whose metastases demonstrate uptake of radioiodine. This is successful because the localization of radioactive iodine in thyroid tissue achieves a high enough target to normal tissue ratio that doses of 30,000 to 40,000 rad can be delivered to the residual thyroid tissue, and local or metastatic disease (16).

More recently, systemic radiotherapy has been utilized for the treatment of patients with metastatic prostate and breast cancer involving bone. Beta-emitting radionuclides linked to phosphate derivatives are useful as palliative agents in the management of pain from bony metastases. ^{89}Sr-chloride (Metastron), [153]Sm-EDTMP (Quadramet), and ^{32}P-orthophosphates are approved for radionuclide therapy. [32]P is no longer utilized because approximately one-third of patients experience clinically significant myelosuppression. Clinical trials in patients with prostate cancer have also shown similar benefit with other agents, including [186]Re-HEDP and [117]Sn-DTPA, although these are not yet FDA approved. A response rate of approximately 80% in terms of decreased pain and increased quality of life has been observed. With ^{89}Sr chloride, the pain relief occurs within 2 weeks, with maximum relief by 6 weeks which is maintained for 4 to 15 months (17).

II. RADIONUCLIDES FOR RIT

The production, cost, availability, and specific activity of the radionuclide must all be considered in chosing the appropriate radionuclide. Most clinical trials have focused on beta-particle emitters because of their suitability for delivering radiation beyond the targeted cell by the crossfire effect, and their widespread availability (Table 1). Several trials using the Auger emitter ^{125}I have also been reported.

Negatively charged electrons are emitted as beta particles from the nucleus in a continuum of energies up to a maximum value. The energy of the beta particle is important because of the range over which the energy is deposited. The average beta particle energy is approximately one-third of its maximum energy. The range of these particles is generally much greater than alpha particles and Auger electrons, and the sparse ionization along their tracks accounts for their low linear energy transfer (LET). The longer range of the beta particle is advantageous

Table 1 Radionuclides for RIT

Radionuclide	Half-life (days)	E beta (max) MeV	X_{90} (mm)	E photon keV (abundance)
[131]I	8	0.81	0.83	364 (81%)
[186]Re	3.7	1.07	1.80	137 (5%)
[90]Y	2.7	2.27	5.34	—
[177]Lu	6.7	0.5	0.6	208 (11%)
[125]I	60	0.03[a]	0.02	3.8

[a] Auger electron.

Table 2 Monoclonal Antibodies Studied in RIT Clinical Trials

Antibody	Antigen	Antibody characteristics	Radionuclide	Tumor types	References
anti-P97	P97 oncofetal glycoprotein	mu IgG1, Fab	I-131	Melanoma	62
NP-4	CEA	mu	I-131	C-R, lung, pancreas, medullary thyroid, breast	63–65
MN-14	CEA	mu and hu intact, fragments	I-131	C-R, lung, pancreas, breast, ovary, medullary thyroid	82,83
COL-1	CEA	mu IgG2a high affinity	I-131	C-R	66
A5-B7	CEA	mu IgG1 high affinity	I-131	C-R	68
cT86.44	CEA	ch IgG1 high affinity	Y-90	C-R	67
NR-CO-02	CEA	mu IgG1	Re-186	C-R lung, ovary	69
NR-LU-10	40-kD surface glycoprotein	mu and ch IgG2b	Re-186	C-R, lung, ovary, renal, gastro-esophageal	69,70
B72.3	TAG-72	mu and ch	I-131	C-R	71,72,73
CC49	TAG-72	mu IgG1, high affinity	I-131	C-R, breast, prostate, ovary	74,75,76,77, 85,86,87, 93,95,96
A33	Colonic cell membrane Ag	mu IgG2a	I-131 I-125	C-R	78 79
17-1A	Cell surface glycoprotein	ch IgG2a	I-125	C-R	80
CYT-356	Prostate membrane Ag	mu IgG1	Y-90	Prostate	83
KC4	High-MW glycoprotein	mu IgG3	I-131	Prostate	84
L6, cL-6	Membrane-bound 24-kD protein Ag	mu IgG2a ch L-6 IgG1	I-131	breast, lung, ovary colon	87–90
BrE-3	Human milkfat globule		Y-90	breast	92
EGFr	Epidermal growth factor	mu	I-131	Astrocytoma, glioblastoma	97
425	Epidermal growth factor	mu IgG2a	I-125	Astrocytoma, glioblastoma	98,99

Abbreviations: mu, murine; ch, chimeric; hu, humanized; C-R, colorectal carcinoma.

because of the inhomogeneous uptake of the antibodies. The high LET of alpha particle emitters and the low energy of short-range Auger-electron emitters are attractive for situations where all cells are targeted. Homogeneous targeting of tumor cells in solid tumors with conventional RIT is unlikely (this volume, Chapter 5).

The presence of gamma emission can be an advantage if the abundance and energy of photon emission are not too high. Since photons in the 75- to 250-KeV range are suitable for detection with standard nuclear medicine gamma cameras, they can be used to follow the localization and pharmacokinetics of the radioimmunoconjugate and estimate the radiation dose from the therapeutic radionuclide. High-energy gamma radiation increases the exposure of normal organs and the medical personnel to radiation and is a significant drawback to the use of ^{131}I for RIT.

The half-life of the radionuclide will have a major influence on the therapeutic ratio of the radioimmunoconjugate. It must be long enough that most of the decay has not occurred before peak tumor uptake occurs. It must not be too long or the normal organs will continue to be radiated after the radioimmunoconjugate has disappeared from the tumor target, thus causing unnecessary toxicity. Half-lives of 3 to 8 days are considered optimal when conjugated to intact monoclonal antibodies. Shorter half-lives are desirable when delivery at the tumor target is more rapid, e.g., with antibody fragments or with pretargeted RIT.

The majority of clinical trials have utilized ^{131}I-labeled murine monoclonal antibodies, in spite of its long half-life and high gamma exposure. This is because of availability, ease of labeling, low cost, and experience in treating thyroid cancer. Beta-emitting radionuclides that appear to have superior properties to ^{131}I for therapy include ^{90}Y, ^{186}Re, and ^{177}Lu, and these have now been evaluated in patients (Tables 1 and 2). More complete discussions of the issues involved in selecting appropriate nuclides for RIT are available in several excellent reviews (18,19; and this volume, Chapter 3).

III. ANTIBODIES FOR RIT

Selection of antibodies for therapeutic applications requires consideration of antigen expression, form, affinity, mass, biological effector functions, and immunogenicity.

A. Antigen

Both cell surface and extracellular antigens can be targeted by monoclonal antibodies. Antigen density $> 10^5$ sites per cell appears to predict for better localization. Extracellular antigens may be in the stromal matrix surrounding tumor cells or in mucin pools. The antigenic target of the antibody must be compatible with the energy of the therapeutic isotope used. For example, Auger emitters such as ^{125}I would be appropriate for internalizing antibodies so that energy will be deposited in the nucleus, whereas antibodies radiolabeled with beta emitters are more suited to cell surface or extracellular antigens where each cell does not need to be targeted because of the crossfire effect. Generally, stable cell surface antigens that internalize slowly offer the best target for therapy with most radionuclides. Tumor-associated antigens are also found in normal tissues. Thus when antibodies are radiolabeled with therapeutic isotopes, localization at these crossreactive normal tissue antigens could potentially cause toxicity. Thus far myelosuppression from exposure of the bone marrow stem cells to blood radioactivity or binding of isotope to bone subsequent to release from the antibody has been the first dose limiting toxicity.

In instances where antigen is released into the circulation, antibody may bind to the circulating antigen, and while this may not necessarily interfere sufficiently to hamper tumor localization, it has been found to influence pharmacokinetics. In a study of pharmacokinetics of the anti-CEA antibody NP-4, for example, Behr et al. reported that higher serum CEA levels resulted in more rapid complexation and clearance from the serum to the liver. Increasing the antibody protein dose in the presence of high-circulating CEA diminished the impact of the rapid complexation. Behr also found that more rapid clearance was seen in patients with colorectal cancer than in patients with other cancer types, perhaps because of differences in chemical structure of the CEA produced in different tumors (20). Elevated serum levels of TAG-72 are found in 60% of patients with colorectal cancer, but this does not interfere with localization as detected by gamma camera. In fact, increased localization may be seen with increased serum levels. Unlike circulating CEA, serum TAG-72 levels do not affect serum clearance of CC49 and complexation over a protein dose 40- to 95-mg range did not occur.

B. Antibody Form

Murine monoclonal antibodies may be utilized as the whole antibody, or fragmented by enzyme digestion to the $F(ab')_2$, Fab', or Fab fragments. Using genetic engineering, domain deletant mutants such as CCC47, CH1, and 2,2 have been developed. These show more rapid tumor accumulation, but appear to show less less absolute accumulation in the tumor (21). Smaller stable Fv fragments (MW 25 kD) have also been produced by recombinant DNA technology. These smaller molecular forms are able to provide a higher tumor-to-nontarget ratio because of the more rapid penetration into tumor and the more rapid disappearance from the serum by renal clearance. Monovalent forms may have comparable affinity to whole antibodies but the retention at tumor tissue is shorter than with bivalent species. Thus they are suitable for imaging application, i.e. RIS, where the tumor-to-nontarget activity ratios are important but are less suitable for therapy.

Using the smaller molecular forms with the lower associated toxicity from more rapid serum clearance, one may be able to exploit the effect of a higher dose rate at earlier times when the tumor-to-normal-tissue radioactivity ratios are increased. Preclinical studies initially suggested that the intact antibody was the optimal form for use in RIT because a greater fraction of the dose of intact antibody is retained in the tumor tissue for longer than with the fragments. Although the majority of the RIT trials have utilized intact antibodies, $F(ab')_2$ fragments have also been examined as a targeting vehicle for therapy (22). In xenograft studies, higher response rates were shown with $F(ab')_2$ fragments (23). However, it is believed the fragments smaller than the $F(ab')_2$ would result in a lower tumor uptake because of the lower circulation time.

C. Affinity

Monoclonal antibodies must have adequate affinities (10^{-8} mol/L or greater) to bind antigen at the tumor site. It was hoped that the recently developed higher-affinity antibodies (10^{-10} mol/L) would show improved kinetics of uptake and greater stability. Beatty had shown, for example, increased uptake of the newer higher affinity antibodies at low doses relative to antigen in xenograft studies (24). However, Weinstein suggested that higher-affinity antibodies may bind more extensively to low levels of antigen in normal tissues and be affected by binding site barriers, limiting penetration into tumors (25).

Behr et al. retrospectively examined data from 275 patients who received NP-4 and its 10-fold higher-affinity anti-CEA antibody, MN-14. Behr reported that the MN-14 antibody showed increased complex formation with deposition in the liver compared with NP-4 at similar levels of circulating CEA, thus potentially reducing the antibody available for tumor targeting. The molar ratio of the CEA to antibody was important in determining whether complex formation would occur (20). No difference was noted in pharmacokinetics or actual tumor uptake of the higher-affinity antibody. This was contrary to the preclinical studies which showed improved tumor targeting of MN-14 to colon cancer xenografts, but the clinical study may have been influenced by the presence of the high serum CEA levels. The serum clearance of the different forms of these two antibodies were also compared; whether the antibody was intact or fragmented, and whether murine or humanized, did not affect clearance. Clearance was mostly affected by circulating CEA level and protein dose.

CC49 is a second-generation B72.3 antibody with affinity eightfold greater than B72.3, directed to a different epitope on the TAG-72 antigen. CC49 exhibits higher reactivity to gastric, pancreatic, and colon cancer. Colcher (26) carried out dual-label studies in tumor xenograft models and showed that ^{131}I-CC49 localization was up to five times greater than coinjected ^{125}I-B72.3. Schlom showed improved therapeutic efficacy with ^{131}I and ^{90}Y CC49 (27). In an intrapatient comparison study in 10 presurgical patients, Divgi reported an improvement in tumor concentration and tumor to serum ratios with the higher-affinity CC49 (28).

D. Antibody Mass

Localization of some antibodies is influenced by the mass of antibody administered (29). A higher mass dose, or unlabeled antibody used as a cold blocker, can be useful in overcoming nonspecific localization in normal organs and allow greater localization at the tumor antigenic sites. For example, DeNardo showed that added unlabeled antibody reduced nonspecific uptake in the lungs when using L-6, an antiadenocarcinoma antibody (30).

E. Effector Function

IgG2a antibodies with biological activity may be able to increase the therapeutic potential of RIT. Increased vascular permeability from antibody-dependent cellular cytotoxicity (ADCC) may increase accumulation of radiolabeled antibody at the tumor site. For example, L-6 is an antibody which demonstrates ADCC and complement dependent cytolysis (CDC). Thus the cold blocker used to saturate antigen in normal tissues may also increase vascular permeability of the radiolabeled antibody at the tumor by activating the host immune effector cells and CDC (31).

F. Immunogenicity

Administration of high doses of intact murine monoclonal antibodies almost invariably leads to the development of human antimouse antibodies (HAMA) in patients with solid tumors. As single-dose therapy is unlikely to generally produce significant responses in treating cancer, HAMA formation must be eliminated or neutralized so that multiple cycles of RIT can be safely and effectively administered. Using genetic engineering, antibody molecules with less immunogenicity have been developed.

In our study of a chimeric derivative of murine NR-LU-10, a pancarcinoma antibody that we have studied extensively, we demonstrated that the chimeric form, called NR-LU-13 (32), had a slower disappearance from the circulation, which resulted in marrow toxicity at lower doses than the murine form, without any gain in tumor dose. Human antichimeric antibodies (HACA) did develop in 75% of patients, but were typically 10- to 1000-fold lower than after administration of intact murine antibody. Thus although less immunogenic than the murine antibody, the chimeric antibody still induced formation of human antibodies which precluded repetitive dose administration.

HACA responses after administration of other chimeric antibodies have been variable. Chimeric L-6 antibody showed weaker immunogenicity than murine L-6 but similar pharmacokinetics (33). This chimeric L-6 also showed greater ADCC and CMC activity when compared to the murine L-6 (34). Weak antiglobulin responses compared to the related murine antibody was also observed following chimeric 17-1A antibody (35).

Ledermann introduced the idea of immunosuppressive agents to be administered in conjunction with RIT to suppress the HAMA response. Cyclosporine A 15 mg/kg 2 days prior until 14 days after administration of antibody was recommended and achieved modest success in his studies with an anti-CEA antibody (36). In our studies reported by Weiden et al., 80% of patients who received cyclosporin A intact murine NR-LU-10 still developed HAMA, but the mean titer was lower than in those who had not received immunosuppression. Lowering of the cyclosporine A dose was necessary in several patients because of toxicity. None of the three patients given 15 mg/kg of cyclosporin A and the murine $F(ab')_2$ fragment of NR-CO-02 developed HAMA (37). Cyclosporine has now been used with several antibodies and the success depends on the immunogenicity of the particular antibody as well as the tolerance for adequate doses. Thus, while both chimeric antibodies or cyclosporin A can reduce the immune response, neither appears to eradicate the human antibody response enough to permit repetitive radioimmunoconjugate administration to patients.

A more recent development has been the engineering of humanized antibodies, i.e., engineered molecules which are almost entirely human except for a small portion of the antigen combining site. We studied two human monoclonal antibodies labeled with ^{186}Re (38). Fourteen patients received up to three infusions of 100 mg ^{186}Re on a human IgM 16.88 antibody, and eight patients received a single dose of 10 or 100 mg 88BV59, a human IgG antibody. Pharmacokinetics showed that 70% of the ^{186}Re IgM antibody and 30% of the ^{186}Re IgG was excreted within 24 hours. Clearance of these radioimmunoconjugates was more rapid than expected of a human antibody (39). There was no evidence of human antihuman antibody formation. However, tumor targeting was suboptimal, indicating that these particular immunoconjugates were likely to be of limited usefulness for intravenous radioimmunotherapy, but establishing that repetitive doses of human monoclonal antibodies can be administered without evidence of alloimmunization. A humanized MN-14 antibody evaluated in six patients with CEA producing tumors showed similar pharmacokinetics and tumor dosimetry to the murine MN-14 antibody but was not immunogenic (40). Thus, it appears that the problem of HAMA may be solvable with human antibodies.

IV. PRECLINICAL RIT STUDIES

In general, preclinical RIT studies in solid tumor models have been considered an important prerequisite required to justify taking a radiolabeled antibody into the clinic. The demonstration of immunospecific localization and retention in tumor, clearance from blood and normal organs, and statistically significant therapeutic responses relative to control have made up an important part of agent workup for clinical trials. Most commonly, a chloramine T ^{131}I-labeled murine monoclonal antibody is tested in a nude mouse human tumor xenograft model system. Typically, the percentage of injected dose per gram in tumor and normal tissues, tumor to blood and tissues ratios, and often dosimetry, including the ratio of tumor to normal organ absorbed dose, and efficacy and toxicity results are reported.

The rodent human tumor xenograft model is valuable but limited: antigen is expressed homogeneously and exclusively in a cloned tumor target; normal tissue is noncrossreactive in animal models; animal body and organ volumes are dosimetrically irrelevant; tumor doubling time is typically very rapid in xenograft models; metabolic and pharmacokinetic distributional and compartmental exchange rates are extremely rapid; mice have a 10-fold higher hematopoietic stem cell concentration than man and an LD_{50} twice that of humans (41); and mice may be given multiple-dose therapy. Nonetheless, the mouse xenograft system is valuable and relevant when μCi/g units are considered (42).

Preclinical work has focused on the performance of new monocloncal antibodies (Mab) of various specificities and affinities; ^{131}I and other beta emitters such as the ^{90}Y, ^{177}Lu, ^{67}Cu, the Auger emitter ^{125}I, and the alpha emitters ^{212}Bi and ^{213}Bi; the chelates and linkages needed to couple these radioisopes to monoclonal antibodies; the evaluation of single and multiple dosing; and the therapeutic consequences of tumor size and antigen expression levels. More recently, recognizing the inability to clinically cure tumors without intolerable hematopoietic toxicity, various combined modality strategies have been explored such as external beam therapy and RIT, and chemotherapy and RIT.

Estaban used ^{131}I B72.3 to treat 5-mm diameter subcutaneous human colon carcinoma LS-174T (43). Ten mice were treated with either 300 or 500 μCi of antibody. At 500 μCi 8 of 10 mice survived and showed a 3.7-fold reduced tumor mass relative to control. Autoradiography demonstrated substantial heterogeneity of radiolabel distribution in tumor cross sections. The authors demonstrated histological areas of therapeutically induced necrosis and drastically reduced mitotic counts, and showed that with time, activity in the tumor periphery declined, suggesting more biological activity in this zone of the tumor.

Sharkey, using ^{131}I-labeled NP-4, treated the human colon carcinoma GW-39 line (44). One mCi given 1 day postimplantation resulted in no tumors in 6 of 11 hamsters at 12 weeks with an absorbed dose estimate to tumor of 2400 rad over 14 days. A 13% drop in body weight was noted by 7 days. Waiting longer postimplant to treat resulted in greatly reduced efficacy, suggesting radio-antibody is more effective when there is a low tumor burden.

Cheung treated human neuroblastoma tumors with [131]I-3F8 specific for the GD2 disialoganglioside antigen (45). Neither nonspecific radiolabeled antibody nor unlabeled specific 3F8 showed therapeutic effect, but 0.25 to 1.0 mCi of [131]I-3F8 effected >95% tumor shrinkage within 2 weeks. Mice with tumors re-ceiving >4200 rad were cured, but 70% of the animals were dead or dying by 40 days posttreatment.

Buchegger used a 1:2 mixture of three anti-CEA Mabs and their $F(ab')_2$ fragments labeled with ^{131}I to treat 0.2 to 1.5 g T380 human colon carcinoma tumor xenografts (46). A total dose of 600 TCi (200 TCi on Mab 400 µCi $F(ab')_2$) fragments resulted in >5000 rad to tumor and a tumor-to-whole-body ratio of 16:1. Groups of mice received radiolabeled specific MAb, control radiolabeled Mab, and Mab only. Specific radiolabeled Mab produced tumor shrinkage which persisted for 4 to 12 weeks posttreatment.

Buchegger (23) demonstrated superior performance of a pool of four [131]I $F(ab')_2$ fragments relative to a pool of the same antibodies as intact antibody in a T380 colon carcinoma model. The $F(ab')_2$ fragment pool deposited almost the same absorbed dose in tumor as the Mab pool but with much lower doses to normal organs and less toxicity. Complete remissions were noted in 8 of 10 mice after $F(ab')_2$ treatment. In contrast, with intact Mabs, tumors responded to treat-ment but recurred in 7/8 mice with considerable associated hematolgical toxicity. Treated animals with peripheral white cell counts falling below 1000 cells/mm^3 were rescued with marrow transplant.

Washburn evaluated the tissue distribution in nude mice bearing 5-mm-diameter colorectal carcinoma xenografts SW-948 with ^{90}Y CO17-1A using the cyclic anhydride DTPA chelation labeling method. The authors found significant bone uptake of ^{90}Y, which was thought to result from radioactivity dissociation of yttrium from the chelate and subsequent uptake in bone of this bone-seeking radiometal (47).

Roselli demonstrated superior stability using the isothiocyanatobenzyl DTPA (SCN-Bz-DTPA) chelate labeling, compared to SCN-EDTA or cyclic an-hydride-DTPA (48). Using [88]Y-labeled B 72.3 in LS-174T, 40% ID/g in tumor at 5 to 7 days vs. 6% to 8% ID/g and a 3% ID/g in bone compared to 11% to 14% ID/g, respectively, was found.

Beaumier treated 65 mm^3 SHT-1 SCLC tumor xenografts with [186]Re-MAG$_2$-GABA NR-LU-10 in a two- and four-dose regimen (days 0, 3, 7, and 10) with total activity of 500 to 600 µCi (49). Complete remissions were attained in 3 of 16 mice (no recurrence to 140 days) with 2000 to 2700 rad estimated deliv-ered to tumor. An LD$_{50}$ of 600 µCi (880 rad whole body) was determined. The

SHT-1 tumor is radiosensitive but highly aggressive, and the NR-LU-10 anibody exhibited peak uptake of only 8.3% ID/g at 2 days, accounting for the modest responses observed.

Schlom treated established LS-174T colon carcinoma tumors with ^{177}Lu-DOTA-CC49 Mab (50). Single doses of 200 or 350 μCi of ^{177}Lu-DOTA-CC49 Mab produced complete regression of established tumors out to 77 days posttreatment, 500 μCi resulted in the death of five of nine mice. Three multiple doses totaling 750 μCi produced complete regressions of 300 mm^3 tumors in 9 of 10 surviving mice. The authors noted that the softer beta of Lu-177 kills over 12 cell diameters compared with more energetic Y-90, which kills over 150 to 200 cell diameters.

Connett used BAT-2IT chelated ^{64}Cu or [67]Cu 1A3 Mab to treat GW39 human colon carcinoma in the hamster thigh model system (51). One to 3 mCi Cu-64 or 0.2 to 0.6 mCi Cu-67 was used to treat 2-day postimplant smaller 0.4-g tumors, and larger, 7-day postimplant, 0.6-g tumors. Almost 90% of the animals with small tumors were cured (no recurrence to 7 months), but only one animal in the larger tumor group was cured (>6 months). The authors suggested that factors such as lower uptake in large tumors, the need for a higher Mab dose to improve uniform distribution, poorer penetration into larger tumors, and the lower absorbed dose contributed to reduced success with larger tumors.

Chaladon evaluated the potentiation of a single 800 μCi dose of [131]I F(ab')$_2$ by 5-fluorouracil (5-FU), a radiosensitizer (52). 5-FU was administered in five daily intraperitoneal doses of 40 mg/kg with RIT in the T380 colon tumor xenograft model. RIT alone produced significant tumor regression; three of eight of the mice treated with RIT alone were cured (tumor free > 300 days). In contrast, 5-FU alone resulted in only minimal tumor growth delay. Combination therapy produced long-term regression, with tumors remaining smaller for longer than with RIT alone. RIT was shown to be more efficacious against this tumor target than 5-FU and potentiation could not be demonstrated. The general conclusion that in animal model systems RIT is more effective and less toxic than chemotherapy was also reached by Beaumier (53) and Blumenthal (54).

Pedley evaluated the effect of a blood flow modifying agent in potentiating RIT with ^{131}I-A5B7 against LS-174T colon carcinoma (55). Five hundred μCi I-131 Mab was administered and allowed to reach peak uptake in tumor. At this time, 48 hours postadministration, 5,6-dimethylxanthenone-4-acetic acid (DMXAA) was given IP resulting in five of six mice cured. Treatment with DMXAA doubled the retention of radioactivity in tumor at 5 days postadministration. The authors point out that compromising tumor vascular supply can lead to the destruction of a whole zone of supplied tumor cells and potentiate other therapies.

DeNardo evaluated the synergy of taxol with Y-90-DOTA chimeric L6 Mab in a nude mouse human breast carcinoma xenograft model, HBT 3477 (56). Mice receiving a single dose of 300 or 600 μg taxol IP or 315 μg chimeric Mab alone showed no response. Mice treated with 260 µCi ^{90}Y chL-6 showed a 79% response but none were cured. When Taxol was administered 1 to 3 days before, 79% of the mice responded and 29% were cured (>84 days). When Taxol was administered 6 to 24 hours after ^{90}Y chL-6, all the mice responded, and 48% were cured without a significant increase in toxicity. The authors suggest that the synergistic effect of postadministered Taxol on RIT efficacy may related to the p53 mutant and BCL2 expression characteristic of this highly anaplastic breast cancer cell line.

Sun (57) studied timing effects of combined RIT and XRT studies using Col12 colon carcinoma xenografts in nude mice receiving 3000 rad in 10 fractions over 12 days combined with three weekly injections of 200 µCi of ^{131}I Mabs (pool of four to independent CEA epitopes). The best result in terms of delay to regrowth of 105 days was observed in mice simultaneously treated with RIT and XRT. Each dose of radioiodinated Mab delivered 1800 rad to tumor. Tumors in these mice shrank to the smallest average minimal volume—4.5% of initial. XRT and RIT alone had much shorter delay of regrowth—34 and 20 days, respectively. There was no substantial increase in toxicity, which the authors attributed to selective effects from each treatment alone. It was proposed that total XRT dose might be reduced by 20% while maintaining the same tumor absorbed dose through the addition of RIT.

The fact that subcutaneous human tumor xenografts, especially well-established, larger tumors are so hard to cure, and even radiosensitive tumors recur, validates the relevance of the model. Histologically, we have found that subcutaneous human tumor xenografts do exhibit an architecture and vascularization very similar to human tumor biopsies. An even more challenging and relevant model is the disseminated metastatic tumor model in which therapy must be successfully delivered to tumors ranging in size and the degree of vascular accessibility.

The most important aspect of preclinical studies is that they are relevant to clinical objectives. Controlled preclinical studies offer a means to develop and test new therapeutic strategies which may be applied in the clinical setting. It seems clear, after almost 20 years of evaluation, that radiolabeled Mabs may be best utilized in an adjuvant setting. Much of the most successful recent work cited above addresses RIT in combination with XRT, chemotherapy, cytokines, or tumor blood supply modification.

V. RIT CLINICAL TRIALS

The modern era of clinical trials of radioimmunotherapy of solid tumors was initiated by Order. Order et al. studied ^{131}I and ^{90}Y-labeled antiferritin *polyclonal* antibodies and showed that ^{131}I-labeled antiferritin polyclonal antiserum could produce regressions of bulky hepatomas (58). Four of 24 patients had partial responses (PR) and one had a complete response (CR). Single doses as high as 150 mCi of ^{131}I antiferritin were given with acceptable hematologic toxicity. Based on the observations by Dillehay and Williams that radiation and adriamycin caused cell shifts to the radiosensitive G2 and M phase of the cell cycle (59), subsequent studies by Order and colleagues combined cytotoxic agents (5-FU and adriamycin) and external beam radiation with lower doses of radiation (50 mCi in divided doses) delivered by polyclonal ^{131}I-radiolabeled antiferritin antibodies. Using this approach, a response rate of 48% (7% CR; 41% PR) in 108 patients was achieved (60). Order and Lenhard reported responses following up to 30 mCi ^{90}Y antiferritin antibodies in patients with both Hodgkin's disease and hepatocellular carcinoma in conjunction with chemotherapy (61).

Radioimmunotherapy trials using *monoclonal* antibodies in patients with solid tumors was initiated by Larson et al. in 1982. A Fab fragment of anti-97.5 was radiolabeled with ^{131}I and administered to in seven patients with melanoma. Despite good localization of the ^{131}I-labeled Fab with estimated doses of 3800 to 8500 rad to tumor, the antitumor effects were few and modest. The bone marrow was the first organ of critical toxicity. One partial response was obtained in a patient who received 374 mCi of ^{131}I Fab (62).

The following section will describe more recent studies that have been reported for patients with solid tumors. The antibodies that have been adminstered systemically are listed in Table 2. Routes of administration other than systemic injection have also been explored with radiolabeled antibodies (see Table 3). Most of the antibodies react with several tumor types, but we have chosen to categorize these studies according to site of primary disease.

A. Gastrointestinal Carcinoma

1. Anti-CEA Antibodies

CEA is a 200-kD glycoprotein antigen expressed by colorectal, lung, pancreatic, and breast cancers, among others. Several anti-CEA antibodies have been radiolabeled for clinical studies of RIS and RIT. In general, anti-CEA antibodies have been studied in cohorts of patients which include all CEA expressing tumors.

^{131}I NP-4 and MN-14. These are specific to the class III epitope of CEA. Rosenblum et al. carried out a dose escalation study of the F(ab')$_2$ fragment of NP-4 in 13 patients with colorectal cancer. A single infusion of 40 to 135 mCi/ m^2 ^{131}I was used, with 2.4 to 8.1 mg/m^2. They found that pharmacokinetics were complex; the serum clearance half-times ranged from 6 to 42 hours (63). This appeared to be unrelated to tumor burden or protein mass, but may have been from antibody complexation with circulating CEA. Hematological toxicity was the major dose-limiting toxicity, with granulocyte and platelet nadirs occurring

Table 3 Compartmental RIT

Antibody	Antigen	Route	Radionuclide	Disease	Ref.
BC-2, BC-4	Antitenascin	Intralesional	I-131	Glioma	100
81C6	Antitenascin	Intralesional/Intrathecal	I-131	Glioma	101/105
ERIC	Neural cell adhesion molecule	Intralesional	I-131, Y-90	Glioma	102,103
Mel-14	Proteoglycan chondroitin-sulfate-associated protein	Intralesional/Intrathecal	I-131	Glioma Melanoma	102,104
HMFG1	Human milk fat globulin	Intrathecal	I-131	Lung, ovary, bladder, breast	104
M340	Neuroectodermal	Intrathecal	I-131	PNETs	104
		Intraperitoneal	I-131	Ovarian	110–113
				Gastrointestinal carcinomatosis	114

at 4 to 5 weeks after infusion. The MTD was between 90 and 115 mCi/m^2. Five patients developed HAMA. No responses were seen, but four patients with stable disease received a second dose.

Behr et al. reported a phase I/II RIT study in 57 patients with ^{131}I NP-4. Dosages ranged from 44 to 268 mCi. Only one PR occurred in 35 assessable patients, but 11 other patients showed minor responses or stabilization of disease (64). Juweid reported a study using the F(ab')$_2$ fragment of NP-4 in patients with small volume disease and in this situation variable serum clearance was not seen, possibly because of lower levels of CEA (65). At the MTD, responses were not observed but stabilization of disease occurred for 3 to 7 months in 6 of 13 patients who previously had progressive disease. HAMA limited the number of infusions that could be given.

^{131}*I-COL-1.* This is a high-affinity anti-CEA murine antibody. Yu et al. studied 18 patients with advanced gastrointestinal malignancies, using increasing doses of ^{131}I-COL-1 (66). Dose levels ranged from 10 to 74 mCi/m^2. Thrombocytopenia was dose limiting at 65mCi/m^2, and was less severe in the patients with high serum CEA and high tumor burden who also showed increased serum clearance. In this study bone marrow aspirates and biopsies were performed in 11 patients at 1 week. No significant correlations were found between the fraction of the injected dose in the marrow and hematological toxicity or pharmacokinetics. No objective responses were seen but four patients had stable disease.

^{90}*Y-T84.66.* Wong et al. evaluated another high affinity, anti-CEA chimeric antibody, T84.66 (67). In a preliminary report, 15 patients received the antibody radiolabeled with ^{111}In, and three had received T84.66 radiolabeled with 5 mCi ^{90}Y DTPA in a Phase I RIT study. Again serum clearance was variable, $T_{1/2}$ beta ranging from 30 to 229 hours. The serum clearance was unrelated to serum CEA and total body tumor burden, but increased serum clearance was related to a high tumor burden in the liver and was inversely proportional to the liver residence time. The tumor targeting was not affected by the variable serum clearance and was comparable to that of the murine T84.66.

^{131}*I A5B7.* Lane undertook a clinical study to assess the differences in tumor uptake and pharmacokinetics using the intact anti-CEA antibody A5B7 and its F(ab')$_2$ fragments (68). Injected dose ranged from 46 to 148 mCi. At the early time point, 4.5 hours, the radioactivity in the tumor from the F(ab')$_2$ was twice that for the intact antibody. Clearance from tumor and blood was highly variable, with no observed difference between the two groups of patients. There was no significant difference in dosimetry, although the early higher uptake of the F(ab')$_2$ would deliver a higher initial dose rate. Typical myelosuppression was seen at 4 to 6 weeks, similar for both groups, indicating a similar exposure to the marrow from both forms of radiolabeled antibodies. One of nine patients achieved a complete response with the fragment, and 1 of 10 patients achieved a partial response with the intact antibody. These authors concluded that the modest increase in tumor localization may have an impact because it is accompanied by an increased dose rate.

^{186}Re-NR-CO-02. We carried out a Phase I trial using the F(ab′)$_2$ fragment of NR-CO-02 in 31 patients, 29 with gastrointestinal cancers. We chose ^{186}Re as the therapeutic radionuclide because it has a higher-energy beta emission than ^{131}I and can be stably conjugated to antibodies with the MAG2-GABA preformed chelate developed by Fritzberg et al. The half-life and photon emission make it a suitable isotope for gamma camera imaging so that we could both confirm that the antibody conjugate localized in tumor tissue and follow biodistribution of ^{186}Re in the normal organs (69). We used the ^{99m}Tc-labeled F(ab′)$_2$ NR-CO-02 as a tumor imaging agent to determine the presence of antigen in tumor. If positive, the ^{186}Re-labeled antibody fragment was administered for therapy. The dose levels studied ranged from 25 to 200 mCi/m^2 ^{186}Re. Clearance of the labeled antibody was variable, but did not correlate with serum CEA or tumor burden. This could have been because the radiolabeled antibody was preceded by cold blocker 5 min prior to injection, which may have complexed circulating CEA. The MTD was 125 mCi/m^2 in patients who were heavily pretreated with radiation or chemotherapy more intensive than antimetabolites (e.g., 5-FU). The MTD was not reached at 200 mCi/m^2 in patients with limited prior therapy (i.e., no chemotherapy or 5-FU only), although toxicity was seen in some patients. HAMA occurred in 86% of these patients.

We also administered the ^{186}Re NR-CO-02 F(ab′)$_2$ by hepatic artery catheter to five patients with metastases from colorectal carcinoma confined to the liver. We evaluated the benefit of this approach by following biodistribution and estimating radiation absorbed dose. We were unable to show any advantage from the first-pass exposure of the liver metastases to the intra-arterially administered radiolabeled antibody, even though one patient with colon carcinoma achieved a PR on two occasions following an intra-arterial dose of 83 and 89 mCi/m^2.

2. Pancarcinoma Antibodies

^{186}Re NR-LU-10. NR-LU-10 is a pancarcinoma antibody reactive with a 40-kD glycoprotein expressed on the surface of most epithelial carcinomas. We conjugated this antibody with ^{186}Re and studied 15 patients with colorectal (10), lung (2), ovary (2), or renal cell (1) carcinoma in a dose escalation study (69). Patients were treated with the ^{186}Re immunoconjugate within 2 weeks of a ^{99m}Tc imaging study using the NR-LU-10 Fab fragment. NR-LU-10 antibody 40 mg was labeled with escalating doses of ^{186}Re, from 25 to 120 mCi/m^2. Responses were not seen in any of the patients on this protocol and all patients developed HAMA.

Because the radiation dose to tumor was insufficient for response, we attempted to increase the MTD of single dose RIT. We continued dose escalation with ^{186}Re-NR-LU-10 using harvested autologous bone marrow or peripheral blood stem cells (PBSC) to manage the marrow toxicity in 14 patients (70). Dose escalation continued up to 300 mCi/m^2 ^{186}Re with reinfusion of marrow or PBSC at day 10 when there was < 25 mCi/m^2 ^{186}Re retained in the whole body. Two PR were seen at the higher dose levels studied. A second organ of dose-limiting toxicity was not identified. Thus, stem cell harvesting and reinfusion did allow increased dose of radioactivity to be administered for RIT of solid tumors, but further modifications still seemed essential in order to administer sufficient radioactivity to achieve responses.

B72.3. B72.3 is an antibody raised against the TAG-72 antigen, a high-molecular-weight glycoprotein (> 1000 kD) which is expressed in colorectal, ovarian, breast, pancreas, lung, and prostate tumors. When murine B72.3 was radiolabeled with ^{131}I or ^{90}Y, no responses were seen even at the MTD (71).

Meredith studied 12 patients with ^{131}I chimeric B72.3, on a dose escalation trial, up to a highest dose level to 36 mCi/m^2 (72) and reported no responses. Meredith then reported a dose-fractionated study in 12 patients receiving 28 or 36 mCi/m^2 ^{131}I chimeric B72.3, given in two or three weekly fractions which showed a modest but significant reduction in myelotoxicity; only one patient had a minor tumor response. In this study, although the incidence of HACA was lower than after the murine antibody, nine patients did develop HACA after the first treatment with this chimeric antibody (73).

CC49. Scott et al. treated 24 heavily pretreated patients with ^{131}I-labeled CC49 on a dose escalation study. The MTD was determined to be 75 mCi/m^2 (74). All patients had HAMA at 4 weeks. One of 24 patients had a PR. This study continued (75) in patients with only minimal prior chemotherapy. In these patients, the dose level was increased to 105 mCi/m^2 without significant toxicity.

Fifteen patients with refractory colon cancer were studied by Murray (76) in a Phase II trial of 75mCi/m^2 ^{131}I CC49. Tumor localization was observed in all patients, but tumor dose estimates were <700 rads. About half the patients had grade 3 to 4 bone marrow toxicity, and nearly all developed HAMA. No responses were seen.

Tempero et al. studied fourteen patients with ^{131}I CC49 at higher dose levels in conjunction with autologous bone marrow or PBSC rescue (77). The therapeutic dose was administered 5 days after the imaging study, and dose levels reached 300 mCi/m^2 ^{131}I. The tumor-to-normal-tissue activity ratios in four biopsy samples ranged from 3 to 19, and tumor dose estimates ranged from 630 to 3300 rads in five patients. Twelve of 14 patients experienced severe marrow toxicity and required marrow or stem cell reinfusion. The highest level was dose limiting because of myelotoxicity; no severe toxicities were observed in other organs.

No objective responses were observed. Because of the heterogeneous uptake of antibody into tumor and the low path length of the ^{131}I, CC49 was thought to be of limited value for RIT in colon cancer, but is still being evaluated for prostate cancer (see below).

^{131}I A33. A33 is an antibody to a cell membrane antigen found in colorectal cancer and in normal small bowel and colon. It is an antibody that internalizes rapidly in cancer cells but not in normal tissue cells. Welt (78) reported on 23 patients with colorectal cancer who received escalating doses of ^{131}I A33 monoclonal antibody. The MTD in heavily pretreated patients was 75 mCi/m². Mild gastrointestinal symptoms were experienced in eight patients, most likely because this antibody crossreacts with normal bowel tissue. Three patients had mixed responses and two without radiological evidence of disease had decreased serum CEA levels.

^{125}I A33. A33 was also studied in 21 patients but with ^{125}I, an auger electron-emitting radioisotope (79). The radioactivity dose was increased to 350 mCi/m² with minimal toxicity to marrow and only mild or absent gastrointestinal symptoms. CEA levels decreased in three patients, one patient had a mixed response, and stable disease was seen in 12 patients. Interestingly, additional significant responses were seen in patients who had subsequent chemotherapy.

^{125}I ch17-1A. Meredith (80) also studied ^{125}I for 28 colorectal cancer patients with another internalizing Ab, chimeric 17-1A. Doses were administered as a single dose of up to 100 mCi, or up to 250 mCi subdivided 4 days apart. Although the beta phase serum clearance of 100 to 190 hours was slow, no toxicity was observed and it was concluded that high-dose ^{125}I was safe. However, no responses were observed either.

Although gastrointestinal malignancies are relatively radioresistant and responses have been infrequent, these patients have been widely studied in Phase I trials. In general they have not been exposed to intensive chemotherapy from myelosuppressive drugs and do not have rapidly progressive disease. Thus they are relatively ideal patients for Phase I studies. Additional strategies will have to be implemented for RIT in these patients to achieve higher response rates. A complicating factor in several of these Phase I trials has been the use of anti-CEA antibodies and their complexation with circulating CEA antigen which alters pharmacokinetics. For example, in both NP-4 and COL-1 studies, complexes were detected within 5 min of injection indicating that antibodies directed against circulating antigen are subject to variable pharmacokinetics related to the level of circulating antigen. In other anti-CEA antibody studies, tumor burden was noted to alter the pharmacokinetics, probably more so than in patients when antibodies to non-shedding antigens are used.

B. Other CEA-Expressing Cancers

Phase I studies with anti-CEA antibodies have also been carried out in patients with ovarian cancer and unresectable or metastatic medullary thyroid cancer.

Juweid et al. reported on a dose ecalation trial in which ^{131}I MN-14, was administered to 11 patients with advanced ovarian cancer. The MTD was 40 mCi/m^2. A clinical response was seen in one patient (81).

Nonmyeloablative doses of ^{131}I-labeled NP-4 and MN-14 intact antibodies and the bivalent fragments have been administered to 17 patients with medullary thyroid cancer (82). Dosages of ^{131}I ranged from 46 to 268 mCi, depending on whether a fragment was administered and whether HAMA was present. Myelotoxicity was the only toxicity observed. Virtually all patients receiving intact antibody and half of those receiving fragments developed HAMA. Minor responses were observed in 5 of 11 evaluable patients, mostly with the F(ab')$_2$ fragments of both antibodies.

C. Prostate Cancer

CYT-356, Prostascint. CYT-356, an antibody directed against a prostate-specific antigen, 7E11-C5.3, has been studied extensively as an imaging agent (83). This antibody has also been radiolabeled with ^{90}Y for a Phase I therapy study. Twelve patients were studied; the maximum tolerated dose was below 12 mCi/m^2, limited by marrow toxicity. The authors believed marrow toxicity to be related to extensive bony involvement and prior marrow irradiation to more than half the marrow. No objective responses were seen, but improvement in symptoms was reported.

KC4. KC4 is a pancarcinoma antibody directed against a high-molecular-weight membrane and cytoplasmic glycoprotein (84). In a dose escalation study, calcium disodium EDTA was administered for 72 hours in conjunction with escalating doses of ^{90}Y KC4 to patients with refractory prostate cancer. Symptomatic improvement was reported again here, but at the low dose of 9 mCi/m^2 severe marrow toxicity was observed.

Meredith has reported on several Phase I trials using ^{131}I-CC49 in prostate cancer patients. A Phase II study with 75 mCi/m^2 ^{131}I-CC49 also showed symptomatic improvement in two-thirds of patients but all patients developed HAMA within 4 weeks (85,86). A trial with a low dose of cyclosporin, 8 mg/kg, and the dose fractionated to 38 mCi/m^2 at 15-day intervals was unsuccessful because HAMA still developed in two-thirds patients. The single dose approach was adopted, with the addition of alpha interferon and the higher 75 mCi/m^2 ^{131}I dose. Again, no objective tumor responses was seen, but there was substantial bone pain relief in several patients. Marrow toxicity was not related to the extent of bony involvement.

A combined modality study is ongoing. Patients have PBSC collected following Cytoxan and G-CSF 16 and 2 days prior to RIT. The initial dose level was 100 mCi/m^2 ^{131}I-CC49 followed by 13.2 Gy total body irradiation given over 4 days, beginning 8 days following RIT. The stem cells and G-CSF are then reinfused. Both patients treated at the first dose level have achieved objective tumor response.

D. Breast Cancer

L-6. L-6 is an adenocarcinoma antibody with biological activity that has been evaluated in breast cancer patients by DeNardo et al. (88). Preliminary work showed that reactive sites in the vascular endothelium of the lungs that were readily available for binding trapped up to 20% of the injected dose immediately following injection. Increasing doses of unlabeled antibody, "cold blocker," 50 to 400 mg, were administered prior to radiolabeled antibody to saturate the antigenic sites in the lung. This successfully reduced lung activity from 19% to 4%, allowing the radiolabeled antibody to be visualized at the tumor sites. The increased antibody also resulted in a slower clearance rate from the serum. In a Phase I study using ^{131}I murine L-6, 200 mg cold blocker was administered. Three to 15 mg L-6 was administered with 10 mCi ^{131}I/mg antibody and the MTD was 60 mCi/m^2. One of 10 patients achieved a temporary complete remission, but 40% of patients developed a HAMA response (87). In a multiple dose protocol, 10 heavily pretreated patients were treated with monthly injections of ^{131}I chL-6. The MTD was 60 mCi/m^2, limited by myelotoxicity. In 6 of the 10 patients, clinically measurable tumor responses were seen (88). In this study, serum levels of IL-2 receptors were measured and and the increase in serum IL-2 was greatest in the patients who responded. The authors speculated that the reason for success with the L-6 antibody is a combination of the increased vascular permeability from the unlabeled biologically active antibody, the radiation, and the activated effector cell mechanism. On other multiple-dose protocols, patients received G-CSF 7 to 20 days following infusion, or underwent immunopheresis using a goat antimouse antibody to reduce the nonbound circulating antibody (89). A high-dose study using 150 mCi/m^2 given at 8-week intervals was initiated. Patients had progenitor stem cells reinfused when circulating radioactivity reached an acceptable level. Thrombocytopenia was successfully managed with this regimen. Multiple doses were limited by HAMA for the first two patients. The third patient was given cyclosporin which prevented HAMA formation even after three doses, and she showed evidence of tumor response (90).

BrE-3. This is an antibody directed against the peptide epitope of (91) human milk fat globule. Schrier (92) treated nine heavily treated patients with stage IV breast cancer with ^{90}Y-labeled BrE-3 antibody. Harvested autologous marrow or PBSC was reinfused at 15 days in conjunction with G-CSF. Fifteen and 20 mCi/m^2 ^{90}Y was administered. Pharmacokinetic data indicated that the ^{90}Y biodistribution was not identical to the ^{111}In biodistribution. Six patients developed transient grade 4 marrow toxicity but all recovered and no other toxicities occurred. The ^{90}Y conjugated with MX-DTPA dissociated from the antibody and deposited in the bone, causing the high incidence of marrow toxicity; bone biopsies confirmed this localization of ^{90}Y in the bone. Based on ^{111}In imaging, tumor doses 35 to 56 rad/mCi were reported. Four of eight evaluable patients achieved a PR, noted in lymph nodes, skin, and marrow lesions, and one achieved a clinical CR. This study is ongoing to define the second organ of toxicity.

CC49. The TAG-72 antigen is expressed in 90% of breast carcinomas. Mulligan studied nine patients with ^{177}Lu DOTA CC49 (five of whom were breast cancer patients). ^{177}Lu was considered an attractive alternative radionuclide with a lower-energy beta emission and longer half-life than ^{90}Y (93). However, ^{177}Lu accumulated in the cells of the reticuloendothelial system and was retained there for a prolonged period. Images demonstrated the tumor uptake as well as activity in the bone marrow. This resulted in myelosuppression at low doses; the MTD was 15 mCi/m^2. Reduction in the RES uptake would be required for this to become a useful radioimmunoconjugate.

The biological response modifier α-interferon is able to increase the antigenic expression of TAG-72 and increase antibody targeting in tumors (94). Murray tested this in 15 patients with breast cancer, assessing TAG-72 expression and ^{131}I CC49 uptake (95). After 3 days of α-interferon, 3 million units daily, 10 or 20 mCi ^{131}I-CC49 was administered and 48 hours later a biopsy was taken and compared with a prestudy biopsy. The TAG-72 expression was increased by 45% following the α-interferon ($P < .05$), and increased ^{131}I CC49 localization in tumor was also present. However, because of intra- and interpatient variability in percentage of tumor cells in the biopsy specimens as well as heterogeneity of TAG-72 expression, this was difficult to evaluate with certainty. Pharmacokinetics and biodistribution were changed with administration of the α-interferon. RIT at the MTD with concurrent α-interferon administration is under investigation. In a preliminary report, one of 15 patients had achieved a PR at the expense of increased marrow toxicity, from a more prolonged serum clearance at the higher doses (96).

E. Glioma

In patients with gliomas, because of the difficulty in interpreting diagnostic imaging scans, and the short survival time in these patients (median 10 months), survival is used as an endpoint. Radiation following surgical resection offers a several-months' advantage in survival time, but is limited by normal brain tolerance. Targeted radiation is therefore an attractive approach to increase radiation dose to tumor and potentially contribute to increased survival.

Kalofonas reported a study with ^{131}I antiepidermal growth factor receptor antibody (EGFr) (97). Ten patients with recurrent gliomas received intravenous or intra-arterial administration of the radioimmunoconjugate; six showed clinical improvement.

Brady treated 101 patients with high-grade gliomas by intravenous or intra-arterial injections of ^{125}I-labeled antiepidermal growth factor receptor antibody, 425. Patients with both primary and recurrent astrocytomas and glioblastoma multiforme were treated with an average total dose of 139 mCi ^{125}I, administered divided into three weekly infusions. Brady reported one CR and two PR of short duration following ^{125}I EGF-425 intravenously The median survival in both groups was improved with these relatively radioresistant tumors. Fifteen of these patients had recurrent malignant astrocytomas and were treated with 25 to 130 mCi intra-arterially. The median survival was 8 ± 7 months (98).

Twenty-five patients with malignant astrocytomas were then treated in a Phase II adjunctive therapy trial (99). Four to 6 weeks following surgical debulking (2) or biopsy (13), and external beam radiation, one to three doses of ^{125}I-labeled antibody 425 were administered intravenously or intra-arterially at 7- to 14-day intervals. Cumulative doses ranged from 40 to 224 mCi. HAMA did not develop in any of these patients. The 1-year survival was 60% with a projected median survival of 15.6 months.

Malignant gliomas tend to spread by local invasion rather than metastases. Thus intralesional, intracavitary or intrathecal administration of the therapeutic radiolabeled antibody may be useful to deliver the therapeutic radiation directly to these solid tumors (Table 3).

Intralesional Injection. One approach is to inject the radioimmunoconjugate through an Ommaya reservoir into the surgical cavity following surgical resection, or directly into a cystic tumor when the lesion has a predominantly cystic component. Here the antibody binding to antigen serves to prolong retention of the radiation at the target, while sparing normal brain tissue.

Initial studies with ^{131}I antibodies into the surgical cavity demonstrated the feasibility of an intralesional or intracavity approach following surgical resection. Riva et al. (100) reported their experience with intralesional administration of ^{131}I-labeled antibodies for treatment of both newly diagnosed and recurrent glioma. Tenascin is a polymorphic extracellular glycoprotein found in the several carcinomas and malignant gliomas. Antitenascin antibodies BC-2 and BC-4 were radiolabeled with up to 65 mCi ^{131}I, and injected into the resection cavity through a catheter. The radioactivity remained at the target site for an effective half-time of 60 hours and thus could deliver high doses to the tumor, on average 42,000 rad/cycle. Up to four cycles were given to 50 patients. Although HAMA developed in some patients, it did not intefere with tumor targeting in subsequent cycles. In all there were three CRs, six PRs, 11 tumor stabilizations, and 19 tumor progressions recorded. Eleven patients with no radiological evidence of disease at the time of treatment remained disease free. In 26 patients the median time to progression was 3 months, and in the group of newly diagnosed patients who were treated time to progression was 7 months. The median survival was 20 months—17 months in patients with bulky disease, and 23 months in patients with minimal or microscopic disease. The median survival of these patients is usually 10 months; thus this study suggests an improved outcome for these patients.

Another anti-Tenascin antibody, 81C6, radiolabeled with up to 100 mCi ^{131}I has been studied in patients with recurrent cystic gliomas and in patients with a surgically created resection cavity from primary or metastatic brain tumor. High retention in the cysts with little systemic dissemination resulted in absorbed dose esimates of 12,700 to 70,300 rad. No hematological toxicity or neurotoxicity was observed. In preliminary results, all five patients with recurrent cystic glioma appeared to benefit from the treatment with an increased survival; partial responses (four) or prolonged stabilization of disease (one) were observed. In the majority of patients with administration into the surgically created cavity, stabilization of disease was observed (101).

ERIC-1 antibody was radiolabeled with up to 60 mCi ^{131}I and administered to nine patients with relapsed glioma who had a cyst or cavity following prior resection (102). In two patients with cystic lesions, the need for aspiration was markedly reduced. The short range of the ^{131}I beta particles delivers a high dose to only a rim of tissue approximately 1 mm thick, around the surgical cavity. In a study with ^{90}Y-labeled ERIC-1, 15 patients were treated with up to 18 mCi, and the cerebral edema that developed was managed successfully with dexamethasone (103). Dose estimates from this treatment ranged from 5500 to 35,100 rad, depending on whether complete binding on antibody occurred. Again in this study, the two patients with cystic tumors required less frequent aspirations. While the overall benefit of the RIT could not be easily determined from this group of patients, median survival was 6 months from treatment.

Intrathecal Injection. In neoplastic meningitis, external beam therapy is limited by dose to the normal nervous system. The average survival of patients with neoplastic meningitis is 3 months from diagnosis. Tumor cells are found floating freely in the CSF or in sheets lining the meninges. Thus an intrathecal route of administration bypasses the problems of access to tumor antigen that are present when radioimmunoconjugates are administered systemically.

Papanastassiou treated patients with diffuse leptomeningeal deposits with intrathecal radiolabeled antibodies administered through an Ommaya reservoir. Patients included those with carcinomatous meningitis (7), primitive neuroectodermal tumors (18), and CNS leukemia (22), with the antibody depending on the disease (104). The radioimmunoconjugate leaves the intrathecal space relatively quickly; peak blood flow levels of 6% to 48% of the injected dose reached the vascular system at 24 to 56 hours following injection. Dosage of ^{131}I ranged from 17 to 90 mCi on 1.7 to 9 mg antibody. Transient aseptic mengitis was common following intrathecal RIT, occurring in approximately 60% of patients. Occasional patients developed seizures. No long-term sequelae have been observed. Significant myelosuppression occurred in several patients who received >54 mCi. Response was difficult to assess and was measured by clearance of cells from the CNS and clinical improvement. Papanastassiou reported a 33% overall response rate. This was poorest in the carcinoma patients. The mean time to relapse in 37% of PNET patients was 10 months. In patients with leukemia, marked responses of clearance of leukemic cells from the CSF were observed, but for only 4 to 8 weeks.

Brown et al. reported on patients with leptomeningeal disease and brain tumor resection cavities with subarachnoid communication. Patients with anaplastic gliomas, ependyomas, medullablastoma, and anaplastic astrocytoma received a single dose of up to 100 mCi of ^{131}I 81C6 antibody administered intrathecally through an Ommaya reservoir (105). No nonhematological toxicity occurred and the MTD was 80 mCi, limited by hematological toxicity. Ten of 24 evaluable patient developed HAMA, but in two patients who were retreated, there was no alteration in biodistribution of radiolabeled antibody. Of 31 patients with malignant gliomas, one showed a radiographic PR and disease stabilization occurred in 42%, representing an apparent increased survival rate although this was difficult to evaluate.

F. Melanoma

Bigner used the (Fab')$_2$ fragment of Mel-14, antimelanoma antibody directed against antiproteoglycan chondroitin sulfate–associated protein, to treat a patient with a brain metastasis from melanoma (103). The patient received Mel-14 F(ab')$_2$ labeled with 37mCi ^{131}I injected into the surgical resection cavity, and achieved a complete local response.

Eleven patients were treated with up to 80 mCi ^{131}I Mel-14 (Fab')2 intrathecally via lumbar puncture. They had melanoma (8), melanosis (1), oligodendroglioma (1) and glioblastoma (1). One patient at 80 mCi had hematological toxicity. After treatment, three patients had complete CSF responses and two had partial responses radiologically; survival ranged from 1 to 11 months, an apparent improvement on the 3-month average survival.

VI. FURTHER STRATEGIES TO IMPROVE OUTCOME OF RIT

It now seems clear that a single dose of conventionally radiolabeled murine monoclonal antibody administered at the maximum tolerated dose is unlikely to provide sufficient radiation to tumor to be effective as therapy for patients with

Table 4 Strategies to Improve Outcome

Increase dose intensity	Increase administered activity	Bone marrow support
		Autologous marrow or PBSC
		Cytokines
		Hematopoetic growth factors
	Increase localization	Non systemic injection: intraperitoneal/ intrathecal/intralesional
		Improve vascular access: external-beam therapy/hyperthermia
		Upregulate antigen expression: interferons
		Higher-affinity antibodies
	Increase dose rate	Smaller molecules
		Radioisotopes
Increase radio-sensitivity	Radiosensitizing chemotherapy	
Reduce marrow exposure	Dose fractionation	
	Remove circulating radiolabeled antibody	Second antibody
		Immunosorption columns
		Pretarget RIT

solid tumors. In Phase I studies with radiolabeled monoclonal antibodies or fragments, bone marrow toxicity has been dose limiting and few complete responses have been seen, even at the MTD. This in part reflects the fact that antibodies are not ideal carriers of radiation to a tumor target. In general, $<0.1\%$ of the injected dose localizes to each gram of tumor. Explanations for this low accretion include the small fraction of the cardiac output that reaches the tumor; poor vascular permeability, because of vascular spasm and high interstitial pressure from decreased lymphatic drainage causing a high-pressure gradient which compromises transport toward the center; and restricted antigen expression on tumor cells.

To increase the radiation absorbed dose to the tumor, one can approach the issue of the therapeutic ratio by either increasing the dose intensity, increasing the radiation sensitivity of the tumor, or alternatively reducing the toxicity and thereby allowing higher doses of radioactivity to be administered (see Table 4).

A. Increasing Dose Intensity

1. Increase Radioactivity Administered

The initial approach to increase the dose intensity was to administer more radioactivity. The MTD was limited by hematological toxicity which can be managed with transfusions or autologous marrow and stem cell harvest. Cytokines act as indirect marrow protective agents by increasing the pool of hematopoietic stem cells. Blumenthal showed that IL-1 and GM-CSF can allow increased doses of radioactivity to be administered in mice (106). The addition of hematopoietic growth factors has aided the recovery of patients undergoing these procedures (107). This approach has increased the MTD but has not consistently resulted in significantly increased response rates; other tactics to achieve tumor regression are necessary.

2. Increasing Tumor Localization

Because of the physical limitation of accessibility of antibodies to tumors, strategies have been developed to increase tumor localization. Increasing the mass amount of antibody and using intra-arterial administration were attempted but did not have a significant impact. Other approaches under investigation are the following.

Compartmental Administration. Intraperitoneal administration of the immunoconjugates for RIT has shown some success because the more prolonged tumor cell exposure results in improved binding (108,109). Several trials have been undertaken in patients with ovarian cancer using IP administration. [131]I-, [90]Y-, [186]Re-, and ^{177}Lu-labeled antibodies have been used. Responses in patients with small-volume peritoneal disease have been observed (110–113). The experience with patients with ovarian cancer is discussed in detail in this volume in Chapter 12.

Riva reported a study of 34 patients with peritoneal gastrointestinal carcinomatosis who received 100 mCi ^{131}I FO23C5 via the intraperitoneal and intravenous route. Therapy was administered in conjunction with cyclosporin A every 3 months with up to four injections. Three complete and six partial responses were observed. Seventeen patients received α-interferon to increase the expression of CEA; this increased the response rate to 59%, compared with 29% without α-interferon (114).

Intratumoral and intrathecal injection for patients with glioma have been described above. A similar approach developed by Order uses ^{32}P administered with albumin as brachytherapy for pancreatic cancer (115). These intralesional approaches are valuable in situations when the tumor is localized and accessible, and local therapy is all that is necessary for tumor control.

Blood Flow Manipulations. RIT may be most effective for small tumors, which are more vascular, but manipulations to improve tumor blood flow to larger tumors may also be worthwhile. Studies to increase vascular flow or permeability at the tumor site using external beam therapy and hyperthermia have been carried out (116,117). The results of the preclinical studies with external beam radiation prior to administering immunoconjugate have varied with tumor type and location (118,119). Combined RIT/external beam therapy is being evaluated in patients (120).

DeNardo reported that IL-2 modified with polyethylene glycol, PEGIL-2, administered before radiolabeled antibody enhanced antibody localization by a factor of 2 in mice by increasing vascular permeability to the antibody (121). DeNardo also showed the rIL-2 increased the response rate in xenografts treated with ^{67}Cu-Lym-1 by about 20% (122). In a preclinical study, when IL-2 was conjugated to an anti-CEA antibody, ZCE025, Nakamura found that the cytokine function of IL-2 was destroyed but that vascular permeability specific to the tumor was increased (123).

Biological Response Modifiers. IL-2 and alpha interferon appear to be successful in upregulating the antigen expression of CEA and TAG-72. In 1990, Murray et al. showed altered biodistribution and an improved relative tumor uptake of ^{111}In antimelanoma antibody 96.5 in patients who had received α-interferon (95). In other clinical studies evaluating the effects of α-interferon, Greiner showed increased serum levels of TAG-72 and CEA antigen (124). Greiner also demonstrated increased levels of both antigens in ascites cells following intraperitoneal injection of γ-interferon to patients with ovarian cancer (125) and increasing targeting in tumors, but whether this will translate into increased tumor response rate is still under investigation. α-Interferon (96) and IL-2 (91) have been studied in RIT clinical trials but definitive results have yet to be published.

Increasing the Dose Rate at the Tumor. This may be achievable by using radiolabeled antibody fragments or small molecules which penetrate the tumor more rapidly. Early preclinical studies supported the theory that total dose delivered is of primary importance. Thus, the belief that greater exposure of tumor to radioactivity as determined by area under the curve led to the use of intact antibodies as the vehicle to carry the therapeutic radiation in the majority of studies. Behr et al. compared response rates of patients with CEA-expressing tumors who received the intact antibodies and the F(ab')$_2$ fragment of NP-4 and MN-14. Their data showed that more frequent responses occurred in patients receiving the radiolabeled fragments, although only minor responses were reported. This will require further investigation. Recently studies of ^{90}Y on a small peptide, octreotide, have shown responses in Phase I RIT studies for patients with neuroendocrine tumors (126).

3. Increasing Radiation Sensitivity

Radiation-sensitizing chemotherapeutic agents such as 5-FU and cisplatin have been used in combination with 3000-rad external beam therapy and have resulted in improved response rates in carcinoma of the esophagus, colon, anus, cervix, bladder, and head and neck compared with chemotherapy alone (127).

Drugs to increase radiation sensitivity to RIT have been studied in mouse xenograft models, and greater tumor growth delays and/or cures have been seen with Taxol and ^{90}Y chimeric L-6 (56), with Topotecan and ^{90}Y human BrE (128), cisplatin with ^{131}I 323/A3 (129), and 5-FU with ^{90}Y CC49 (130) and ^{131}I A33 (131). The effects of these combination approaches are dependent on the timing and dosing of the chemotherapeutic agents, and will require considerable study in clinical trials.

Another approach to increase radiation sensitization is to use halogenated pyrimidines as radiation sensitizers. 5-Iododeoxyuridine (IudR) and bromodeoxyuridine (BudR) have been most widely studied (132–134). These act as a thymidine analog which is incorporated into DNA via the thymidine salvage pathway. This appears to increase DNA susceptibility to radiation and inhibits DNA repair. In vitro studies and xenograft studies of these pyrimidines in conjunction with RIT have shown increased tumor growth delay (135,136). Clinical studies using BudR and external-beam therapy have shown a survival advantage in patients with anaplastic astrocytoma (137).

4. Reducing the Exposure to Normal Tissues

Several strategies have been proposed to reduce the exposure of normal tissues to radiation.

Dose fractionation appears to have an impact on reducing marrow toxicity but repeated fractions are limited by the formation of HAMA with murine antibodies. We attempted to reduce toxicity by fractionating IP ^{186}Re NR-LU-10 and administering a second dose of IP ^{186}Re NR-LU-10 7 days after the first dose (138). At the highest dose level of 90 mCi/m^2 twice, i.e., 180 mCi/m^2, there was severe marrow toxicity in one of three patients. In contrast, similar toxicity was seen in two of three patients in the single-dose study at only 150 mCi/m^2. Meredith et al. have incorporated this strategy into several clinical trials with B72.3 in patients with colorectal cancer and with CC49 in patients with colon and prostate cancer, and have confirmed a reduction in myelotoxicity but the number of infusions was still limited by HAMA (139).

To address the HAMA problem with murine antibodies, immunosuppression was attempted with cyclosporine. This approach appears to have some efficacy in reducing immunogenecity but does not appear to be sufficient to permit administration of multiple doses of antibodies. With modern genetic engineering, chimeric antibodies were produced in an attempt to overcome HAMA. The HACA was still a problem in several clinical trials. Richman et al. successfully used cyclosporin in studies of chimeric L-6 to reduce HACA formation in patients with breast cancer (91). Low-dose cyclosporin, however, as used by Meredith with the highly immunogenic CC49 antibody, was unable to significantly reduce HAMA (86).

Several human antibodies have now been studied in clinical trials and have established that repetitive doses of human monoclonal antibodies can be administered without evidence of alloimmunization. Thus, it appears that the problem of HAMA may be solvable with human antibodies, and dose fractionation is becoming more feasible.

Another approach is to remove the circulating activity that has not localized at the tumor site. In 1982, Begent described a method that used a liposomally entrapped second antibody directed at the labeled antitumor antibody to accelerate clearance of the non-tumor-bound antibody without affecting clearance from the tumor. This was never used on a large scale in patients, but formed the basis of ideas to clear circulating activity. Such a clearing agent could either be administered intravenously or be extracorporeal. Candidate clearing agents include anti-antibodies directed at the Fc portion of the immunoconjugate or the avidin/biotin system with one component linked to the immunoconjugate and the other to the clearing agent (140).

The extracorporeal approach is being evaluated with external immunoadsorption columns (141). In this procedure, the patient's blood is separated into cells and plasma by a cell separator, phereis machine, and the plasma is then circulated through a column which specifically removes the radiolabeled antibody either by another antibody, e.g., goat antimouse antibody as used by DeNardo, or by avidin removing a biotinylated radiolabeled antibody as performed by Strand as discussed in Chapter 9.

The specificity of the antibody may be better exploited by a pretargeted approach. This approach delays the delivery of the radioactivity to a time when the ratio of tumor-bound to non-tumor-bound antibody has reached its highest value. After attaining an optimal antibody concentration at the tumor and simultaneous clearance of unbound antibody, a subsequently administered radioisotope bound to a small molecule can be captured by the tumor-bound antibody (142). The radionuclide administered clears rapidly from the whole body, thus minimizing the radiation dose to radiosensitive bone marrow and other normal tissues. Pretargeting has been discussed in this volume in Chapter 8. In our preliminary work, we have demonstrated that 110 mCi/m^2 can be safely administered to patients, and tumor regressions have been observed.

VII. SUMMARY

RIT is a complex, multidisciplinary effort which still faces many challenges. We have come to understand these obstacles and have realized that a single high dose of a radiolabeled antibody administered systemically is unlikely to be successful in curing cancer. In most of the trials, radiation-absorbed doses higher than 3000 rad are only infrequently reported, and with these doses, responses cannot be induced in the relatively resistant solid tumors. However, with modifications of the initial approaches, RIT may yet have a role in the management of patients with solid tumors. Preclinical studies suggest that RIT used as adjuvant therapy in patients with cancer may play an important role, but these clinical trials have not yet been completed.

Wessels has proposed that an additional 1500 to 2000 rad delivered by RIT as a boost to external beam therapy may have an effect on local control after external-beam therapy—for example, in patients with lung cancer or rectal cancer (143). Preclinical studies with external-beam therapy and RIT of liver metastases suggest that toxicities are additive; thus, for example, RIT with a radioimmuno-conjugate that does not localize in normal liver tissue may be beneficial to treat hepatic metastases while sparing the normal liver tissue.

The tumor regressions observed in preclinical studies and in patients with B-cell lymphoma and leukemia have encouraged investigators to pursue antibodies as vehicles for targeted therapy. Disappointing results overall may be due in part to the selection of advanced-stage patients with bulky disease who have failed prior treatments. The most encouraging studies in the patients with solid tumors receiving systemic RIT have been the breast cancer studies with ^{131}I chimeric L-6 antibody and its associated effector functions, and ^{90}Y-labeled BrE antibody. The compartmental approach has also shown encouraging results, and several Phase II studies are ongoing. Progress has been made in reducing the incidence of HAMA formation and in decreasing marrow toxicity. Genetically engineered chimeric antibodies have shown a reduction of the antiantibody response, and clinical trials with human and humanized antibodies indicate no immunogenicity. With the reduction in the incidence of HAMA, multiple dosing will be possible. By radiolabeling the antibody directly, marrow toxicity limited the amount of radioactivity that could be administered to less than that required to cause significant responses in most situations. Injected doses up to 300 mCi/m^2 [186]Re in our own studies and 300 mCi/m^2 ^{131}I have been administered, but marrow rescue was necessary at these high dose levels. It appears that reduction in exposure to the marrow is essential to be able to deliver higher radiation doses to tumor. Pretargeting the antibody prior to injection of the radioisotope is one strategy that seems to offer promise for achieving that goal.

REFERENCES

1. Pressman D, Keighley G. The zone of activity of antibodies as determined by the use of radioactive tracers: the zone of activity of nephrotoxic antikidney serum. J Immunol 1948; 59:141–146.

2. Pressman D. The use of paired labeling in the determination of tumor-localizing antibodies. Cancer Res 1957; 17:845–850.
3. Bale WF, Centeras MA, Goody ED. Factors influencing localization of antibodies in tumors. Cancer Res 1980; 40:2965–2972.
4. Spar IL, Bale WF, Manach D. ^{131}I-labeled antibodies to human fibrinogen: diagnostic studies and therapeutic trials. Cancer 1969; 78:731–759.
5. McCardle RJ, Harper PV, Spar IL. Studies with iodine-131-labeled antibody to human fibrinogen for diagnosis and therapy of tumors. J Nucl Med 1966; 7:837–847.
6. Vial AB, Callahan W. Univ Mich Med Bull 1956; 20:284–286.
7. Ghose T, Guclu A. Cure of a mouse lymphoma with radio-iodinated antibody. Eur J Cancer 1974; 10:787–791.
8. Kohler G, Milstein C. Continuous cultures of fused cells secreting antibody of predefined specificity. Nature 1975; 256:495–497.
9. Ballou B, Levine G, Hakala RR, Soltei D, et al. Tumor localization detected with radioactivity labeled monoclonal antibody and external scintigraphy. Science 1979; 206:844–847.
10. Breitz HB, Sullivan K, Nelp WB. Imaging lung cancer with radiolabeled antibodies. Semin Nucl Med 1993; 23(2):127–132.
11. Collier BD, Abdel-Nabi H, Doerr RJ, et al. Immunoscintigraphy performed with In-111-labeled CYT-103 in the management of colorectal cancer: comparison with CT. Radiology 1992; 185(1):179–186.
12. Surwit EA, Childers JM, Krag DN, Katterhagen G, Gallion H, Waggoner S, Mann WJ Jr. Clinical assessment of ^{111}In-CYT-103 immunoscintigraphy in ovarian cancer. Gynecol Oncol 1993; 48:285–292.
13. Moffat FL, Pinsky CM, Hammershaimb L, et al. Clinical utility of external immunoscintigraphy with the IMMU-4 technetium-99m Fab' antibody fragment in patients undergoing surgery for carcinoma of the colon and rectum: results of a pivotal, phase III trial. J Clin Oncol 1996; 14(8):2295–2305.
14. Chengazi VU, Feneley MR, Ellison D, Stalteri M, Granowski A, Granowska M, Nimmon CC, Mather SJ, Kirby RS, Britton KE. Imaging prostate cancer with technetium-99m-7E11-C5.3 (CYT-351). J Nucl Med 1997; 38:675–682.
15. Arnold MW, Schneebaum S, Berens A, Mojzisik C, Hinkle G, Martin EW Jr. Radioimmunoguided surgery challenges traditinal decision making in patients with primary colorectal cancer. Surgery 1992; 112:624–630.
16. Mazzaferri EL. Radioiodine and other treatments and outcomes. In: Braverman LE, Utiger RD, eds. The Thyroid: A Fundamental and Clinical Text. Philadelphia: Lippincott, 1991:1138–1165.
17. Laing AH, Ackery DM, Bayly J, et al. Strontium-89 chloride for pain palliation in prostatic skeletal malignancy. Br J Radiol 1991; 64:816–822.
18. Volkert WA, Goeckeler WF, Ehrhardt GJ, Ketring AR. Therapeutic radionuclides: production and decay property considerations. J Nucl Med 1991; 32:174–185.
19. Fritzberg AR, Wessels BW. Therapeutic radionuclides. In: Wagner HN, ed. Principles of Nuclear Medicine, 2nd ed. Philadelphia: Saunders, 1995:229–234.
20. Behr TM, Sharkey RM, Juweid MI, et al. Factors influencing the pharmacokinetics, dosimetry, and diagnostic accuracy of radioimmunodetection and radioimmuno-

therapy of carcinoembryonic antigen-expressing tumors. Cancer Res 1996; 56: 1805–1816.

21. Slavin-Chirorini DC, Kashmiri SVS, Schlom J, et al. Biological properties of chimeric domain-deleted anticarcinoma immunoglobulins. Cancer Res Suppl 1995; 55(23):5957–5967.

22. Pedley RB, Boden JA, Boden RW, Dale R, Begent RHJ. Comparative radioimmunotherapy using intact or F(ab')₂ fragments of ¹³¹I anti-CEA antibody in a colonic xenograft model. Br J Cancer 1993; 68(1):69–73.

23. Buchegger F, Pelegrin A, Delaloye B, Bischof-De-Laloye A, Mach JP. Iodine-¹³¹labelled MAb F(ab')₂ fragments are more efficient and less toxic than intact anti-CEA antibodies in radioimmunotherapy of large human colon carcinoma grafted in nude mice. J Nucl Med 1990; 31(6):1035–1044.

24. Beatty BG, Beatty JD, Williams LE, Paxton RJ, Shively JE, O'Connor-Tressel M. Effect of specific antibody pretreatment on liver uptake of ¹¹¹In-labeled anticarcinoembryonic antigen monoclonal antibody in nude mice bearing colon cancer xenografts. Cancer Res 1989; 49:1587–1594.

25. Weinstein JN, Eger RR, Covell DG, et al. The pharmacology of monoclonal antibodies. Ann NY Acad Sci 1987; 507:199–210.

26. Colcher D, Minelli MF, Roselli M, Muraro R, Simpson-Milenic D, Schlom J. Radioimmunolocalization of human carcinoma xenografts with B72.3 second generation (CC) monoclonal antibodies. Cancer Res 1988; 48:4597–4603.

27. Schlom J, Eggensperger D, Colcher D, et al. Therapeutic advantage of high-affinity anticarcinoma radioimmunoconjugates. Cancer Res 1992; 52:1067–1072.

28. Divgi CR, Scott AM, McDermott K, et al. Clinical comparison of radiolocalization of two monoclonal antibodies against the TAG-72 antigen. Nucl Med Biol 1994; 21:9–15.

29. Carrasquillo JA, Abrams PG, Schroff RW, Reynolds JC, et al. Effect of ¹¹¹In-9.2.27 monoclonal antibody dose on the imaging of metastatic melanoma. J Nucl Med 1987; 26:67.

30. DeNardo SJ, O'Grady LF, Macey DJ, et al. Quantitative imaging of mouse L-6 monoclonal antibody in breast cancer patients to develop a therapeutic strategy. Nucl Med Biol 1991; 18(6):621–631.

31. Hellstrom I, Beaumier P, Hellstrom KE. Antitumor effects of L-6, and IgG2a antibody that reacts with most carcinomas. Proc Natl Acad Sci USA 1986; 83:7059–7063.

32. Weiden PL, Breitz HB, Seiler CA, et al. Rhenium-186-labeled chimeric antibody NR-LU-13: pharmacokinetics, biodistribution and immunogenicity relative to murine analog NR-LU-10. J Nucl Med 1993; 34:2111–2119.

33. Goodman GE, Hellstrom I, Yelton DE, et al. Phase I trial of chimeric (human-mouse) monoclonal antibody L6 in patients with non-small cell lung, colon, and breast cancer. Cancer Immunol Immunother 1993; 36:267–273.

34. Adams GP, DeNardo SJ, Amin A, Kroger LA, DeNardo GL, Hellstrom I, Hellstrom KE. Comparison of the pharmacokinetics in mice and the biological activity of murine L6 and human-mouse chimeric Ch-L6 antibody. Antib Immunoconj Radiopharm 1992; 5(1):81–95.

35. LoBuglio AF, Wheeler RH, Trang J, et al. Mouse/human chimeric antibody in

man: kinetics and immune response. Proc Natl Acad Sci USA 1989; 86:4220–
4224.

36.   Ledermann JA, Begent RHJ, Massof C, Kelly AMB, Adam T, Bagshawe KD. A
      phase-I study of repeated therapy with radiolabed antibody to carcinoembryonic
      antigen using intermittent or continuous administration of cyclosporin A to suppress
      the immune response. Int J Cancer 1991; 47:659–664.

37.   Weiden PL, Wolf SB, Breitz HB, et al. Human anti-mouse antibody suppression
      with cyclosporin A. Cancer 1994; 73(3):1093–1097.

38.   Breitz HB, Seiler C, Weiden P, Appelbaum J, Ratliff B, Stiekema J, Klein J, Ruppel
      S, DeJager R. Re-186 16.88 IgM and 88BV69 IgG human antibody studies to assess
      potential for radioimmunotherapy. J Nucl Med 1994; 34(5):100P.

39.   Waldmann TA, Strober W. Metabolism of immunoglobulin. Prog Allergy 1969;
      13:1–10.

40.   Sharkey RM, Juweid M, Shevitz J, et al. Evaluation of a complementarity-determin-
      ing region-grafted (humanized) anti-carcinoembryonic antigen monoclonal anti-
      body in preclinical and clinical studies. Cancer Res Suppl 1995; 55(23):5935s–
      5945s.

41.   Hall EI. Radiobiology for the Radiologist, 4th ed. Philadelphia: Lippincott, 1994:317.

42.   Behr TM, Goldenberg DM, Becker WS. Radioimmunotherapy of solid tumors: a
      review "of mice and men." Hybridoma 1997; 16:101–107.

43.   Estaban JM, Schlom J, Mornex F, Colcher D. Radioimmunotherapy of athymic
      nude mice bearing human colon carcinomas with monoclonal antibody B72.3: his-
      torical and autoradiographic study effects on tumors and normal organs. Eur J Can-
      cer Clin Oncol 1987; 23:643–655.

44.   Sharkey RM, Pykett MJ, Siegel JA, Alger, EA, Primus FJ, Goldenberg DM. Radio-
      immunotherapy of the GW-39 human colonic tumor xenograft with I-131 labeled
      murine monoclonal antibody to carcinoembryonic antigen. Cancer Res 1987; 47:
      5672–5677.

45.   Cheung NK, Landmeier B, Neely J, et al. Complete tumor ablation with iodine-131
      radiolabeled disialoganglioside GD2-specific monoclonal antibody against human
      neuroblastoma xenografted in nude mice. J Natl Cancer Inst 1986; 77:739–745.

46.   Buchegger F, Vacca A, Carrel S, Schreyer M, Mach J-P. Radioimmunotherapy of
      human colon carcinoma by I-131 labeled monoclonal anti-CEA antibodies in a
      nude mouse model. Int J Cancer 1988; 41:127–134.

47.   Washburn LC, Lee Y-CC, Sun TTH, Byrd B, Crook JE, Stabin MG, Steplewski
      Z. Preclinical assessment of Y-90 labeled monoclonal antibody CO17-1A, a poten-
      tial agent for radioimmunotherapy of colorectal carcinoma. Nucl Med Biol 1988;
      15:707–711.

48.   Roselli M, Schlom J, Gansow OA, Raubitschek A, Mirzadeh S, Brechbiel MW,
      Colcher D. Comparative biodistributions of yttrium- and indium-labeled mono-
      clonal antibody B72.3 in anthymic mice bearing human colon carcinoma xeno-
      grafts. J Nucl Med 1989; 30:672–682.

49.   Beaumier PL, Venkatesan P, Vanderheyden J-L, et al. Re-186 radioimmunotherapy
      of small cell lung carcinoma xenografts in nude mice. Cancer Res 1991; 51:676–
      681.

50.   Schlom J, Siler K, Milenic D, et al. Monoclonal antibody-based therapy of a human

tumor xenograft with a lutetium-177-labeled immunoconjugate. Cancer Res 1991; 51:2889–2896.

51. Connett JM, Anderson CJ, Guo L-W, et al. Radioimmunotherapy with a Cu-64-labeled monoclonal antibody: a comparison with Cu-67. Proc Natl Acad Sci USA 1996; 93:6814–6818.

52. Chalandon Y, Mach J-P, Pelegrin A, Folli S, Buchegger F. Combined radioimmunotherapy and chemotherapy of human colon carcinoma grafted on nude mice, advantages and limitations. Anticancer Res 1992; 12:1131–1140.

53. Beaumier PI, Vanderheyden J-L. Venkatasen P, et al. Concurrent Re-186 radioimmunotherapy and chemotherapy of experimental small cell lung carcinoma. Antibod Immunoconj Radiopharm 1991; 4:735–744.

54. Blumenthal RD, Sharkey RM, Natale AM, Kashi R, Wong G, Goldenberg DM. Comparison of equitoxic radioimmunotherapy and chemotherapy in the treatment of human colonic cancer xenografts. Cancer Res 1994; 54:142–151.

55. Pedley RB, Boden JA, Boden R, Dale R, Begent RHJ. Ablation of colorectal xenografts with combined radioimmunotherapy and tumor blood flow-modifying agents. Cancer Res 1996; 56:3293–3300.

56. DeNardo SJ, Kukis DL, Kroger LA, et al. Synergy of taxol and radioimmunotherapy with yttrium-90-labeled chimeric L6 antibody: efficacy and toxicity in breast cancer xenografts. Proc Natl Acad Sci USA 1997; 94:4000–4004.

57. Sun L-Q, Vogel C-A, Mirimanoff R-O, Coucke P, Slosman DO, Mach J-P, Buchegger F. Timing effects of combined radioimmunotherapy and radiotherapy on a human solid tumor in nude mice. Cancer Res 1997; 57:1312–1319.

58. Order SE, Klein JL, Leichner PK. Radiation therapy of hepatoma with I-131 and Y-90 labeled antiferritin antibodies. Int Conf Monoclonal Antib Immunoconj Cancer 1986; 1:27–28.

59. Dillehay LE, Williams JR. Radiobiology of dose-rate patterns achievable in radioimmunoglobulin therapy. Front Radiat Ther Oncol 1990; 24:96–103.

60. Order SE, Stillwagon GB, Klein JL, et al. [131]I antiferritin. A new treatment modality in hepatoma. An RTOG study. J Clin Oncol 1985; 3:1573–1582.

61. Order SE, Vriesendorp HM, Klein JL, Leichner PK. A phase I study of [90]yttrium antiferritin: dose escalation and tumor dose. Antibod Immunoconj Radiopharm 1988; 1(2):163–168.

62. Larson SM, Carrasquillo JA, McGuffin RW, et al. Preliminary clinical experience using an I-131 labeled, murine Fab against a high molecular weight antigen of human melanoma. Radiology 1985; 155:487–492.

63. Rosenblum MG, Macey D, Podoloff D, et al. A phase I pharmacokinetic, toxicity and dosimetry study of ^{131}I labeled IMMU-4 F(ab')$_2$ in patients with advanced colorectal carcinoma. Antibod Immunoconj Radiopharm 1993; 6(4):239–255.

64. Behr TM, Sharkey RM, Juweid ME, et al. Phase I/II clinical radioimmunotherapy with an iodine-131-labeled anti-carcinoembryonic antigen murine monoclonal antibody IgG. J Nucl Med 1997; 38:858–870.

65. Juweid ME, Sharkey RM, Behr T, Swayne LC, Dunn R, Siegel J, Goldenberg DM. Radioimmunotherapy of patients with small-volume tumors using iodine-131-labeled anti-CEA monoclonal antibody NP-4 F(ab')$_2$. J Nucl Med 1996; 37(9): 1504–1510.

66. Yu B, Carrasquilo J, Milenic D, et al. Phase I trial of iodine-131-labeled COL-1 in patients with gastrointestinal maliganacies: influence of serum carcinoembryonic antigen and tumor bulk on pharmacokinetics. J Clin Oncol 1996; 6:1798–1809.
67. Wong JYC, Williams LE, Yamauchi DM, et al. Initial experience evaluating [90]yttrium-radiolabeled anti-carcinoembryonic antigen chimeric T84.66 in a Phase I radioimmunotherapy trial. Canc Res (Suppl) 1995; 55:5929s–5934s.
68. Lane DM, Eagle KF, Begent RHJ, et al. Radioimmunotherapy of metastatic colorectal tumours with iodine-131-labeled antibody to carcinoembryonic antigen: phase I/II study with comparative biodistribution of intact and F(ab')$_2$ antibodies. Br J Cancer 1994; 70:521–525.
69. Breitz HB, Weiden PL, Vanderheyden J-L, et al. Clinical experience with Re-186-labeled monoclonal antibodies for radioimmunotherapy: results of phase I trials. J Nucl Med 1992; 33:1099–1112.
70. Su F-M, Lyen L, Breitz HB, Weiden PL, Fritzberg AR. [186]Rhenium MAG2GABA antibody radiolabeling for high dose radioimmunotherapy studies. In: Nicolini M, Bandoli G, Mazzi U, eds. Technetium and Rhenium in Chemistry and Nuclear Medicine. Padua: SC Editorial, 1995.
71. Haller D, Cannon L, Alavi A, Guifo J. A phase I trial of ^{90}Y-labeled monoclonal antibody (MoAb) B72/3 (CYT-103-^{90}Y) administered with concurrent EDTA in refractory adenocarcinomas. Antibod Immunoconj Radiopharm 1992; 5:142.
72. Meredith RM, Khazaeli MB, Plott WE, et al. Phase I trial of iodine-131-chimeric B72.3 in metastatic colorectal cancer. J Nucl Med 1992; 33:23–29.
73. Meredith RF, Khazaeli MB, Liu T, Plott G, et al. Dose fractionation of radiolabeled antibodies in patients with metastatic colon cancer. J Nucl Med 1992; 33(9):1648–1653.
74. Scott AM, Divgi CR, Kemeny N, et al. Radioimmunotherapy with I-131 labeled monoclonal antibody CC49 in colorectal cancer. Eur J Nucl Med 1992; 8:709.
75. Larson SM, Divgi CR, Scott A, et al. Current status of radioimmunotherapy. Nucl Med Biol 1994; 21(5):785–792.
76. Murray JL, Macey JD, Kasi LP, et al. Phase II radioimmunotherapy trial with ^{131}I-CC49 in colorectal cancer. Cancer 1994; 73:1057–1066.
77. Tempero M, Leichner P, Dalrymple G, et al. High-dose therapy with iodine-131-labeled monoclonal antibody CC49 in patients with gastrointestinal cancers: a phase I trial. J Clin Oncol 1997; 15(4):1518–1528.
78. Welt S, Divgi CR, Kemeny N, Finn RD, et al. Phase I/II study of iodine-131-labeled monoclonal antibody A33 in patients with advanced colon cancer. J Clin Oncol 1994; 12(8):1561–1571.
79. Welt S, Scott AM, Divgi CR, Kemeny NE, et al. Phase I/II study of iodine-125-labeled monoclonal antibody A33 in patients with advanced colon cancer. J Clin Oncol 1996; 14(6):1787–1797.
80. Meredith RF, Khazaeli MB, Plott WE, et al. Initial clinical evaluation of iodine-125-labeled chimeric 17-1A for metastatic colon cancer. J Nucl Med 1995; 36(12):2229–2233.
81. Juweid M, Sharkey RM, Swayne LC, et al. Phase I dose-escalation trial of ^{131}I-labeled MN-14 anti-carcinoembryonic antigen (CEA) monoclonal antibody in patients with epithelial ovarian cancer. Tumor Targeting 1996; 2(3):189.

82. Juweid M, Sharkey RM, Behr T, et al. Targeting and initial radioimmunotherapy of meduallary thyroid carcinoma with ^{131}I-labeled monoclonal antibodies to carcinoembryonic antigen. Cancer Res Suppl 1995; 55(23):5946s.
83. Deb N, Goris M, Trisler K, et al. Treatment of hormone-refractory prostate cancer with ^{90}Y-CYT-356 monoclonal antibody. Clin Cancer Res 1996; 2:1289–1297.
84. Abdel-Nabi HH, Spaulding M, Farrell E, Derby L, Lamonica D. Treatment of refractory prostate carcinoma with Y-90 KC4. J Nucl Med (suppl) 1995; 36: 213P.
85. Meredith RF, Bueschen AJ, Khazaeli MB, et al. Treatment of metastatic prostate carcinoma with radiolabeled antibody CC49. J Nucl Med 1994; 35:1017–1022.
86. Meredith RF, Khazaeli MB, Carabasi MH, LoBuglio AF. Radioimmunotherapy of prostate cancer. In: Riva P, ed. Therapy of Malignacies with Radioconjugate Monoclonal Antibodies: Present Possibilities and Future Perspectives. Harwood, U.K.: Academic Press, 1998.
87. Goodman GE, Hellstrom I, Yelton DE, et al. Phase I trial of chimeric (human-mouse) monoclonal antibody L6 in patients with non-small cell lung, colon, and breast cancer. Cancer Immunol Immunother 1993; 36:267–273.
88. DeNardo SJ, O'Grady LF, Richman CM, Goldstein D, O'Donnell RT, DeNardo DA, Kroger LA, Lamborn KR, Hellstrom KE, Hellstrom I, DeNardo GL. Radioimmunotherapy for advanced breast cancer using I-131-ChL6 antibody. Anticancer Res 1997; 17:1745–1752.
89. DeNardo SJ, O'Grady LF, Warhoe KA, Kroger LA, Hellstrom I, Hellstrom KE, Maddock SW, et al. Radioimmunotherapy in patients with metastatic breast cancer. J Nucl Med 1992; 33(5):862. Abstract.
90. Richman CM, DeNardo SJ, O'Grady LF, Valk PE, DeNardo GL. Radioimmunotherapy for breast cancer using escalating fractionated doses of I-131 chimeric (Ch) L6. J Immunother 1994; 16(2):161. Abstract.
91. Blank EW, Pant KD, Chan CM, Peterson JA, Ceriani RL. A novel anti-breast epithelial mucin MoAb (BrE-3). Cancer 1992; 5:38–44.
92. Schrier DM, Stemmer SM, Johnson T, et al. High-dose [90]Y Mx-diethylenetriaminepentaacetic acid (DPTA)-BrE-3 and autologous hematopoietic stem cell support (AHSCS) for the treatment of advanced breast cancer: a phase I trial. Cancer Res Suppl 1995; 55(23):5921s.
93. Mulligan T, Carrasquillo JA, Chung Y, et al. Phase I study of intravenous ^{177}Lu-labeled CC49 murine monoclonal antibody in patients with advanced adenocarcinoma. Clin Cancer Res 1995; 1447–1454.
94. Murray JL, Zukiwski AA, Mujoo K, et al. Recombinant alpha-interferon enhances tumor targeting of an anti-melanoma monoclonal antibody in vivo. J Biol Response Mod 1990; 4:556–563.
95. Murray JL, Macey DJ, Grant EJ, et al. Enhanced TAG-72 expression and tumor uptake of radiolabeled monoclonal antibody CC49 in metastatic breast cancer patients following I-interferon treatment. Cancer Res Suppl 1995; 55(23):5925s.
96. Murray JL, Macey DJ, Grant EJ, et al. Phase II trial of ^{131}I-CC49 Mab plus alpha interferon in breast cancer. J Immunother 1994; 16(2):162. Abstract.
97. Kalofonas HP, Pawlikowska TR, Hemingway A, et al. Antibody guided diagnosis and therapy of brain gliomas using radiolabeled monoclonal antibodies against epi-

dermal growth factor receptor and placental alkaline phosphatase. J Nucl Med 1989; 30:1636–1645.

98. Brady L, Woo D, Markoe A, et al. Radioimmunotherapy with ^{125}I-EGF-425 in patients with brain tumors: preliminary results of a phase II clinical trial. Antibod Immunoconj Radiopharm 1990; 3:169–179.

99. Brady LW, Miyamoto C, Woo DV, et al. Malignant astrocytomas treated with iodine-125 labeled monoclonal antibody 425 against epidermal growth factor receptor: a Phase II trial. Int J Radiat Oncol Biol Phys 1991; 22:225–230.

100. Riva P, Arista A, Franceschi G, et al. Local treatment of malignant gliomas by direct infusion of specific monoclonal antibodies labeled with [131]I: comparison of the results obtained in recurrent and newly diagnosed tumors. Cancer Res Suppl 1995; 55(23):5952s.

101. Bigner DD, Brown M, Coleman RE, et al. Phase I studies of treatment of malignant gliomas and neoplastic meningitis with ^{131}I-radiolabeled monoclonal antibodies anti-tenascin 81C6 and anti-chondroitin proteoglycan sulfate me1-14 F(ab')$_2$—a preliminary report. J Neuro-Oncol 1995; 24:109–122.

102. Papanastassiou V, Pizer BL, Coakham HB, Bullimore J, Zananiri T, Kemshead JT. Treatment of recurrent and cystic malignant gliomas by a single intracavity injection of ^{131}I monoclonal antibody: feasibility, pharmacokinetics and dosimetry. Br J Cancer 1993; 67:144–151.

103. Hopkins K, Chandler C, Bullimore J, Sandeman D, Coakham H, Kemshead JT. A pilot study of the treatment of patients with recurrent malignant gliomas with intratumoral yttrium-90 radioimmunoconjugates. Radiother Oncol 1995; 34:121–131.

104. Papanastassiou V, Pizer BL, Chandler CL, Zananiri, Kemshead JT, Hopkins KI. Pharmacokinetics and dose estimates following intrathecal administration of ^{131}I-monoclonal antibodies for the treatment of central nervous system malignancies. Int J Radiat Oncol Biol Phys 1995; 31(3):541–552.

105. Brown, MT, Coleman RE, Friedman AH, et al. Intrathecal ^{131}I-labeled antitenascin monoclonal antibody 81C6 treatment of patients with leptomeningeal neoplasms or primary brain tumor resection cavities with subarachnoid communication: phase I trial results. Clin Cancer Res 1996; 2:963–972.

106. Blumenthal RD, Sharkey RM, Forman D, Wong G, Goldenberg DM. Cytokine intervention permits dose escalation of radioantibody. Cancer Suppl 1994; 73(3): 1083–1092.

107. DeNardo GL, DeNardo SJ, Kukis D, et al. Strategies for enhancement of radioimmunotherapy. Nucl Med Biol 1991; 18:633–640.

108. Colcher D, Esteban J, Carrasquillo JA, et al. Complementation of intracavitary and intravenous administration of a monoclonal antibody (B72.3) in patients with carcinoma. Cancer Res 1987; 47:4218–4224.

109. Epenetos AA, Snook D, Durbin H, et al. Limitations of radiolabeled monoclonal antibodies for localization of human neoplasms. Cancer Res 1986; 46:3183–3191.

110. Jacobs AJ, Fer M, Su F-M, et al. A phase I trial of a rhenium-186-labeled monoclonal antibody administered intraperitoneally in ovarian carcinoma: toxicity and clinical response. Obstet Gynecol 1993; 82:586–593.

111. Hird V, Stewart JSW, Snook D, et al. Intraperitoneally administered ^{90}Y-labeled monoclonal antibodies as a third line of treatment in ovarian cancer, a phase 1-2 trial: problems encountered and possible solutions. Br J Cancer 1990; 10: 48–51.

112. Stewart JSW, Hird V, Snook D, et al. Intraperitoneal radioimmunotherapy for ovarian cancer: pharmacokinetics, toxicity, and efficacy of I-131 labeled monclonal antibodies. Int J Radiat Oncol Biol Phys 1989; 16:405–413.

113. Alvarez RD, Partridge EE, Khazaeli MB, Plott G, Austin M, Kilgore L, Russell CD, Liu T, Grizzle WE, Schlom J, LoBuglio AF, Meredith RF. Intraperitoneal radioimmunotherapy of ovarian cancer with ^{177}Lu-CC49: a phase I/II study. Gynecol Oncol 1997; 65:94–101.

114. Riva P, Tison G, Franchesci N, Casi M, Moscatelli G. Successful treatment of metastatic gastrointestinal cancer by means of radioimmunotherapy. J Nucl Med 1992; 33(5):863. Abstract.

115. Order SE, Siegel JA, Principato R, Zeiger LE, Johnson E, Lang P, Lustig R, Wallner PE. Selective tumor irradiation by infusional brachytherapy in nonresectable pancreatic cancer: a phase I study. Int J Radiat Oncol Biol 1996; 36(5):1117–1126.

116. Misrikale JS, Iein JL, Schroeder J, Order SE. Radiation enhancement of radiolabelled antibody deposition in tumors. Int J Radiat Oncol Biol 1987; 3:1839–1844.

117. Stickney DR, Gridley DS, Kirk GA, Slater JM. Enhancement of monoclonal antibody binding to melanoma with single dose radiation or hyperthermia. J Natl Cancer Inst Monogr 1985; 3:47–52.

118. Kalofonos HP, Rowlinson G, Epenetos AA. Enhancement of antibody uptake in human colon xenografts following irradiation. Cancer Res 1990; 50:159–163.

119. Warhoe KA, DeNardo SJ, Wolkov HB, Doggett EC, Kroger LA, Lamborn KR, DeNardo GL. Evidence for external beam irradiation enhancement of radiolabeled monoclonal antibody uptake in breast cancer. Antibod Immunoconj Radiopharm 1992; 5(2):227–235.

120. Epenetos AA. Combined radiolabeled antibodies and radiotherapy for the treatment of head and neck cancer. J Immunother 1994; 16(2):163. Abstract.

121. DeNardo GL, DeNardo SJ, Lamborn KR, et al. Enhanced tumor uptake of monoclonal antibody in nude mice with PEG IL-2. Antibod Immunocon Radiopharm 1991; 4:859–870.

122. DeNardo GL, Kukis DL, DeNardo SJ, Shen S, Mausner LF, O'Donnell R, Srivastava SC, Miers LA, Meares CF. Enhancement of Cu-67-2IT-BAT-LYM-1 therapy in mice with human Burkitt's lymphoma (RAJI) using interleukin 2 (rIL-2). Tumor Targeting 1996; 2(3):150.

123. Nakamura K, Kubo A. Biodistribution of I-126-labeled monoclonal antibody/IL-2 immunoconjugate in athymic mice bearing human tumor xenograft. Tumor Targeting 1996; 2(3):153.

124. Greiner JW, Guadagni F, Goldstein D, Smalley RV, Borden EC, Simpson JF, Molinolo A, Schlom J. Evidence for the evaluation of serum carcinoembryonic antigen and tumor associated glycoprotein-72 levels in patients administered interferons. Cancer Res 1991; 51:4155–4163.

125. Greiner JW, Ullman CD, Nieroda C, Qi C-F, Eggensberger D, Shimada S, Steinberg

SM, Schlom J. Improved radioimmunotherpeutic efficacy of an anticarcinoma monoclonal antibody (^{131}I-CC49) when given in combination with gamma-interferon. Cancer Res 1993; 53:600–608.

126. Krenning EP, Valkema R, Kooij PPPM, Breeman WAP, Bakker WH, deHerder WW, vanEijck CHJ, Kwekkeboom DJ, deJong M, Pauwels S. Peptide receptor radionuclide therapy with In-111-DTPA-D-Phe-octreotide. J Nucl Med 1997; 38(5):47P. Abstract.

127. Rotman M, Kuruvilla AM, Choi K, Bhutani I, Aziz H, Rosenthat J, Braverman A, Marti J, Brandys M. Response of colorectal hepatic metastases to concomitant radiotherapy and intravenous infusion 5 fluouracil. Int J Radiat Oncol Phys 1986; 12:2179–2187.

128. Ng B, Liebes L, Kramer EL, Wasserheit C, Hochster H, Blank E, Ceriani R, Furmanski P. Synergistic activity of radioimmunotherapy with Y-90 MX-DTPA Hu-Bre-3 and prolonged Topotecan infusion in human breast cancer xenografts. J Nucl Med 1997; 38(5):46P.

129. Kievit E, Pinedo HM, Schluper HMM, Boven E. Improvement of the therapeutic efficacy of monoclonal antibody [131]I-323/A3 by the addition of cisplatin in experimental human ovarian cancer. Proc AACR 1996; 37:609.

130. Remmenga SW, Colcher D, Gansow O, Pippen G, Raubitschek A. Continuous infusion chemotherapy as a radiation-enhancing agent for yttrium-90-radiolabeled monoclonal antibody therapy of a human tumor xenograft. Gynecol Oncol 1994; 55:115–122.

131. Tschmelitsch J, Barendswaard E, Williams C, Yao T-J, Cohen AM, Old LJ, Welt S. Enhanced antitumor activity of combination radioimmunotherapy (^{131}I-labeled monoclonal antibody A33) with chemotherapy (fluorouracil). Cancer Res 1997; 57: 2181–2186.

132. Clifton KH, Szybalski W, Heidelberger C, Gollin FF, Ansfield FJ, Vermund H. Incorporation of I-125 labeled iodoxyuridine into the deoxyribonucleic acid of murine and human tissues following therapeutic doses. Cancer Res 1963; 23:1715–1723.

133. Kinsella TJ, Mitchell JB, Russo A. Continuous intravenous infusion of bromodeoxyuridine as a clinical radiosensitizer. J Clin Oncol 1984; 2(10):1144–1150.

134. Buchsbaum DJ, Khazaeli MB, David MA, Lawrence TS. Sensitization of radiolabeled monoclonal antibody therapy using bromodeoxyuridine. Cancer 1994; 73: 999–1005.

135. Morstyn G, Miller R, Russi A, Mitchell J. 131-Iodine conjugated antibody cell kell enhanced by bromodeoxyuridine. Int J Radiat Oncol Biol Phys 1994; 10:1437–1440.

136. Santos O, Pant KD, Blank EW, Ceriani RL. 5-Iododeoxyuridine increases the efficacy of the radioimmunotherapy of human tumors growing in nude mice. J Nucl Med 1992; 33:1530–1534.

137. Philips TL, Prados MD, Bodell WJ, et al. Rationale for and experience with clinical trials of halogenated pyrimidines in malignant gliomas: the UCSF/NCOG experience. In: Dewey WC, Edington M, Fry RJ, et al., eds. Radiation Research: A Twentieth Century Perspective. San Diego: Academic Press, 1991:191, 601.

138. Breitz HB, Durham JS, Fisher DR, Weiden PL. Radiation absorbed dose estimates

in normal organs following intraperitoneal [186]Re-labeled monoclonal antibody: methods and results. Cancer Res Suppl 1995; 55:5817s–5822s.

139. Meredith RF, Khazaeli MB, Liu T, Plott G, Wheeler RH, Russell C, Colcher D, Schlom J, Shochat D, LoBuglio AF. Dose fractionation of radiolabeled antibodies in patients with metastatic colon cancer. J Nucl Med 1992; 33(9):1648–1653.

140. Goodwin DA. Tumor pretargeting: almost the bottom line. J Nucl Med 1995; 36(5): 876–879.

141. DeNardo GL, Maddock SW, Sgouros G, Scheibe PO, DeNardo SJ. Immunoadsorption: an enhancement strategy for radioimmunotherapy. J Nucl Med 1993; 34(6): 1020–1027.

142. Breitz HB, Ratliff B, Reno J, Axworthy D, Fritzberg A, Su F-M, Appelbaum J, Kunx S, Seiler C, Weiden P. Performance of antibody streptavidin pretargeting in patients initial results. J Nucl Med 1995; 36(5):225P.

143. Wessels BW. Current status of animal radioimmunotherapy. Cancer Res 1990; 50: 970s–973s.

12

Intraperitoneal Radioimmunotherapy of Ovarian Cancer

Konstantinos N. Syrigos
University of Athens Medical School,
Athens, Greece

Agamemnon A. Epenetos
Antisoma Research Laboratories, St. George's Hospital Medical
School, London, England

I. INTRODUCTION

Although the management of cancer by exploiting the differences between neo-plastic and normal cells has always been an attractive concept, it was the develop-ment of hybridoma technology and the resulting tumor-associated monoclonal antibodies (Mabs) that offered new prospects on that strategy. Twenty years later some of the applications of Mabs to oncology are now part of the everyday diag-nosis and treatment (i.e., immunohistochemistry, radioimmunodetection), while others, including radioimmunotherapy (RIT), remain an area of intensive investi-gation. Over the last decade the use of Mabs as carriers of high-activity radionu-clides for the treatment of malignant diseases spurred an unprecedented effort in oncology and nuclear medicine research. The Mab-isotope conjugate, after bind-ing to the target cell and delivering a lethal radiation dose, could offer the advan-tage of killing many untargeted cells through ''crossfire irradiation'' (1).

This distribution of the cytotoxic activity by the radiolabeled Mab could, in theory, be the solution to the considerable problem of tumour heterogeneity in antigen expression. Unfortunately, but not surprisingly, the clinical application of the above model proved to be rather more complicated and the initial enthusiasm was replaced by skepticism and disappointment, as the hopes of decreasing the side effects by increasing the specificity of tumour localization remained unfulfilled.

Since access to the tumor site is the main limiting factor in the targeting of solid tumours, nonsystemic routes of administration have been considered for the regional delivery of the radioconjugate. Routes such as the intrathecal for meningeal carcinomatosis, the intravesical for superficial bladder carcinoma, the intraperitoneal for ovarian and colorectal carcinomas, and the intratumoral routes of administration have been tried in experimental and clinical situations (2).

Being the most common cause of death from gynecological tumors (52%) and the fourth leading cause of cancer death in women (5%) (3), ovarian cancer (OC) is an attractive target for the application of regional radioimmunotherapy, because of the clinical features and natural history of the disease. Epithelial ovarian tumors express high levels of many antigens (4), including the polymorphic epithelial mucin (PEM) (5), to which several Mabs have been raised (6,7). As the tumor remains primarily within the peritoneal cavity, the regional delivery of radiolabeled Mabs could be tested whether it could achieve better access of tumor sites and higher therapeutic ratio, compared with the systemic route of administration. Furthermore, as patients with OC often undergo laparotomy as part of the standard management of their disease, the study of Mabs' distribution, monitoring of recurrence or the response to therapy, and the overall survival can be estimated. More than 3500 women in England and Wales and 12,500 women in the United States die of this disease each year, mainly of uncontrolled locoregional intraperitoneal spread (3). As there is not currently available an effective method of identifying patients with asymptomatic early stages, at diagnosis most OC patients present at an advanced stage, with the disease spread beyond the ovary, usually on the peritoneal surface. The combination of surgical debulking and platinum-based chemotherapy (8) has resulted in increased overall response rates (60% to 80%) (9,10), although the overall long-term survival is still poor (30% 5-year survival for all stages) (11,12), indicating that the effectiveness from the combination of traditional therapeutic schemes has reached a plateau (13) and the need for novel therapeutic strategies is apparent. All the above make the ovarian cancer patients ideal candidates for intraperitoneal (IP) RIT.

II. THE RADIOCONJUGATE

A. The Mab

Since the development of the hybridoma technology for producing monoclonal antibodies, several animal models have been studied to explore the pharmacokinetics of Mabs and to optimize their therapeutic efficacy in IP RIT.

The choice of the antibody to be radiolabeled greatly depends on the tumor antigenic expression and the accessibility, the macro- and microdistribution, the kinetics, and the in vivo stability of the Mab. When an antibody is administered, only 0.007% to 0.01% of it finally targets to the tumor, regardless of the route of administration. The rest of it, passing through the body compartments (vascular network, organs, and body fluid) is catabolized and excreted. Furthermore, some Mabs bind to tumor antigen present in normal organs, such as the liver. Other factors interfering with Mab targeting include the antigen size, density, location, and accessibility (14). Tumor size also influences the uptake of Mabs, since inadequate blood supply, necrosis, and elevated interstitial pressure (15–17) decrease the tumor uptake: the best targeting of tumor is observed in tumors <2 cm, while there is virtually no uptake in tumour masses >8 g (18). Finally, the dense cellularity and the lack of lymphoid vessels of the malignant lump may further decrease the Mab penetration (18). Table 1 presents the most commonly used Mabs for the IP RIT of ovarian cancer.

B. The Isotope

The choice of the optimal radionuclide for IP RIT, which would deliver the maximum possible dose to the tumor, respecting the normal tissues, has been and continues to be the issue of intensive study. Some of the isotope selection criteria include:
1.   The physical characteristics of the radionuclide half-life and type of energy produced. Alpha particles, although more lethal for the cell, and active even in the presence of hypoxia, have short range of 50 to 100 mm in the tissue and are suitable to kill only very small volume tumors. Short-range beta emitters (I-131, Re-186) can effectively sterilize micrometastases, but underdose tumors

Table 1 Most Commonly Used Mabs for Radioimmunotherapy

Antibody	Antigen
HMFG1	PEM
HMFG2	PEM
AUA1	40-kDa gp
OC 125	CA-125
OV-TL-3	OA3
MOV 18	38-kDa gp
B72.3	TAG-72
H17E2	PLAP

higher than 1 cm in diameter. High-energy beta particles (Y-90), which travel a much greater distance within the tumor, can circumvent the heterogeneous distribution of the radioconjugate within the tumor, but if the tumor is too small, then too much activity is delivered outside the tumor. The problematic gamma component (I-131) adds little to the tumor delivered dose, but significantly to the bone marrow toxicity and must be avoided.

2.   The availability and cost of the isotope, the convenience and efficiency of the labeling technique, and the stability of the radioconjugate in vivo (19).

3.   The specific activity of the isotope per amount of Mab (MBq/mg), which mainly depends on the method of radiolabeling.

4.   The ideal isotope should have decay compatible with the carrier Mab's biological half-life in the peritoneal cavity, since, when the antibody targeting (tumor-to-normal tissue) is maximum at 2 to 4 days, a radionuclide with much shorter half-life is at a disadvantage.

Iodine-131, with proven efficacy in the treatment of thyroid malignancies, was the first applied in OC RIT not only because of its availability and low cost, but also because the I-131-immunoconjugate could be safely given, since the myelosuppression following its administration is directly correlated to the radiation dose received and therefore predictable. Significant but reversible toxicity was observed at doses of 150 mCi, while activities of I-131 up to 100 mCi can be administered with negligible toxicity (20). Unfortunately, radioconjugates with I-131, which are usually made by oxidizing a tyrosine residue (21), are susceptible to in vivo dehalogenation. Furthermore, the emission of unwanted γ-radiation and its low-energy β-particles made it less than ideal for RIT (22,23) and led to the use of other isotopes. Metal isotopes conjugated to Mabs through chelating agents are more stable in vitro, although they may be released and catabolized by the liver and kidneys to free degradation products comprising the chelate ring or the chelate and a protein fragment (24). There is also the rare possibility that the isotope may leach from the ring. Some of the metal isotopes investigated for IP RIT are Y-90, Sm-153, Rh-166, Rh-168, At-111, P-32, Au-199, and Bi-212.

Yttrium-90 labeling of Mabs can be achieved with the use of bifunctional chelating agents, such as DTPA, but its administration is followed by severe myelotoxicity even at activities as low as 15 mCi (25) due to the in vivo instability of Y-90 chelation by DTPA, consequent release of the isotope, and the deposition of this "bone seeking" metal to the patients' bone marrow (26). To circumvent that problem, patients were given intravenously calcium disodium EDTA, which can chase complex free Y-90, and promote its urine excretion (27,28).

Of particular interest is the clinical use of new, more stable chelating agents, such as the macrocycle DOTA. Phase I/II clinical trials showed better in vivo stability of the radioimmunoconjugate when DOTA was used instead of DTPA (29,30). In addition, the myelotoxicity observed was of minor significance at activities of 15 to 20 mCi Y-90 (31). Unfortunately, the application of DOTA

Table 2 Isotopes Most Commonly Used in
Intraperitoneal Radioimmunotherapy of Ovarian
Cancer

Isotope	Decay Mode	Half-life
Rhenium-186	beta	3,5 days
Yttrium-90	beta	2,5 days
Iodine-131	beta	8 days
Iodine-125	electron capture	60 days

was implicated with serum-sickness-like reactions, since it proved to be immunogenic, producing raised titers of anti-DOTA antibodies (32,33). To surmount the
above difficulties, alternative chelating agents such as CITC and TETA or other
β-emitters such as Sm-153, Re-186, and Co-67 have been investigated (34). Both
options have been tried for the intraperitoneal RIT of OC with promising preliminary results, although CITC-DTPA has also been shown to have immunogenic
properties after IP administration (35). The isotopes most commonly used in radioimmunotherapy of ovarian cancer are listed on Table 2.

Concluding, one must always bear in mind that the nonuniform tumor uptake and the poor tumor blood supply may intervene with the distribution of the
radioimmunoconjugate within the malignant mass. Research efforts are still in
progress for the development of the ideal radioconjugate which should be stable
and with an isotope, for which the pharmacokinetics, physical half-life, and emission are matched with the Mab used, in order to achieve the best possible therapeutic ratio (19).

III. BIODISTRIBUTION AFTER IP ADMINISTRATION

The best experimental model that could be used as a simplistic analog of the
peritoneal cavity in ovarian cancer patients is that of the multicellular microspher-
oids (36). With the use of that model it is now recognized that penetration of
whole IgG immunoglobulin is about 3 to 4 cell diameters deep and is a time-
dependent procedure, taking 3 days to uniformly infiltrate a tumor nodule of
1 mm (15,16). Better penetration can be achieved with the smaller antibody fragments F(ab')2 and Fab, with Fab having the best uniformity and penetration
(37,38). Although the spheroids model helped us to understand the biodistribution
of the radioimmunoconjugate after IP administration, cavitary fluid circulation
in vivo is much more complicated, making the above artificial model inaccurate.
Clearance from the cavity has been shown to be a size-dependent process (39),

and the use of antibody fragments with their more rapid clearance (and therefore less residence time in the cavity) will not necessarily result in better tumor penetration. On the other hand, there are patients with large amounts of soluble IP antigen form high-molecular-weight immune complexes that delay removal from the cavity. In addition ovarian cancer patients usually undergo large surgical procedures that often involve omentectomy and result in formation of adhesions. The above factors make the estimation of biodistribution of radioimmunoconjugates after IP administration difficult in ovarian cancer patients (Fig. 1).

Despite the above-described difficulties, there is now adequate evidence that the IP route of administration seems to offer an advantage for RIT, when compared with IV administration. Although the absolute uptake of antibody by the tumor is approximately equal for IV and IP routes, the latter offers better pharmacokinetics, which results to a better tumor-to-normal ratio (40–43), allowing the administration of higher activity with relatively low toxicity. When Ward et al. compared these two routes of administration in ovarian cancer patients, the maximum localization of the radioimmunoconjugate was on free-floating cells of the ascitic fluid, resulting in a tumor cell-to-normal tissue ratio of 100/1. With regard to the tumor nodules, maximum localization was achieved by those with "free" access to the peritoneal cavity. The authors concluded that there is a 4-to 70-fold advantage of the IP route over the IV route (44). When

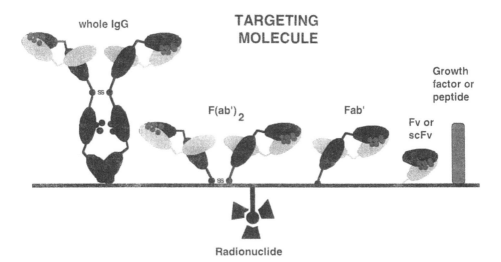

Figure 1   Molecular biology cloning techniques present the possibility of creating new molecules, more suitable for radioimmunotherapy. (Reprinted by permission from Dr. Mahendra Deonarain.)

F(ab')2 fragments were studied, intraperitoneal administration resulted in lower estimated radiation dose to blood as compared with IV administration, and in lower systemic toxicity. It has also been shown that further tumor radiation deposit can be achieved if ascitic fluid is evacuated prior to the radioconjugate injection (45). However, it is now recognized that retroperitoneal, hematogenous, and lymph node metastases are not successfully targeted via IP administration (46).

IV. CLINICAL EVALUATION

Over the last decade a number of clinical studies with IP RIT in ovarian cancer patients have been reported with the use of the Mabs HMFG1, HMFG2, AUA1, H17E2, and others. The Mabs have been labeled with I-131, Y-90, and Re-186 and injected through a peritoneal dialysis catheter into the peritoneal cavity under local anesthetic and after any ascites had been drained off. The volume injected ranged from 1 to 2 L of normal saline and the specific activity was 4 to 8 mCi/mg (47).

When I-131 is used, the patient is given potassium iodinate or iodide for 2 days before and for 1 month after therapy to protect the thyroid gland. The effective dose of the isotope is thought to be 150 mCi. After intraperitoneal injection, the mean peak radioactivity in serum is at 44 h and corresponds to 26% of the injected dose. Most of the radioactivity given (80%) is found as free iodine in the urine. Urinary excretion results in reduction of normal tissue irradiation, while frequent bladder emptying and high fluid intake decrease absorption by the bladder wall. When Y-90 is used, the mean peak radioactivity in serum is 23%, and only 8% to 11% of the injected dose is released in the urine after 72 h (48).

From review of the relevant clinical trials, it is clear that IP RIT is of benefit mainly to patients with small-volume disease. All the studies performed agree that patients with lesions <2 cm had a prolonged disease-free period when compared with historical control group (49). In addition, in the same group of patients, some investigators observed tumor regression in a number of cases (50,51); others demonstrated a decrease in the tumour size (52). On the contrary, the results are rather poor in patients with nodules >2 cm in diameter (53), since at that size both the Mab penetration and the high-energy beta particles reach the limit of their potential.

Patients with negative second-look laparotomy who received IP RIT as an adjuvant treatment also had increased disease-free survival, when compared to historical control group (49). Patients with minimal residual disease (microscopic disease <5 mm or positive peritoneal washing) also achieved complete response after IP RIT, as confirmed on third-look surgical evaluation and/or clinical follow-up (54). In ovarian cancer patients IP RIT seems to have a palliative role as well; it has a beneficial effect for palliation of recurrent ascites (44) and symptomatic, chemotherapy-resistant ascites (55).

The above observations, although interesting and promising, give rise to many questions regarding the potential mechanisms involved, since in most cases the radioactivity administered is not tumoricidical, according to our models. As explained, the models we currently use to study the peritoneal environment bear little correlation with what really happens in vivo and our dosimetry calculations are not accurate. An attractive explanation of the above results could be that the antibody itself may exert antitumor effect through an anti-idiotype immunizing mechanism (56). It has been shown that when HMFG1 is administered via the IP route into humans it can initiate a cascade of immunological reactions leading to both humoral and cellular activation (57,58).

The above theory is further supported by the observation that ovarian cancer patients who developed high titers of anti-idiotype reactions after repeated administrations of Mabs had prolonged survivals, in comparison with historical controls (59). Furthermore, there are observations indicating direct cellular toxicity mediated by antibodies. The mechanisms implicated include complement activation (58), antibody-dependent cell cytotoxicity (56,57), and induction of apoptosis. The involvement of the above mechanisms to the tumoricidal effect of the IP administration of Mabs is under investigation.

In conclusion, cumulative clinical observations suggest that IP RIT has a role in the treatment of small-volume lesions and minimal residual disease. It is also of benefit as an adjuvant or palliative treatment in OC patients. The above promising data are now being tested vigorously in Phase III clinical trials.

V. TOXICITY

Intraperitoneal radiotherapy is usually well tolerated. Although the IP route of administration is 4- to 70-fold more advantageous than the IV route for the targeting of the tumor site (44,60), a high percentage of the injected activity still localizes in normal tissues. The dose-limiting organ is the bone marrow. Myelosuppression arises 4 to 6 weeks after the initial injection. Grade 3 platelet and granulocyte toxicity was observed at a total dose of 20 mCi with Y-90 and 160 mCi with I-131 (25,27,51), while grade 3 and 4 hematologic toxicity was observed at a total dose of 150 mCi with Re-186 (52). The IV administration of EDTA after the IP infusion of Y-90-DTPA reduces the bone marrow toxicity by chelating Y-90 and facilitating its urine excretion.

Hypersensitivity reactions due to HAMA Production are mild and usually well tolerated. Ten percent of the patients may develop fever, chills, pruritus, and urticaria. More sever reactions, such as anaphylaxis and bronchospasms, are rare but may occur even in patients with previously negative skin tests (61). HAMA reactions usually occur 10 days to 3 weeks after the initial injection and are unrelated to the rate and dose of immunoconjugate administration. In addition HAMA production may interfere with the treatment, since in the presence of HAMA the effective half-life of the antibody is reduced (62) and antibody-to-tumor binding is decreased, resulting to increased toxicity (63). Furthermore, the follow-up of ovarian cancer patients may become problematic since the presence of HAMA can cause false-positive CA-125 values (59). It is of particular interest that the likelihood of HAMA formation is reduced when patients had recently undergone chemotherapy before IP RIT (63).

Finally, elevation of hepatic enzymes has also been described, but this has not reached clinically significant levels (52).

VI. TWO- AND THREE-STEP APPROACH

To amplify the tumoricidal effect and limit the toxic effects of RIT, a novel therapeutic approach has been introduced. It consists of the separate administration of the Mab and the radioisotope. The tumor-associated antibody is first administered IP, without the radionuclide but being conjugated with biotin. It binds the tumor, where it remains for a long period, while the unbound Mab is removed from the circulation. The first step is followed by administration of radiolabeled streptavidin (second step) which, owing to its extremely high affinity for biotin $(Kd = 10^{-15} M)$, binds to biotinylated antibody at the tumor sites. The unconjugated radioactive streptavidin is cleared quickly by the kidneys, owing to its small molecular size. The system is flexible, and several alternative methods of tumor pretargeting can be used for the radioactivity administered to be bound mainly at tumor sites.

A more complicated, three-step technique has also been introduced. The biotinylated Mab is infused (first step), followed by the infusion of a 10-fold excess of streptavidin (second step), which chases the antibody from the circulation, as the liver clears the antibody-biotin-streptavidin complexes. When tumor uptake is maximum (48 h), labeled biotin is administered which is localized in the tumor sites and quickly cleared by the circulation because of its small molecular size (64–68). This novel strategy results in decreased irradiation of normal tissues by improving the tumor-to-nontumor ratios, but has little additional benefit in the absolute amount of radioactivity delivered to the tumour (69). Although it has already been introduced in the systemic RIT, its effectiveness in the intraperitoneal RIT of OC needs further evaluation. In addition, if multiple administrations are required, one must take under consideration that avidin and streptavidin are immunogenic molecules (70).

VII. FUTURE DEVELOPMENTS

Nonspecific uptake in normal tissues and high background activity levels in blood and other organs remain a significant problem of IP RIT. To extend the acquisition of the conjugate in the tumor sites without increasing toxicity, several approaches are under investigation including the use of hyperthermia and vasoactive substances that promote tissue perfusion (71–73). Optimization of IP RIT can be achieved by an initial injection of IFN-gamma and TNFa. These two cytokines synergistically upregulate the antigen expression and may result to up to 1.5-fold increase in cytotoxicity (74–78). Plasmapheresis has also been shown to permit an increase the amount of antibody administered and achieve a more uniform distribution of the immunoconjugate within the tumor (79).

The possibility of increased tumor radioactivity when IgM Mabs are used has also been investigated. Preliminary results of animal studies suggest that IgM radioconjugates, when administered IP, have an early and high (29% ID/g) tumor uptake as well as prolonged retention, with a biological half-life of 4 days. Furthermore, as the peritoneal membrane acts as a barrier, delaying the diffusion of the large IgM molecule in the circulation, the uptake by the normal organs is reduced and the toxicity is significantly less. Unfortunately, the above advantages are offset by the impaired penetration of the large IgM (900 Kd) molecule (80).

Other techniques that have been used to amplify the benefit of IP RIT include the concomitant application of radiation-enhancing agents, such as 5-FU (81) and the combination of RIT and external-beam radiotherapy, which seems to have an additive effect (82). As has already been explained, retroperitoneal, hematogenous, and lymph node metastasis are not successfully targeted via IP administration. Investigations are being carried out to examine whether this problem can be circumvented by the simultaneous use of both IP and IV routes.

VIII. CONCLUSIONS

Therapy with radiolabeled Mabs appears promising for establishing itself as an important part of the treatment of ovarian cancer. Clinical data presented in this review suggest an encouraging outlook. Peritoneal delivery of the radioimmunoconjugate is being evaluated in Phase III clinical trials. The production of chimeric or human antibodies and of immunoreactive fragments or peptides, as well as the introduction of two- and three-step pretargeting techniques, show promise for solving some of the present weaknesses of intraperitoneal RIT and lead to its more widespread applications.

REFERENCES

1. Britton KE, Mather SJ, Granowska M. Radiolabelled monoclonal antibodies in oncology. III. Radioimmunotherapy. Nucl Med Commun 1991; 12:333.
2. Syrigos KN, Epenetos AA. Achievements, failings and promises of radioimmunotherapy. In: Klapdor R, ed. Current Tumor Diagnosis: Applications, Clinical Relevance, Research, Trends. Munich: W Zuckschwerdt Verlag, 1994.
3. Silverberg E, Boring CC, Squires TS. Cancer statistics 1990. Cancer J Clin 1990; 40:318.
4. Bast RC, Knauf S, Epenetos AA, Dhokia B, Daly L, Tanner M, Soper J, Creasman W, Gall S, Knapp RC. Coordinate elevation of serum markers in ovarian cancer but not in benign disease. Cancer 1991; 68:1758.
5. Gendler SI, Burchell JM, Duhing T, Lamport D, White R, Parker M, Taylor-Papadimtriou J. Cloning of partial cDNA encoding differentiation and tumour associated mucin glycoproteins expressed by human mammary epithelium. Proc Natl Acad Sci USA 1987; 84:6060.
6. Epenetos AA, Britton K, Mather S, Shepherd J, Granowska M, Taylor-Papadimitriou J, Nimmon C, Durbin- H, Hawkins LR, Malpas JS, Bodmer WF. Targeting of ^{123}I-labelled tumour associated monoclonal antibodies to ovarian, breast and gastrointestinal tumours. Lancet 1982; ii:999.
7. Colcher D, Zalutsky M, Kaplan W, Kufe D, Austin F, Schlom J. Radiolocalisation of human mammary tumors in athymic mice by a monoclonal antibody. Cancer Res 1983; 43:736.
8. Ozols RF. Ovarian cancer: new clinical approaches. Cancer Treat Rep 1991; 18:77.
9. Ozols RF, Hamilton TC, Hoskins WJ, Bast RC Jr, Young RC. Biology and therapy of ovarian cancer. Semin Oncol 1991; 18:297.
10. Neijt JP, ten Bokkel Huinink WW, Van der Burg MEL, van Oosterom AT, Vriesendorp, R, Kooyman CD, van Lindert AC, Hamerlynck JV, van Lent M, van Houwelingen JC. Randomised trial comparing two combination chemotherapy regimens in advanced ovarian carcinoma. Lancet 1984; 2:594.
11. Ozols RF, Young RC. Ovarian cancer: where to next? Semin Oncol 1991; 18:307.
12. Perez RP, Godwin AK, Hamilton TC, Ozols RF. Ovarian cancer biology. Semin Oncol 1991; 18:186.
13. Marsoni S, Torri V, Valsecchi M, Belloni C, Bianchi U, Bolis G, Bonazzi C, Colombo N, Epis A, Favalli G. Prognostic factors in advanced epithelial ovarian cancer. Br J Cancer 1990; 62:444.
14. Epenetos AA, Snook D, Durbin H, Johnson PM, Taylor-Papadimitriou J. Limitations of radiolabelled monoclonal antibodies for localisation of human neoplasms. Cancer Res 1986; 46:3183.
15. Jain RK. Physiological barriers to delivery of monoclonal antibodies and other macromolecules in tumors. Cancer Res 1990; 50:814.

16. Jain RK. Vascular and interstitial barriers to delivery of therapeutic agents in tumors. Cancer Metast Rev 1990; 9:253.

17. Jain RK, Baxter LT. Mechanisms of heterogeneous distribution of monoclonal antibodies and other macromolecules in tumors: significance of elevated interstitial pressure. Cancer Res 1988; 48:7022.

18. Klein JL, Kopher KA, Rostock RA. Ferritin concentration and ^{131}I-antiferritin tumor localisation in experimental hepatome. Int J Radiat Oncol Biol Phys 1986; 12:137.

19. Mausner LF, Srivastava SC. Selection of radionuclides for radioimmunotherapy. Med Phys 1993; 20:503.

20. Stewart JS, Hird V, Snook D, Sullivan M, Hooker G, Courtenay-Luck N, Sivolapenko G, Griffiths M, Myers MI, Lambert HE. Intraperitoneal radioimmunotherapy for ovarian cancer pharmacokinetics, toxicity and efficacy of I-131 labeled monoclonal antibodies. Int J Radiat Oncol Biol Phys 1989; 16:405.

21. Fraker PJ, Speck JC Jr. Protein and cell membrane iodinations with a sparing soluble chloramide 1,3,4,6-tetrachloro-3a.6a-diphenyl-glyoluril. Biochem Biophys Res Commun 1978; 80:849.

22. Buchsbown D, Randall B, Hanna D, Chandler R, Loken M, Johnson E. Comparison of the distribution and binding of monoclonal antibodies labeled with ^{131}I and [111]In. Eur J Nucl Med 1985; 30:398.

23. Leichner PK, Klein JL, Garrison JB, Jenkins RE, Nickoloff EL, Ettinger DS, Order SE. Dosimetry of ^{131}I labelled anti-ferritin in hepatoma. A model for radioimmunoglobulin dosimetry. Int J Radiat Oncol Biol Phys 1981; 7:323.

24. Sands H, Jones PL. Methods for the study of the metabolism of radiolabelled monoclonal antibodies by liver and tumour. J Nucl Med 1987; 28:390.

25. Stewart JSW, Hird V, Snook D, Sullivan M, Meyers MJ, Epenetos AA. Intraperitoneal I-131 and Y-90 labeled monoclonal antibodies for ovarian cancer: pharmacokinetics and normal tissue dosimetry. Int J Cancer 1988; 3(suppl):71.

26. Sharkey R, Kaltovich FA, Shih LB, Fand I, Govelitz G, Goldenberg DM. Radioimmunotherapy of human colonic cancer xenografts with yttrium-90 labeled monoclonal antibodies to CEA. Cancer Res 1988; 48:3270.

27. Stewart JS, Hird V, Snook D, Dhokia B, Sivolapenko G, Hooker G, Papadimitriou JT, Rowlinson G, Sullivan M, Lambert-HE. Intraperitoneal yttrium-90 labelled monoclonal antibody in ovarian cancer. J Clin Oncol 1990; 8:1941.

28. Rowlinson-Busza G, Snook D, Epenetos AA. ^{90}Y-labeled antibody uptake by human tumor xenografts and the effect of systemic administration of EDTA. Int J Radiat Oncol Biol Phys 1994; 28:1257.

29. Deshpande SV, DeNardo SJ, Kukis DL, Moi MK, McCall MJ, DeNardo GL, Meares CF. Yttrium-90-labeled monoclonal antibody for therapy: labeling by a new macrocyclic bifunctional chelating agent. J Nucl Med 1990; 31:473.

30. Meares C, Moi M, Diril H, DeNardo SJ, Snook D, Epenetos AA. Macrocyclic chelates of radiometals for diagnosis and therapy. Br J Cancer 1990; 62:21.

31. Hird V, Snook D, Kosmas C. Intraperitoneal radioimmunotherapy with yttrium-90 labelled immunoconjugates. In: Epenetos AA, ed. Monoclonal Antibodies. London: Chapman and Hall, 1991: 267.

32. Syrigos KN, Epenetos AA. Radioimmunotherapy of ovarian cancer. Hybridoma 1995; 14:121.

33. Kosmas C, Snook D, Gooden C, Courtenay-Luck NS, McCall MJ, Meares CF, Epenetos AA. Development of humoral immune responses against a macrocyclic chelating agent (DOTA) in cancer patients receiving radioimmunoconjugates for imaging and therapy. Cancer Res 1992; 52:904.
34. Boniface GR, Izard M, Walker KZ, McKay DR, Sorby PJ, Turner JH, Morris JG. Labeling of monoclonal antibodies with samarium-153 for combined radioimmunoscintigraphy and radioimmunotherapy. J Nucl Med 1989; 30:683.
35. Kosmas C, Maraveyas A, Gooden CS, Snook D, Epenetos AA. Anti-chelate antibodies after intraperitoneal Y-90-labeled monoclonal antibody immunoconjugates for ovarian cancer therapy. J Nucl Med 1995; 36:746.
36. Sutherland RM. Cell and environment interactions in tumour microregions: the multicell spheroid model. Science 1988; 240:177.
37. Sutherland R, Buchegger F, Schreyer M, Vacca A, Mach JP. Penetration and binding of radiolabeled anti-carcinoembryonic antigen monoclonal antibodies and their antigen binding fragments in human colon multicellular tumor spheroids. Cancer Res 1987; 47:1627.
38. Langmuir V, McCann JK, Buchegger F, Sutherland RM. The effect of antigen concentration, antibody valency and size, and tumour architecture on antibody binding in multicell spheroids. Nucl Med Biol 1991; 18:753.
39. Sivolapenko GB, Kalofonos HP, Stewart JSW, Hird JV, Epenetos AA. Pharmacokinetics of radiolabelled murine monoclonal antibodies administered intravenously and intraperitoneally to patients with cancer for diagnosis and therapy. J Pharm Med 1992; 2:155.
40. Haisma H, Moseley K, Battaile B, Griffiths TC, Knapp RC. Distribution and pharmacokinetics of radiolabeled monoclonal antibody OC 125 after intravenous and intraperitoneal administration in gynecologic tumors. Am J Obstet Gynecol 1987; 159:4218.
41. Hnatowich DJ, Chinol M, Siebecker DA, Gionet M, Griffin T, Doherty PW, Hunter R, Kase KR. Patient biodistribution of intraperitoneally administered yttrium-90-labeled antibody. J Nucl Med 1988; 29:1428.
42. Malamitsi J, Skarlos D, Fotiou S, Papakostas P, Aravantinos G, Vassilarou D, Taylor-Papadimitriou J, Koutoulidis K, Hooker G, Snook D. Intracavitary use of two radiolabeled tumor-associated monoclonal antibodies. J Nucl Med 1988; 29:1910.
43. Colcher D, Esteban J, Carrasquillo JA, Sugarbaker P, Reynolds JC, Bryant G, Larson SM, Schlom J. Complementation of intracavitary and intravenous administration of a monoclonal antibody (B72.3) in patients with carcinoma. Cancer Res 1987; 47:4218.
44. Ward BG, Mather SJ, Hawkins LR, Crowther ME, Shepherd JH, Granowska M, Britton KE, Slerin ML. Localization of radioiodine conjugated to the monoclonal antibody HMFG2 in human ovarian carcinoma: assessment of intravenous and intraperitoneal routes of administration. Cancer Res 1987; 47:4719.
45. Tibben JG, Massuger LF, Boerman OC, Borm GF, Claessens RA, Corstens FH. Effect of the route of administration on the biodistribution of radioiodinated OV-TL 3 F(ab')2 in experimental ovarian cancer. Eur J Nucl Med 1994; 21:1183.
46. Perkins AC, Symonds IM, Pimm MV, Price MR, Wastie ML, Symonds EM. Immunoscintigraphy of ovarian carcinoma using a monoclonal antibody (^{111}In-NCRC48)

defining a polymorphic epithelial mycin (PEM) epitope. Nucl Med Commun 1993; 14:578.

47. Epenetos AA, Muto MG, Kassis AI. Antibody-guided irradiation of advanced ovarian cancer with intraperitoneally administered monoclonal antibodies. J Clin Oncol 1987; 5:1890.

48. Rosenblum MG, Kavanagh JJ, Burke TW, Wharton JT, Cunningham JE, Shanken LJ, Silva EG, Thompson L, Cheung L, Lamki L. Clinical pharmacology, metabolism and tissue distribution of Y-90-labeled monoclonal antibody B27.3 after intraperitoneal administration. J Natl Cancer Inst 1991; 83:1629.

49. Hird V, Maraveyas A, Snook D, Dhokia B, Soutter WP, Meares C, Stewart JS, Mason P, Lambert HE, Epenetos AA. Adjuvant therapy of ovarian cancer with radioactive monoclonal antibody. Br J Cancer 1993; 82:586.

50. Epenetos AA, Courtenay-Luck N, Snook E. Antibody guided irradiation of malignant lesions: three cases illustrating a new method of treatment. Lancet 1984; i: 1441.

51. Maraveyas A, Snook D, Hird V, Kosmas C, Meares CF, Lambert HE, Epenetos AA. Pharmacokinetics and toxicity of an yttrium-90-CITC-DPTA-HMFG1 radioimmunoconjugate for intraperitoneal radioimmunotherapy of ovarian cancer. Cancer 1993; 73:1067.

52. Jacobs AJ, Fer M, Su FM, Breitz H, Thompson J, Goodgold H, Cain J, Heaps J, Weiden J. A phase I trial of a renium 186-labeled monoclonal antibody administered intraperitoneally in ovarian carcinoma: toxicity and clinical response. Obstet Gynecol 1993; 82:586.

53. Ward B, Mather E, Shepherd J, Crowther M, Hawkins L, Britton K, Slevin ML. The treatment of intraperitoneal malignant disease with monoclonal antibody guided ^{131}I radiotherapy. Br J Cancer 1988; 58:658.

54. Crippa F, Bolis G, Seregni E, Gavoni N, Scarfone G, Ferraris C, Buraggi GL, Bombardieri E. Single-dose intraperitoneal radioimmunotherapy with the murine monoclonal antibody I-131 MOv18: clinical results in patients with minimal residual disease of ovarian cancer. Eur J Cancer 1995; 31:686.

55. Buchman R, De Angelis C, Shaw P, Covens A, Osborne R, Kerr I, Reed R, Michaels H, Woo M, Reilly R. Intraperitoneal therapy of malignant ascites associates with carcinoma of ovary and breast using radioiodinated monoclonal antibody 2G3. Gynecol Oncol 1992; 47:102.

56. Courtenay-Luck NS, Epenetos AA, Larche M, Pectasides D, Dhokia B, Ritter MA. Development of primary and secondary immune responses to mouse monoclonal antibodies used in the diagnosis and therapy of malignant neoplasms. Cancer Res 1986; 46:6489.

57. Kosmas C, Epenetos AA, Courtenay-Luck NS. Patients receiving murine monoclonal antibody therapy for malignancy develop T cells that proliferate in vitro in response to these antibodies as antigens. Br J Cancer 1991; 64:494.

58. Berek JS, Hacker NF, Lichtenstein A, Jung T, Spina C, Knox RM, Brady J, Greene T, Ettinger LM, Lagasse LD. Intraperitoneal recombinant alpha-interferon for ''salvage'' immunotherapy in stage III epithelial ovarian cancer: a Gynecologic Oncology Group study. Cancer Res 1985; 45:4447.

59. Baum RP, Niesen A, Hertel A, Nancy A, Hess H, Donnerstag B, Sykes TR,

Sykes CJ, Suresh MR, Noujaim AA. Activating anti-idiotypic human anti-mouse antibodies for immunotherapy of ovarian carcinoma. Cancer 1994; 73:1121.

60. Ward BG, Mather SJ, Granowska M. Radiolabelled monoclonal antibodies in oncology. III. Radioimmunotherapy. Nucl Med Commun 1991; 12:333.
61. Bruland OS. Cancer therapy with radiolabeled antibodies: an overview. Acta Oncol 1995; 34:1085.
62. Riva P, Marangolo M, Lazzari S, Agostini M, Sarti G, Moscatelli G, Franceschi G, Spinelli A, Vecchietti G. Locoregional immunotherapy of human ovarian cancer: preliminary results. Int J Radiat Appl Instrum B 1989; 16:659.
63. Muto MG, Finkler NJ, Kassis AI, Lepisto EM, Knapp RC. Human anti-murine antibody responses in ovarian cancer patients undergoing radioimmunotherapy with the murine monoclonal antibody OC-125. Gynecol Oncol 1990; 38:244.
64. Hnatowich DJ, Virzi F, Ruschkowski M. Investigations of avidin and biotin for imaging application. J Nucl Med 1987; 28:1294–1302.
65. Goodwin DA, Meares CF, McCall MJ, McTigue M, Chaovapong W. Pre-targeted immunoscintigraphy of murine tumors with indium-111-labelled bifunctional haptens. J Nucl Med 1988; 29:225.
66. Le Doussal JM, Martin M, Gautherot E, Delaage M, Barber J. In vitro and in vivo targeting of radiolabelled monovalent and divalent haptens with dual specificity monoclonal antibody conjugates: enhanced divalent hapten affinity for cell bound antibody conjugate. J Nucl Med 1989; 30:1358.
67. Paganelli G, Belloni C, Magnani P, Zito F, Pasini A, Sassi I, Meroni M, Mariano M, Vignali M, Siccardi AG, Fazio F. Two-step tumour targeting in ovarian cancer patients using biotinylated monoclonal antibodies and radioactive streptavidine. Eur J Nucl Med 1992; 19:322.
68. Paganelli G, Magnani P, Zito F. Three-step monoclonal antibody tumour targeting in carcinoembryonic antigen-positive patients. Cancer Res 1991; 51:5960.
69. Peltier P, Curter C, Chatal JF. Radioimmunodetection of medullary thyroid cancer using a bispecific anti-CEA/anti-indium-DTPA antibody and an indium-111-labeled DTPA dimer. J Nucl Med 1993; 34:1267.
70. Marshall D, Pedley RB, Boden JA, Boden R, Melton RG, Begent RH. Polythylene glycol modification of a galactosylated streptavidin clearing agent: effects on immunogenicity and clearance of a biotinylated anti-tumour antibody. Br J Cancer 1996; 73:562.
71. Burton MA, Gray BN, Coletti A. Effect of angiotensin II on blood flow in the transplanted sheep squamous cell carcinoma. Eur J Cancer Clin Oncol 1998; 24:699.
72. Gilgien W, Bischof Delaloye A, Pettavel J. Enhancement of tumor/parenchyma perfusion ratio by betablockage in liver metastases. Eur J Nucl Med 1988; 24:245.
73. Wilder RB, Langmuir VK, Mendona HL, Goris ML, Knox SJ. Local hyperthermia and SR 4233 enhance the antitumor effects of radioimmunotherapy in nude mice with human colonic adenocarcinoma xenografts. Cancer Res 1993; 53:3022.
74. Greiner JW, Shimada S, Gudagni F. Cytokine-based modalities to enhance monoclonal antibody mediated tumor cell killing. In: Goldenberg, ed. Cancer Therapy with Radiolabeled Antibodies. Boca Raton: CRC Press, 1987: 283.
75. Folli S, Pelegrin A, Chalandon Y, Yao X, Buchegger F, Lienard D, Lejeune F, Mach JP. Tumor necrosis factor can enhance radio-antibody uptake in human colon

carcinoma xenografts by selective increase of vascular permeability. Int J Cancer 1993; 53:829.

76. Imbert-Marcille BM, Berreur M, Thedrez P, Riet A, Devys A, Chatal JF, Pradal G. Effects of interferon gamma (IFN gamma) and tumor necrosis factor alpha (TNF alpha) association in intraperitoneal radioimmunotherapy: studies on an in vitro micrometastasis model. Anticancer Drug Des 1995; 10:491.

77. Imbert-Marcille BM, Thedrez P, Sai-Maurel C, Francois C, Auget JL, Benard J, Jacques Y, Imai S, Chatal JF. Modulation of associated ovarian carcinoma antigens by 5 cytokines used as single agents or in combination. Int J Cancer 1994; 57:392.

78. Oettgen HF. Cytokines in clinical cancer therapy. Curr Opin Immunol 1991; 3:699.

79. Sgouros G. Plasmapheresis in radioimmunotherapy of micrometastasis: a mathematical modeling and dosimetrical analysis. J Nucl Med 1992; 33:2167.

80. Quadri SM, Malik AB, Tang YZ, Patenia R, Freedman RS, Vriesendorp HM. Preclinical analysis of intraperitoneal administration of ^{111}In-labeled human tumour reactive monoclonal IgM AC6C3-2B12. Cancer Res 1995; 55:5736s.

81. Remmenga SW, Colcher D, Gansow O, Pippen CG, Raubitschek A. Continuous infusion chemotherapy as a radiation-enhancing agent for yttrium-90-radiolabeled monoclonal antibody therapy of a human tumour xenograft. Gynecol Oncol 1994; 55:115.

82. Buchegger F, Rojas A, Bischof Delaloye A, Vogel CA. Combined radioimmunotherapy and radiotherapy of human colon carcinoma grafted in nude mice. Cancer Res 1995; 55:83.

13

Targeted Radiotherapy in the Treatment of Osteosarcoma
Radiobiological Basis, Clinical Status, and Future Prospects

Øyvind S. Bruland and Alexander Pihl
Norwegian Radium Hospital, Oslo, Norway

I. INTRODUCTION

Targeted radiotherapy, alone or in combination with external radiation therapy, may become an important addition to our therapeutic armamentarium against osteosarcoma (OS). Potential applications of this approach are to combat lung and skeletal micro-metastases not eliminated by chemotherapy, and to eradicate remaining tumor cells of a primary tumor, not amenable to complete surgical removal.

II. CLINICAL AND BIOLOGICAL FEATURES

Recently we have discussed some of the dilemmas and challenges confronting the clinician treating patients with OS (1). This disease has several unique features. We shall briefly review some of its salient characteristics and point out why targeted radiotherapy may be particularly useful in this disease.

Osteosarcoma is a rare disorder which primarily strikes children and adolescents (2,3) and develops from neoplastic mesenchymal cells which undergo osteoblastic differentiation. The disease displays considerable heterogeneity and appears in clinical entities having different prognoses (1–5). The most common form, "classical OS," strikes people below the age of 30 years with a primary tumor localized in the long bones of the extremities, predominantly in the meta-physeal regions. By definition overt metastases are not detectable at initial presentation. In another OS-entity the primary tumor emerges in the bones of the axial skeleton. This is more often seen in elderly patients and carries a much poorer prognosis (5,6).

An important feature of OS is its propensity for early hematogenic dissemination. Thus, after surgical removal of the primary tumor as the sole treatment, about 80% of patients with classical OS eventually die from metastatic disease developing from micrometastases that must already have been present at presentation (1). The vast majority of the metastases develop in the lungs; progressive, uncontrollable metastatic lung disease is the most frequent cause of death.

The cornerstones in the current therapy of OS are radical surgery combined with heavy adjuvant polydrug chemotherapy. Conventional external radiotherapy has contributed little to the improved survival (7). Surgical removal of the primary tumor is an essential step in treatment with curative intent. A limb–salvage procedure is feasible in the majority of cases, under the protective umbrella of chemotherapy. Moreover, surgical extirpation of isolated lung metastases has curative potential in certain patients (8–12). During the past two decades the survival of young, nonmetastatic patients has been raised by about 40% to at least 60% (13–16), primarily achieved by the use of adjuvant chemotherapy to eradicate micrometastases. However, the prognosis is still grave (1), especially in patients with overt metastases at presentation (17–19) and in patients where the OS is located in the bones of the axial skeleton (6).

Adjuvant chemotherapy is today most often given preoperatively as so-called neoadjuvant chemotherapy (20–22). This allows subsequent histological examination of the tumor specimens and permits an early assessment of the drug responsiveness of the tumor and the patient's prognosis. Hence, in cases where the response to chemotherapy is inadequate, alternative treatments may be initiated at an early stage.

Only in rare cases does OS present with lymph node metastases, in contrast to the situation in many other solid cancers. This is partly due to the fact that bony tissue is devoid of a draining lymphatic system. The presence of lymph node metastases invariably heralds a dismal prognosis. Locoregional radiation therapy is not a curative treatment in such cases; probably the lymph node metastases represent secondary sites associated with extensive systemic disease.

In spite of the treatment progress made during the past decades, even today about half of an unselected OS population eventually succumb to the disease (1). In several centers increasingly toxic combination chemotherapy is now used in attempts to further raise the survival rate, but the consequent side effects are serious and the net gain is questionable (1,23). There is no consensus as to the future strategy to be followed. Clearly, there is a strong need for novel approaches and to explore new avenues.

III. RADIOSENSITIVITY

The limited clinical role of external radiotherapy in the curative treatment of OS may partly be due to inherent low radiosensitivity of the tumor cells, but is also a result of the predominant localization of metastases within radiosensitive lung tissue. Furthermore, primary tumors, not amenable to complete surgical removal, are most often localized to the pelvis, spine, and basis of the skull, adjacent to and invading radiosensitive structures (6).

The early radiation studies in OS contain significant observations that should not be disregarded. Before the advent of modern chemotherapy, the principal treatment was radical surgery only, in most cases involving amputation of the affected limb. In attempts to avoid overtreatment of young people doomed to die from micrometastases already present in the lungs, the English physician Sir Stanford Cade introduced a significant modification of the then-current treatment (24). To spare the patients with systemic disease from fruitless mutilation, he postponed the operation for 4 to 6 months, a "holding action," and treated the primary tumor initially with irradiation only. In the course of 7 to 8 weeks a radiation dose of 70 to 90 Gy was given—i.e., doses above the long-term tolerance of the normal tissues within the field of irradiation. By this strategy rapid pain relief and tumor growth delay were consistently achieved. Patients who developed manifest metastases were merely given further palliative treatment. In those who remained free of metastases, he then offered radical surgery, now with a curative aim. It is noteworthy that some of the nonmetastatic patients who refused amputations later turned out to be cured by the radiation treatment alone (24,25). That local control of OS can be achieved by radiotherapy, at least in some cases, has also been found in some recent studies (7,26).

The results of the early radiation studies indicated that a dose-effect relationship obtains also in OS. In one series none of the patients attained control of their disease at tumor doses <30 Gy, whereas >90 Gy all tumors were sterilized (27). The aggregate experience from a number of studies indicated that even large OS tumors could indeed be sterilized by external radiation at doses >80 to 90 Gy (7,28). However, when large tumors were irradiated to sterilizing doses, unacceptable damage to surrounding normal tissues too often ensued among long-term survivors.

Since then, the technology has been considerably improved, and high radiation doses can now be delivered to better-defined target volumes with less damage to normal tissues. However, even today radiation doses >70 Gy to large volumes cannot be administered with impunity by external irradiation only.

The effects of prophylactic external lung irradiation have been explored in several studies (7,29,30). Since in OS the lung metastases are usually distributed throughout the lungs, both lungs must be irradiated. To avoid disabling lung fibrosis the radiation dose must be limited to 20 Gy (1.5 Gy $\times$ 13). Theoretically, this may prevent further growth of metastases containing $<10^4$ to 10^5 tumor cells. This view is supported by some studies in which such doses have indeed shown therapeutic effects, expressed as delayed appearance of a reduced number of lung metastases (31). However, in most instances the clinical benefits have not been convincing, and prophylactic, external total lung irradiation is no longer in general use (2,3,7). Apparently, the doses required to reliably sterilize the whole spectrum of lung metastases are higher than those that can be safely given by external radiation alone.

IV. RATIONALE FOR TARGETING

The main shortcoming of external radiotherapy is its lack of selectivity for the cancer cells. Normal cells within the target volume receive the same dose as the tumor cells, and since the radiosensitivity of the latter is usually not much higher than that of the normal cells, the therapeutic index is low. In contrast, by targeted radiation in which a radionuclide is brought to the surface or the vicinity of the tumor cells, preferential destruction of cancer cells can be accomplished.

To achieve optimal results with external irradiation it is necessary to know the exact location and extent of the tumorous foci; this is not a prerequisite with radiopharmaceuticals capable of binding selectively to the tumor cells wherever they are. Because of the range of the ionizing particles that expose the tumor cells to "cross fire," valuable clinical results may be obtained without absolute tumor cell specificity, as well as when some tumor cells fail to express the binding sites. In contrast, when drugs or toxins are used in targeting, cure usually requires that the effector-molecules be internalized by every cancer cell.

The targeting process is a dynamic, complex interaction involving three players: the target proper, the effector moiety, and the targeting vehicle. In the case of OS, the targets are expressed either on the surface of the tumor cells or in the intercellular matrix.

In targeted radiotherapy proper microdosimetry adapted to the specific clinical situation is essential. Optimal destruction of micrometastases may require different strategies depending on whether they consist primarily of single cells, microscopic clusters of cells, or subdiagnostic tumor foci. Microdosimetry is a complex field which is extensively covered elsewhere in this treatise.

V. TARGETS AND LIGANDS

For targeting of OS, two types of ligands are available, viz. Mabs, which bind to specific epitopes on cell surface antigens, and synthetic bone-seeking pharmaceuticals, such as bis- and polyphosphonates adsorbing to osteoid and bony elements produced by the osteosarcoma cells. The Mabs and the bone-seeking pharmaceuticals have widely different, but complementary properties and applications. Both types can serve as carriers of radionuclides.

The Mabs are particularly suitable for targeting single cells and small clusters of cells. Several antigens, more or less specific for osteosarcoma cells, have been identified, and Mabs directed against these have been prepared. We have recently reviewed their properties (32,33). These Mabs have been extensively studied in vitro (34), in immunodeficient rodents carrying human OS xenografts (35), in pigs (36), and in dogs with spontaneous OS (37,38), but so far only to a limited degree clinically (39).

Osteogenic sarcoma cells produce excessive amounts of mesenchymal matrix containing primitive bony elements, so-called osteoid. Moreover, the osteoid produced by tumor cells embedded in this matrix differs, both qualitatively and quantitatively, from that found in mature, normal bone. The osteoid produced by OS cells resembles primitive woven bone insofar as it contains a larger number of more accessible binding sites for bis- and polyphosphonates. These substances bind to and are rapidly incorporated into the hydroxy-apatite moiety of the anorganic scaffold of the intercellular matrix. They also bind, but to a lesser degree, to sites possessing proliferating normal osteoblasts.

In bisphosphonates the oxygen atom in a pyrophosphate linkage is replaced by a carbon atom, rendering such molecules resistant to the hydrolyzing enzymes. Hence, they are retained in the bone matrix with a very long biological half-life. After IV injection of bis- and polyphosphonates a high percentage of the injected dose per gram tumor is rapidly deposited in OS tumors (40). Bisphosphonates are nontoxic substances that are efficient inhibitors of osteoclast-mediated bone destruction. They have recently been approved for the treatment of tumor-induced hypercalcemia, skeletal metastases, and osteoporosis (41).

VI. RADIOPHARMACEUTICALS

The therapeutic efficacy of radiolabeled targeting compounds depends on the chemical properties of the vehicle as well as the physical properties of the radionuclide, such as its half-life and the nature of the emitted particles, their energies, and ionization density (the linear energy transfer, LET).

As vehicles for radionuclides, most targeting studies so far have employed Mabs. We have previously reviewed the clinical results of cancer therapy with radiolabeled antibodies (42). Impressive complete response rates have been reported in patients with non-Hodgkin's lymphoma resistant to combination chemotherapy by the use of ^{131}I-anti-CD-20 (43,44). In patients with solid cancers the results so far have been disappointing.

The efficacy of antibody-mediated targeting of radionuclides to tumor sites depends on a number of factors, the most important of which are the degree and heterogeneity of the antigen expression on the tumor cells, the specificity and affinity of the antibody for unique epitopes on antigens, and the vascularization of the tumor. A major limitation of intact antibodies as vehicles is the low penetration of such macromolecules into solid tumor tissues (42,45,46), usually resulting in inadequate tumor radiation doses following IV administration. The extent of targeting can be improved by using antibody fragments, produced either by enzymatic cleavage or by recombinant technology. However, the fragments also have their shortcomings.

The in vivo stability of the Mab/effector complex and its immunoreactivity depend on the method used to couple the radionuclide to the antibody. The biodistribution of [131]I- and ^{125}I-labeled intact IgG of TP-1 and TP-3, as well as of their Fab and $F(ab')_2$ fragments, labeled in their tyrosine-residues by means of Iodogen, has been studied in our laboratory using a nude mouse model with human OS xenografts grown SC (35). The highest degree of targeting, expressed in percent of injected dose per gram tumor, was obtained with intact IgG, whereas the fragments gave the highest target/nontarget ratios. In both cases the ratios increased with time postinjection, but a significant loss of radioactivity from tumor sites occurred, probably due to dehalogenation. The use of a different coupling method which links halogens to lysine residues on the Mabs (47) resulted in improved tumor retention of radioactivity as compared to that obtained after labeling of tyrosine (48).

To our knowledge the TP-Mabs are the only ones with a sarcoma-restricted specificity that have been radio-labeled and injected into OS patients and shown to localize specifically to the tumor tissue. In a study of diagnostic immunoscintigraphy, TP-1-Mab was injected IV into six patients with primary and/or metastatic bone sarcomas (39). A fixed dose of 1 mg $F(ab')_2$, Iodogen labeled with ^{131}I was used. A considerable loss of radioactivity from a primary tumor site was observed. However, despite the low image resolution afforded by ^{131}I, lung metastases were also detected and in one case a small lesion not found by x-ray and CT examination was disclosed by the immunoscintigraphy and later removed surgically (39). The extent of tumor targeting achieved in our study, measured as radioactivity content in tissue specimens, was in the same range as that obtained in colorectal, melanoma and ovarian cancer. Unfortunately, we have not so far had access to sufficient quantities of GMP quality TP antibodies to pursue therapeutic studies in patients.

In dogs with spontaneous OS, the biodistribution of ^{18}F-labeled TP3-FAB fragments was explored by the use of PET scanning. Rapid and selective localization to tumorous sites was observed and small lung metastases were visualized. However, the radioactivity retained, expressed in percent of injected dose per gram in the target tissue, was low (38).

The polyphosphonates are chelators capable of stably binding different metals and their radioactive isotopes (49). [153]Sm forms stable complexes with EDTMP, emits medium-energy beta-particles effective for therapy and 105-keV photons suitable for high-resolution gamma camera imaging (50). Bis- and polyphosphonates, radiolabeled with different radionuclides, have been developed for the purpose of palliation of pain from bone metastases (51–54). In the case of prostate and breast cancer, these radiopharmaceuticals are concentrated in the layer surrounding the metastases where there is a reactive proliferation of normal osteoblasts. In OS tissue the situation is more favourable as the tumors cells proper synthesize the target, the primitive bone matrix, often throughout the entire metastatic lesion.

A majority of OS tumors, including metastases, produce primitive bone matrix and give intense "hot spots" on conventional diagnostic bone scans following injection of the diagnostic bone-seeking radiopharmaceutical ^{99m}Tc-MDP. Biodistribution data obtained in OS patients undergoing surgery showed that metastatic OS foci often accumulate and retain substantial amounts of the injected radioactivity (40). In fact, tumor/normal lung radioactivity ratios as high as 100 to 300 and tumor/normal bone ratios of 5 to 10 were obtained. The chemotherapy, routinely given to all OS patients, may induce partial or almost complete response of the metastases, often resulting in augmented bone formation, rendering previously undetected metastases visible on X-ray examination. Despite a cytotoxic response of the tumor cells the metastases may not shrink due to the rigid structure of the intercellular matrix. Surviving tumor cells may dwell as multiple, small chemotherapy-resistant clusters scattered throughout this scaffold. We have found (unpublished) that such lesions are able to accumulate significant concentrations of [153]Sm-EDTMP.

Most of the clinical therapeutic studies employing targeted radiotherapy have utilized beta-emitting radionuclides as the effector arm. Beta particles are sparsely ionizing (low LET) and have low radiobiological efficiency. A promising development is to exploit densely ionizing alpha particles (high LET) such as [211]At and [212]Bi. Both can be stably conjugated to Mabs (47,55). TP-3 IgG has been conjugated with [211]At and tested both in vitro (56,57) and in preclinical animal models (48,58). Exquisite and specific OS cytotoxicity was observed.

Recently, a novel alpha-emitting polyphosphonate, [212]Bi-DOTMP (59), and the bisphosphonate pamidronate labeled with [211]At via an aromatic intermediate

(60), have been developed. Both possess strong bone-targeting capability and in vivo stability comparable to that of ^{153}Sm-EDTMP.

VII. CLINICAL THERAPEUTIC STUDIES

Based on the biodistribution data mentioned above we have explored the therapeutic use of ^{153}Sm-EDTMP in patients with advanced OS (61,62). This radiopharmaceutical had previously been shown to have therapeutic effects in dogs with spontaneous OS (63,64).

Ten patients with OS, suffering from either local recurrences or metastatic disease, all having failed conventional treatment modalities, were given IV infusions of 25 to 52 MBq/kg body weight of ^{153}Sm-EDTMP on one to three occasions. Since all OS patients had been heavily pretreated with chemotherapy, the question arose whether their bone marrow would tolerate additional systemic treatment with samarium ^{153}Sm-EDTMP, known to be toxic to the bone marrow. The treatments were therefore given 6 weeks apart, an interval sufficient to restore the hematological parameters to normal values.

The toxicity was mild with no subjective side effects. Transient leukopenia and trombocytopenia occurred in all patients except one. In all patients the blood parameters returned to normal values following treatment, usually after 4 to 6 weeks. In none of the cases did neutropenic fever or bleeding occur. The nadir values of leucocytes and trombocytes were not clearly related to the amount of injected radioactivity, but seemed to depend primarily on the age of the patient and the severity of previous chemotherapy regimens (unpublished results).

Three patients suffered from serious pain which was significantly relieved by ^{153}Sm-EDTMP-treatment. In one patient, bedridden with paraparesis and impaired bladder function due to a vertebral lesion, the pareses gradually subsided after two radionuclide administrations (61). Six months after the last treatment the patient had no objective neurological symptoms, and no detectable metastases. However, he then relapsed with increasing pain, was reoperated, but died 2 months later from purulent meningitis.

In five other patients significant growth delays were observed, lasting for up to 18 months. Significant growth delays of metastases, in one patient located in the right lung and in another in the spine, were observed. However, one patient with massive disease, including malignant ascites and lymph node metastases, showed progressive tumor growth, despite good uptake of the radiopharmaceutical in most of the metastatic lesions. Three other OS patients, with tumors of chondroblastic or fibrobroblastic histology, all showed relatively low tumor uptake of ^{153}Sm-EDTMP and, as expected, did not respond to the treatment (unpublished results).

Alkaline phosphatase is produced by the OS tumor cells. Interestingly, in all patients where responses to treatment were documented, the elevated serum levels of alkaline phosphatase were normalized upon treatment.

In some patients the absorbed radiation doses were calculated by the attenuation-corrected conjugated view technique combining the use of CT information and data from whole-body scanning with a dual-head gamma camera (65). By repeated gamma camera imaging the effective half-life of ^{153}Sm-EDTMP in OS lesions was found to be equal to the physical half-life of ^{153}Sm, confirming stable retention of the radioactivity in the tumors. The calculations indicated that tumor doses as high as 60 Gy may be obtained after a single injection of ^{153}Sm-EDTMP.

A new strategy is to use ^{153}Sm-EDTMP in the primary treatment of osteoblastic OS as a boost to conventional external radiotherapy and as an adjunct to chemotherapy in patients with poor prognosis. In one patient with an inoperable primary tumor in the thoracic spine, the radiopharmaceutical was infused intra-arterially in combination with conformal external radiotherapy (66). Gamma camera scintigraphy using ^{99m}Tc-MDP showed that, as expected, the extraction of radiopharmaceutical was greater after IA than after IV administration. The patient remains asymptomatic after 38 months. This attractive treatment is now beeing further explored.

VIII. FUTURE ROLE OF TARGETED RADIOTHERAPY

The results reviewed in this paper show that targeted radiation therapy employing ^{153}Sm-EDTMP can be used in heavily pretreated OS patients without undue toxicity, and that in some cases beneficial therapeutic results such as pain relief and even objective remissions are seen. In our initial clinical study we chose, from a safety point of view, to allow an interval of 6 weeks between injections of the radiopharmaceutical to ensure complete recovery of the bone marrow before the second dose was given. It can be calculated, however, that after an IV injection of ^{153}Sm approximately 90% of the tumor dose is deposited in the course of the first 5 days; during the subsequent 5 weeks the tumor will receive virtually no radiation, allowing surviving tumor cells to repopulate. Thus, dosimetric and radiobiological considerations indicate that the dose schedule used in our preliminary Phase I study was far from optimal. Because the toxicity observed in our study was low, we have now started a dose-escalation trial in patients with advanced bone sarcoma, having autologous hematopoietic stem cells cryo preserved as back up. Our aim is to improve the dose deposition by giving, already at the outset, infusions of ^{153}Sm-EDTMP, in some of the patients concomitant with external irradiation. This schedule is supported by findings in an experimental rat sarcoma model showing that the addition of a radiation boost to external fractionated radiotherapy is most effective when given initially (67).

In relapsing patients, previously quiescent malignant cells resume growth, induce neovascularization, and invade the surrounding lung tissue. We have demonstrated by immunohistochemistry (39) that in such instances the accumulation of the radioactivity occurs in a narrow rim of viable tumor cells strongly expressing the relevant epitope, probably rendering these foci susceptible to radioimmunotherapy. Preclinical studies employing alpha emitters coupled to Moabs seem promising (56,57), and efforts are being made to exploit these in OS patients having failed conventional treatment.

In conclusion, the available evidence indicates that targeted radiotherapy in OS may be useful in the following circumstances:

1. As a concomitant boost to external irradiation in patients
   a. With primary tumors in the axial skeleton not amenable to complete removal by surgery without unacceptable mutilation
   b. Where histological examination of the tumor specimen shows inadequate surgical margins
2. Together with total lung external irradiation in high-risk patients such as
   a. Those presenting with overt metastases
   b. Those relapsing and not responding to second-line chemotherapy and who cannot be salvaged by surgical metastasectomy

REFERENCES

1. Bruland ØS, Pihl A. On the current management of osteosarcoma. A critical evaluation and a proposal for a modified treatment strategy. Eur J Cancer 1997; 33:1725–1731.
2. Malawer MM, Link MP, Donaldson SS. Sarcomas of bone. In: Devita VT, Hellman S, Rosenberg SA, eds. Cancer: Principles & Practice of Oncology, 5th ed. Philadelphia: Lippincott-Raven, 1997:1789–1852.
3. Souhami R, Cannon SR. Osteosarcoma. In: Peckham M, Pinedo HM, Veronesi U, eds. Oxford Textbook of Oncology. Oxford: Oxford University Press, Oxford, 1995: 1969–1976.
4. Dahlin D, Unni K, Osteogenic sarcoma of bone and its important recognizable varieties. Am J Surg Pathol 1977; 1:61–72.
5. Huvos AG. Osteogenic sarcoma. In: Huvos AG, ed. Bone Tumors. Diagnosis, Treatment and Prognosis. Philadelphia: W.B. Saunders, 1991:85–155.
6. Sæter G, Bruland ØS, Follerås G, Boysen M, Høie J. Extremity and non-extremity high grade osteosarcoma. The Norwegian Radium Hospital experience during the modern chemotherapy era. Acta Oncol 1996; 35(s8):129–134.

7. Harter KW. Osteosarcoma and less common sarcomas of childhood. In: Cassady JR, ed. Radiation Therapy in Pediatric Oncology. New York: Springer-Verlag, 1994: 305–317.
8. Sutow WW, Herson J, Perez C. Survival after metastasis in osteosarcoma. Natl Cancer Inst Monogr 1981; 56:227–231.
9. Beattie EJ, Harvey JC, Marcove R, Martini N. Results of multiple pulmonary resections for metastatic osteogenic sarcoma after two decades. J Surg Oncol 1991; 46: 154–155.
10. Roth JA, Putnam JBJ, Wesley MN, Rosenberg SA. Differing determinants of prognosis following resection of pulmonary metastases from osteogenic and soft tissue sarcoma patients. Cancer 1985; 55:1361–1366.
11. Van Rijk Zwikker GL, Nooy MA, Taminiau A, Kappetein AP, Huysmans HA. Pulmonary metastasectomy in patients with osteosarcoma. Eur J Cardiothorac Surg 1991; 5:406–409.
12. Pastorino U, Gasparini M, Tavecchio L, Azzarelli A, Mapelli S, Zucchi V, Morandi F, Fossati Bellani F, Valente M, Ravasi G. The contribution of salvage surgery to the management of childhood osteosarcoma. J Clin Oncol 1991; 9:1357–1362.
13. Meyers PA, Heller G, Healey J, Huvos A, Lane J, Marcove R, Applewhite A, Vlamis V, Rosen G. Chemotherapy for nonmetastatic osteogenic sarcoma: the Memorial Sloan-Kettering experience. J Clin Oncol 1992; 10:5–15.
14. Sæter G, Alvegård TA, Elomaa I, Stenwig AE, Holmström T, Solheim ØP. Treatment of osteosarcoma of the extremities with the T-10 protocol, with emphasis on the effects of pre-operative chemotherapy with single agent high-dose methotrexate. A Scandinavian Sarcoma Group study. J Clin Oncol 1991; 9:1766–1775.
15. Bacci G, Picci P, Ferrari S, Ruggieri P, Casadei R, Tienghi A, Brach del Prever A, Gherlinzoni F, Mercuri M, Monti C. Primary chemotherapy and delayed surgery for nonmetastatic osteosarcoma of the extremities: results in 164 patients preoperatively treated with high doses of methotrexate followed by cisplatin and doxorubicin. Cancer 1993; 72:3227–3238.
16. Winkler K, Bielack S, Delling G, Salzer-Kuntschik M, Kotz R, Greenshaw C, Jurgens H, Ritter J, Kusnierz-Glaz C, Erttmann R. Effect of intraarterial versus intravenous cisplatin in addition to systemic doxorubicin, high-dose methotrexate, and ifosfamide on histologic tumor response in osteosarcoma (study COSS-86). Cancer 1990; 66:1703–1710.
17. Meyers PA, Heller G, Healey JH, Huvos A, Applewhite A, Sun M, LaQuaglia M. Osteogenic sarcoma with clinically detectable metastasis at initial presentation. J Clin Oncol 1993; 11:449–453.
18. Bacci G, Briccoli A, Picci P, Ruggieri P, Avella M, Gnudi S, Dallari O, Biagini R, Rizzente AG, Galletti S, Prasad R, Campanacci M. Osteosarcoma of the extremities metastatic at presentation: results obtained with primary chemotherapy followed by simultaneous resection of the primary and metastatic lesions. Cancer J 1990; 3:213–218.
19. Morgan E, Baum E, Bleyer WA, Movassaghi N, Provisor A, Lampkin B, Lukens J, Griffin T, White H, Fryer C, Telander R, Sather H, Hammond D. Treatment of patients with metastatic osteogenic sarcoma: a report from the Childrens Cancer Study Group. Cancer Treat Rep 1984; 68:661–664.
20. Rosen G, Suwansirikul S, Kwon C, Tan C, Wu SJ, Beattie Jr EJ, Murphy ML.

High-dose methotrexate with citrovorum factor rescue and adriamycin in childhood osteogenic sarcoma. Cancer 1974; 33:1151–1163.

21. Rosen G, Marcove RC, Caparros B. Primary osteogenic sarcoma: the rationale for preoperative chemotherapy and delayed surgery. Cancer 1979; 43:2163–2177.

22. Rosen G. Preoperative (neoadjuvant) chemotherapy for osteogenic sarcoma: a ten year experience. Orthopedics 1985; 8:659–664.

23. Bruland ØS, Sæter G, Pihl A. Dilemmas and challenges in the current management of osteosarcoma. A plea for more individualized treatment. Anticancer Res 1995; 15:1798.

24. Cade S. Osteogenic sarcom: a study based on 133 patients. J R Coll Surg (Edinb) 1955; 1:79–111.

25. Poppe E, Liverud K, Efskind J. Osteosarcoma. Acta Chir Scand 1968; 134:549–556.

26. Lombardi F, Gandola L, Fossati-Bellani F, Gianni MC, Rottoli L, Gasparini M. Hypofractionated accelerated radiotherapy in osteogenic sarcoma. Int J Radiat Oncol Biol Phys 1992; 24:761–765.

27. Gaitan-Yanguas M. A study of the response to osteogenic sarcoma and adjacent normal tissues to radiation. Int J Radiat Oncol Biol Phys 1981; 7:593–595.

28. Allen SEV, Stevens KR. Preoperative irradiation for osteogenic sarcoma. Cancer 1973; 31:1364–1366.

29. Breur K, Cohen P, Schweisguth O, Hart AMM. Irradiation of the lungs as an adjuvant therapy in the treatment of osteosarcoma of the limbs. An EORTC randomized study. Eur J Cancer 1978; 14:461–471.

30. Burgers JM, van Glabbeke M, Bussan A, Cohen P, Mazabraud AR, Abbatucci JS, Kalifa C, Tubiana M, Lemerle JS, Vaute PA. Osteosarcoma of the limbs. Report of the EORTC-SIOP 03 trial 20781 investigating the value of adjuvant treatment with chemotherapy and/or prophylactic lung irradiation. Cancer 1988; 45:1024–1031.

31. Lougheed MN, Palmer JD, Henderson I, McIntyre JM. Radiation and regional chemotherapy in osteogenic sarcoma. Exerpta Med Int Cong Ser 1965; 105:1124–1128.

32. Bruland ØS, Pihl A. Immunoscintigraphy and radioimmunotherapy. Useful approaches in the management of osteogenic sarcoma? In: Novak J, ed. Frontiers of Osteosarcoma Research. London: Hogrefe & Huber, 1993:149–159.

33. Larsen RH, Bruland ØS, Zalutsky MR. Radioimmunotherapy of osteosarcoma: future prospects. In: Riva P, ed., Cancer Therapy with Monoclonal Antibodies. Canada: Harwood Academic Publishers, 1999:209–229.

34. Bruland ØS, Fodstad Ø, Stenwig E, Pihl A. Expression and characteristics of a novel human osteosarcoma-associated cell surface antigen. Cancer Res, 1988; 48:5302–5309.

35. Bruland ØS, Fodstad Ø, Skretting A, Pihl A. Selective radiolocalization of two radio-labelled anti-sarcoma monoclonal antibodies in human osteosarcoma xenografts. Br J Cancer 1987; 56:21–25.

36. Fjeld JG, Bruland ØS, Benestad HB, Schjerven L, Stigbrand T, Nustad K. Radioimmunotargeting in immunocompetent animals using intraperitoneal diffusion chambers containing human tumor cells. Br J Cancer 1990; 62:573–578.

37. Haines DM, Bruland ØS, Matte G, Wilkinson AA, Meric SM, Fowler JD. Immuno-scintigraphic detection of primary and metastatic canine osteosarcoma with F(ab')$_2$ fragments of osteosarcoma-associated monoclonal antibody TP-1. Anticancer Res 1992; 12:2151–2158.

38. Page RL, Garg PK, Garg S, Archer GE, Bruland ØS, Zalutsky MR. Positron emission tomographic imaging of osteosarcoma in dogs using an ^{18}F-labeled monoclonal antibody Fab fragment. J Nucl Med 1994; 35:1506–1513.

39. Bruland ØS, Aas M, Fodstad Ø, Solheim ØP, Høie J, Skretting A, Michaelsen T, Pihl A. Immunoscintigraphy of bone sarcomas. Results in five patients. Eur J Cancer 1994; 30:1484–1489.

40. Bruland ØS, Aas M, Solheim ØP, Winderen M, Høie J. Treatment of metastatic disease in osteosarcoma patients. New applications of radiolabelled poly- and bis-phosphonates. Bone Miner 1994; 25:78.

41. Fleisch H. Bisphosphonates in Bone Disease. London: Parthenon Publishing Group, 1997.

42. Bruland ØS. Cancer therapy with radiolabeled antibodies. An overview. Acta Oncol 1995; 34:1085–1094.

43. Press OW, Eary JF, Appelbaum FR, et al. Phase II trial of ^{131}I-B1 (anti-CD20) antibody therapy with autologous stem cell transplantation for relapsed B cell lymphomas. Lancet 1995; 346:336–340.

44. Kaminski MS, Zasadny KR, Francis IR, et al. Radioimmunotherapy of B-cell lymphoma with (I-131) anti-B1 (anti-CD20) antibody. N Engl J Med 1993; 329:459–465.

45. Jain RK. Physiological barriers to delivery of monoclonal antibodies and other macromolecules in tumors. Cancer Res 1990; 50:814–819.

46. Hjelstuen MH, Rasch-Halvorsen K, Brekken C, Bruland ØS, Davis C. Penetration and binding of monoclonal antibody in human osteosarcoma multicell spheroids. Comparison of confocal laser scanning microscopy and autoradiography. Acta Oncol 1996; 35:273–279.

47. Zalutsky MR, Garg PK, Friedman HS, Bigner DD. Labelling of monoclonal antibodies and F(ab')$_2$ fragments with the alpha-particle emitting nuclide astatine-211: preservation of immunoreactivity and in vivo localizing capacity. Proc Natl Acad Sci USA 1989; 86:7149–7153.

48. Larsen RH, Hoff P, Alstad J, Bruland ØS. Preparation and quality control of [211]At-labelled and ^{125}I-labelled monoclonal antibodies. Biodistribution in mice carrying human osteosarcoma xenografts. J Labelled Compds Radiopharm 1994; 34:773–785.

49. Goeckeler WF, Edwards B, Volkert WA, Holmes RA, Simon J, Wilson D. Skeletal localization of samarium-153 chelates: potential therapeutic bone agents. J Nucl Med 1987; 28:495–504.

50. Bayouth JE, Macey DJ, Leela PK, Fossella FV. Dosimetry and toxicity of samarium-153-EDTMP administered for bone pain due to skeletal metastases. J Nucl Med 1994; 35:63–69.

51. Lewington VJ. Cancer therapy using bone-seeking isotopes. Phys Med Biol 1996; 41:2027–2042.

52. Maxon HR III, Schroder LE, Hertzberg VS, Thomas SR, Englaro EE, Samaratunga R, Smith H, Moulton JS, Williams CC, Ehrhardt GJ, Schneider HJ. Rhenium-

186(Sn)HEDP for treatment of painful osseous metastases: results of a double-blind crossover comparison with placebo. J Nucl Med 1991; 32:1877–1881.

53. Farhanghi M, Holmes RA, Volkert WA, Logan KW, Singh A. Samarium-153-EDTMP: pharmacokinetics, toxicity and pain response using an escalating dose schedule in treatment of metastatic bone cancer. J Nucl Med 1992; 33:1451–1458.

54. Collins C, Eary JF, Donaldson G, Vernon C, Bush NE, Petersdorf S, Livingston RB, Gordon EE, Chapman CR, Appelbaum FR. Samarium-153-EDTMP in bone metastases of hormone refractory prostate carcinoma: a phase I/II trial. J Nucl Med 1993; 34:1839–1844.

55. Kozak RW, Atcher RW, Gansow OA, Friedman AM, Hines JJ, Waldman TA. Bismuth-212-labelled anti-Tac monoclonal antibody: alpha-particle emitting radionuclides as modalities for radioimmunotherapy. Proc Natl Acad Sci USA 1986; 83: 474–478.

56. Larsen RH, Bruland ØS, Hoff P, Alstad J, Lindmo T, Rofstad EK. Inactivation of human osteosarcoma cells in vitro by [211]At-TP-3 monoclonal antibody: comparison with [211]At-labeled bovine serum albumin, free [211]At, and external beam X-rays. Radiat Res 1994; 139:178–184.

57. Larsen RH, Bruland ØS, Hoff P, Alstad J, Rofstad EK. Analysis of the therapeutic gain in the treatment of human osteosarcoma microclonies in vitro with [211]At-labelled monoclonal antibodies. Br J Cancer 1994; 69:1000–1005.

58. Larsen RH, Bruland ØS. Intratumor injection of immunoglobulins labelled with the alpha-emitter [211]At: analyses of tumor retention, microdistribution and growth delay. Br J Cancer 1998; 77(7):1115–1122.

59. Hassfjell S, Bruland ØS, Hoff P. [212]Bi-DOTMP—an alpha particle emitting bone seeking agent for targeted radiotherapy. Nucl Med Biol 1997; 24(3):231–237.

60. Larsen RH, Bruland ØS. Initial evaluation of a new radiolabeled bisphosphonate. J Labelled Compds Radiopharm 1998; 51:823–830.

61. Bruland ØS, Skretting A, Solheim ØP, Aas M. Targeted radiotherapy of osteosarcoma using [153]Sm-EDTMP. A new promising approach. Acta Oncol 1996; 35:381–384.

62. Bruland ØS, Skretting A, Sæter G, Solheim ØP, Aas M. Targeted internal radiotherapy in osteosarcoma patients using [153]Sm-EDTMP. Med Pediatr Oncol 1996; 27: 215.

63. Lattimer JC, Corwin LA, Stapleton J, Volkert WA, Ehrhardt GJ, Ketring AR, Anderson SK, Simon J, Goeckeler WF. Clinical and clinicopathologic response of canine bone tumors patients to treatment with samarium-153-EDTMP. J Nucl Med 1990; 31:1316–1325.

64. Moe L, Boysen M, Aas M, Lønnaas L, Gamlem H, Bruland ØS. Maxillectomy and targeted radionuclide with [153]Sm-EDTMP in a recurrent canine osteosarcoma. J Small Anim Pract 1996; 37:241–246.

65. Skretting A, Bruland ØS, Aas M. Absorbed dose estimation by combined use of CT information and whole body scanning with a dual head gamma camera in patients with osteosarcoma treated with [153]Sm-EDTMP. In: Bergmann, Kroiss, Sinzinger, eds. Radioactive Isotopes in Clinical Medicine and Research. Basel: Birkhauser Verlag, 1997:383–386.

66. Monge O, Følling M, Hordvik M, Hafslund R, Lilleng P, Bruland ØS. Neoadjuvant chemotherapy, conformal radiotherapy and intra-arterial [153]samarium-EDTMP as primary treatment of high grade osteosarcoma of the spine. Acta Orthop Scand 1996; 67:48.
67. Dubben HH, Beck-Bornholdt HP. Influence of the timing of a concomitant boost during fractionated irradiation of a rat rhabdomyosarcoma R1H. Acta Oncol 1993; 32(1):79–82.

14
Targeted Radiotherapy of Neuroblastoma

Cornelis A. Hoefnagel
Netherlands Cancer Institute, Amsterdam, The Netherlands

I. INTRODUCTION

Neuroblastoma is a malignant tumor of the sympathetic nervous system, occurring most frequently in early childhood. The tumor originates from the neural crest: the cells that form the sympathetic nervous system, called sympathogonia, migrate from the neural crest to the adrenal medulla, the paraganglion of Zuckerkandl, and a large number of paraganglia retroperitoneally along the aorta down into the pelvis. The pluripotential sympathogonia differentiate into ganglion, neurofibrous, and chromaffin cells, and tumors arising from these cells can be classified as neuroblastoma (sympathicoblastoma), ganglioneuroma, neurofibroma, and pheochromocytoma, respectively. Because of this development neuroblastoma has the potential ability to mature into ganglioneuroma, ganglioma and pheochromocytoma (1). Interacting with characteristic features of these neuroendocrine tumors, specific targeting of radiopharmaceuticals may be achieved via the metabolic route (MIBG), receptor binding (peptides), or the immunological route (antibodies).

Newly developed radiopharmaceuticals such as ^{131}I-metaiodobenzylguanidine (MIBG) and ^{111}In-pentetreotide (octreotide) are currently used for diagnostic scintigraphy of neuroblastoma (2). In addition to octreotide several other peptides are emerging for potential use in nuclear medicine (3), of which ^{123}I-labeled vasoactive intestinal peptide (VIP) is being explored in clinical medicine (4). By autoradiography somatostatin and VIP receptors have been demonstrated in neuroblastoma in 86% and 57% of cases, respectively (3).

In comparison to antibodies, peptides, typically consisting of 14 to 28 amino acids, are relatively small molecules targeting receptors at the cell membrane. MIBG is an even smaller molecule, which was formed by combining the benzyl group of bretylium and the guanidine group of guanethidine; it is concentrated intracellularly.

Unlike MIBG and antibodies directed against neuroblastoma, ^{111}In-pentetreotide is not specific for neural crest tumors, as scintigraphy is also positive in many other tumors, granulomas, and autoimmune diseases (5). Although the high uptake of ^{111}In-pentetreotide in the kidneys, liver, and spleen is less favorable for radionuclide therapy using beta emitters, attempts of radiolabeled peptide therapy using high doses of ^{111}In-pentetreotide or ^{90}Y-DOTA-lanreotide/octreotide are being made in patients with neuroendocrine tumors other than neuroblastoma, despite the unfavorable physical characteristics and biodistribution (6). Therefore, after a brief description of the disease, this chapter will review the current role of both MIBG therapy and radioimmunotherapy of neuroblastoma, as well as the new developments in these areas.

II. NEUROBLASTOMA—PRESENTATION AND CLINICAL MANAGEMENT

A. Presentation of Disease

Neuroblastoma occurs predominantly in children with a reported incidence in U.S. children of around five per million population per year. Fifty percent of neuroblastoma patients are <2 years old, 75% <4, and the disease is rare after the age of 14. The site of the primary tumor varies: 70% of all cases originate in the retroperitoneal region, including around 30% in the adrenal gland and 10% in the abdominal sympathetic side chain, and 8% occur in the cervical, 17% in the thoracic, and 5% in the pelvic sympathetic side chain (1). This is in contrast to the distribution of pheochromocytoma, of which extra-adrenal occurrence is reported in only 10% of adults and 25% of children with this tumor.

Metastases may present in two patterns: diffuse metastases in the liver (Pepper type), as are seen in the youngest patients with stage IVs disease and may be accompanied by subcutaneous metastatic nodules, and metastases to the regional lymph nodes, bone, bone marrow, and soft tissues (Hutchison type). Other organs, like brain, heart, and lungs, are rarely affected.

The symptomatology of this disease is variable and depends on the site and size of the primary tumor and its metastases and the excessive production and excretion of catecholamines.

More than 90% of neuroblastomas produce the catecholamines dopamine, norepinephrine, and epinephrine in excess; these products and their metabolites can be monitored in serum and urine. The degree of malignancy and the prognosis are correlated with the pattern and rate of excretion. Other tumor markers in serum are neuron-specific enolase (NSE), ferritin; and ganglioside G_{D2}; serum lactodehydrogenase (LDH) may also be elevated (7). The diagnosis of neuroblastoma is established by surgical pathology or tumor biopsy, using standard techniques of chromaffin staining and electron microscopy revealing the characteristic ultrastructure of the cells (neurotubules and neurosecretory granules). Alternatively the diagnosis may rely on bone marrow trephines showing unequivocal tumor cells in combination with increased levels of catecholamine metabolites (VMA/HVA) in urine.

B. Procedures for Staging and Follow-up

For the staging of disease the Evans criteria, TNM classification and, more recently, the International Neuroblastoma Staging System (INSS) apply.

For both staging and follow-up a number of diagnostic procedures are used. Plain x-rays of the thorax and abdomen may show the primary tumor by the finding of calcifications. Intravenous pyelography may show displacement of the kidney and ureter. Ultrasonography is a most informative, noninvasive, and inexpensive method to visualize pediatric tumors and to monitor the tumor size during treatment. Computerized tomography (CT) and magnetic resonance imaging (MRI) are more invasive techniques for young children, but provide better anatomical detail and information about the tumor's attachment to surrounding tissue. This is essential for the determination of resectability/operability. Myelography should be done, when intraspinal extension of the tumor is suspected. Bone scintigraphy, using ^{99m}Tc-diphosphonates, has always been the most sensitive technique to detect skeletal metastases, although in children discrete lesions near the epiphyses may be more difficult to interpret, and its findings lack the specificity of scintigraphy using radioiodinated metaiodobenzylguanidine (MIBG) (8). Occasionally also the primary tumor may be visualized on the bone scintigram. Total body scintigraphy using ^{123}I- or ^{131}I-MIBG is a very sensitive and highly specific noninvasive technique to demonstrate both the primary tumor and its metastases, regardless of their localization, in a single procedure (see below). Bone marrow aspiration, together with ^{131}I-MIBG scintigraphy, remains the most reliable proof of bone marrow infiltration, especially if multiple samples are taken by trephine and immunohistochemical staining techniques are applied (9).

C. Treatment

Prognostic factors in the treatment of neuroblastoma are stage of disease, patient's age, site of the primary tumor, pattern and rate of catecholamine excretion, serum ferritin and lactodehydrogenase (LDH) levels at diagnosis, tumor histology, and genetic parameters such as the amplification of the myc-N oncogene (10) and chromosome 1p36 deletion (11).

The choice of treatment for neuroblastoma depends on the stage of disease: localized disease without distant metastases (TNM stage I and II) is treated by complete surgical excision and has a good prognosis (2-year survival rates of 90%); lymph node metastases and spread to other organs (TNM stage III-V) is correlated with a poor prognosis and is treated by combination chemotherapy preceding surgery for the primary tumor. This is followed by postoperative chemotherapy, sometimes including high-dose chemotherapy requiring allogenic or autologous bone marrow transplantation. Radiation therapy may be added to these regimens. Despite a high initial response rate to the combination of these treatment modalities, most patients will have a recurrence of disease before or after completion of therapy, which is likely to reflect multiple drug resistance (MDR), and the 5-year survival remains only 10% to 20% (12). New therapeutic approaches include targeting of radionuclides via the immunological (monoclonal antibodies) and metabolic (MIBG) route.

III. TARGETED RADIOTHERAPY USING RADIOIODINATED META-IODOBENZYLGUANIDINE (MIBG)

A. Radiopharmaceutical and Targeting Mechanism

After studies in dogs at the University of Michigan had demonstrated a strong affinity of ^{131}I-meta-iodobenzylguanidine (^{131}I-MIBG) for the adrenal medulla (13), the agent has been successfully applied in humans for the localization of pheochromocytoma (14) and other tumors derived from the neural crest (15). These tumors characteristically present an active uptake-1 mechanism at the cell membrane and neurosecretory storage granules in the cytoplasm, responsible for the uptake and retention of ^{131}I-MIBG, respectively. Although the radiopharmaceutical may be released from the granules, reuptake through this specific mechanism maintains prolonged intracellular concentration, in contrast to nonadrenergic tissues which rely on passive diffusion only, resulting in high tumor/nontumor ratios. More recently, also ^{123}I-MIBG has been used for diagnostic scintigraphy of pheochromocytoma and neuroblastoma. Due to its relatively short physical half-life (13.2 hours) and the lack of beta particles, the radiation dose per MBq to the patient is lower than with [131]I. However, a higher dose of ^{123}I is administered. A clear advantage, however, is the greater photon flux at a photon energy peak of 159 keV, enabling images of superior quality as well as single-photon emission tomography.

Cumulative findings of ^{131}I-MIBG scintigraphy reported in the world literature, concerning 776 patients, indicate that 91.5% of neuroblastomas concentrate ^{131}I-MIBG (2), making ^{131}I-MIBG scintigraphy together with the urinalysis for catecholamine metabolites to be the most sensitive and specific indicators of neuroblastoma. This has the following implications for clinical management of the disease (16):

1. The uptake of ^{131}I-MIBG is so tissue-specific that in a child presenting with a tumor of unknown origin, ^{131}I-MIBG scintigraphy can noninvasively establish the diagnosis of neuroblastoma and rule out differential diagnoses such as Wilms' tumor, Ewing sarcoma, rhabdomyosarcoma, osteosarcoma, and malignant lymphoma.

2. The enhanced detection of metastases anywhere in the body in a single procedure influences the staging of disease, frequently by upgrading it.

3. The findings of postoperative or postchemotherapy ^{131}I-MIBG scintigraphy should be included in the criteria of response.

4. The good concentration and the relatively long biologic half-life of ^{131}I-MIBG at tumor sites in comparison to normal tissues enable therapy with this radiopharmaceutical; ^{131}I-MIBG tracer studies are used to identify patients who are likely to benefit from this form of treatment.

B. Therapeutic Procedure

The basis for successful treatment is a high and selective tumor uptake together with prolonged retention of MIBG. As a systemic treatment, ^{131}I-MIBG therapy will be directed at both the primary tumor and its distant metastases.

Contraindications for ^{131}I-MIBG therapy, as for other forms of radionuclide therapy, are severe myelosuppression and renal failure and, in adults, pregnancy or continued breast feeding. In addition, an unstable condition of the patient that does not allow isolation therapy is a relative contraindication.

In the workup of a patient for ^{131}I-MIBG therapy, the extent of disease must be determined and the parameters for monitoring the tumor response and side effects must be identified. Attention must be paid to the medication the patient is using, as many drugs are known or may be expected to interfere with the uptake and/or retention of ^{131}I-MIBG by the tumor cells (17). Harvesting of bone marrow prior to ^{131}I-MIBG therapy may be considered. To protect the thyroid from free ^{131}I-iodide, 100 mg potassium iodide is used orally daily (200 mg for adults).

An adequate infusion line must be in place, through which, in general, a fixed dose of 3.7 to 7.4 GBq (100 to 200 mCi) of ^{131}I-MIBG with a high specific activity (up to 1.48 GBq/mg) is administered over a 1- to 4-hour period using a lead-shielded infusion pump. An alternative approach is to administer a varying, calculated dose, as assessed by a prior tracer study, aiming for the maximal acceptable 2 Gy bone marrow dose (18). The treatment may be repeated at not less than 4-week intervals.

To prevent acute effects from excess catecholamines in circulation during or shortly after ^{131}I-MIBG infusion administration of dibenilene (alpha-blockade) and/or propanolol (beta blockade) may occasionally be indicated.

Patients need to be isolated according to local legislation, and encouraged to drink large volumes of fluid. Isolation may present practical difficulties when treating young children. Problems can be minimized by parents or other relatives becoming involved in their child's care. They need to be instructed in issues of radiation protection. Under these conditions participation of parents in patient care is both feasible and safe (19).

Before the administration of a therapeutic-dose quality control, checking both the radionuclide and radiochemical purity may be desirable, as impurities will not contribute to the tumor targeting but may add to the side effects of the treatment. High doses of ^{131}I-MIBG with a high specific activity undergo autoradiolysis, which is dependent on the temperature, volume, and presence of stabilizers in the formulation (20).

C. Clinical Results

1. ^{131}I-MIBG Therapy After Conventional Treatment

Since 1984 therapeutic doses of ^{131}I-MIBG have been administered to children failing conventional treatment with metastatic or recurrent neuroblastoma. After initial reports had indicated the feasibility and effectiveness of this treatment (15), several small series of patients treated in this way were reported (21–24). In a Phase II study, carried out in 53 such patients at the Netherlands Cancer Institute (25), the following response was observed: 7 complete and 23 partial remissions with a duration of 2 to 38 months; in 10 other patients progressive disease was arrested. Apart from objective response, the palliative effect of the treatment under these conditions was impressive, often leading to complete pain relief within days after treatment. The best results were obtained in patients with bulky soft-tissue disease (Fig. 1). Similar results of ^{131}I-MIBG treatment were recorded by Troncone et al. (26) and in a German multicenter study involving 47 patients with stage III or IV neuroblastoma (27); in the latter study nine children reached a complete or very good partial remission, and 13 a partial remission (47% objective response).

In 1991 pooled results of the major centers in a total of 273 neuroblastoma patients (predominantly children) indicated an overall objective response rate of 35%. Most of these patients had stage IV, progressive, and intensely pretreated disease, and were treated with ^{131}I-MIBG only after other treatment modalities had failed. In addition MIBG therapy provided valuable palliation and improved quality of life in most patients (28). For patients with recurrent and progressive disease after conventional treatment ^{131}I-MIBG therapy is probably the best palliative treatment, as the invasiveness and toxicity of this therapy compare favourably with that of chemotherapy, immunotherapy, and external-beam radiotherapy.

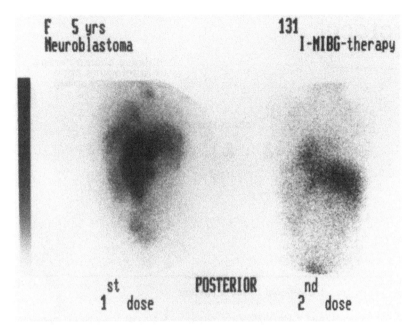

Figure 1 Posttherapy scintigrams (posterior view) of a 5-year-old girl with recurrent neuroblastoma after conventional therapy, presenting as a large abdominal mass (left). Four weeks following treatment using 3.7 GBq (100 mCi) ^{131}I-MIBG, only a small residual tumor in the left upper abdomen is shown (right).

2. ^{131}I-MIBG Therapy at Diagnosis

Based on the observed response to ^{131}I-MIBG therapy in advanced neuroblastoma after conventional therapy and the noninvasiveness of this therapeutic modality, ^{131}I-MIBG therapy was integrated in the treatment protocol instead of preoperative combination chemotherapy in children with advanced disease/inoperable neuroblastoma (29). The objective of introducing ^{131}I-MIBG therapy as the first therapy was to reduce the tumor volume, enabling adequate surgical resection and to avoid toxicity and the induction of early drug resistance. An additional advantage of this approach was that the child's general condition is unaffected or improved before undergoing surgery. Chemotherapy was reserved to treat minimal residual disease postoperatively (Fig. 2). Improvement in the overall outcome was attempted by integrating these three effective treatment modalities in a more optimal order.

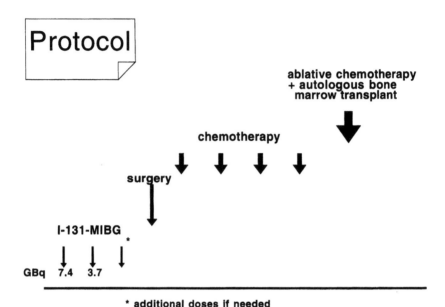

Figure 2   Protocol used since 1989 at the Netherlands Cancer Institute for inoperable (stage III/IV) neuroblastoma, introducing ^{131}I-MIBG therapy at diagnosis, followed by surgery and chemotherapy.

Initial results of preoperative ^{131}I-MIBG therapy in 31 children who presented with inoperable neuroblastoma demonstrated the feasibility and effectiveness of this approach (30). The objective response rate of ^{131}I-MIBG at diagnosis was better (>70%) than after conventional treatment, and 19 of 27 evaluable patients (70%) had complete or >95% resection of the primary tumor or did not require surgery at all (Fig. 3). Only 11 patients developed isolated thrombocytopenia and moderate myelosuppression occurred in only two cases, despite the fact that the bone marrow was invaded in 16 patients.

In 1996 the follow-up of these and eight additional patients was reported. By then, 21 patients had died, 12 within the first year; 6 patients died due to complications of surgery, chemotherapy, or autologous bone marrow transplant unrelated to ^{131}I-MIBG or the disease. Fifteen patients died due to recurrent or progressive disease, 13 of whom had unfavorable prognostic factors. The survival was 25/38 (66%) at 1 year, 16/31 (52%) at 2 years, 13/27 (48%) at 3 years; of 13 patients with >5 years follow-up, five survive (31). It was concluded that I-131 MIBG therapy at diagnosis to attain operability is at least as effective as combination chemotherapy but is associated with considerably less toxicity, and does not negatively affect the overall outcome.

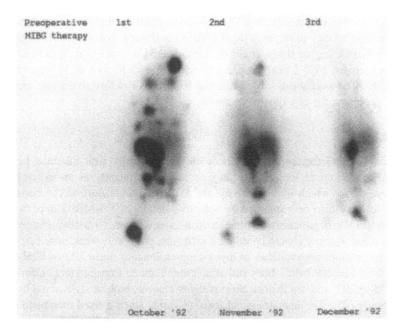

Figure 3 ^{131}I-MIBG therapy at diagnosis in a 14-month-old girl presenting with an inoperable neuroblastoma in the abdomen, metastatic to lymph nodes, bone, bone marrow, and lungs (stage IV). Total-body scintigraphy (posterior view) following three consecutive treatments at 4-week intervals demonstrate the excellent response of the metastases and the shrinkage of the primary tumor, enabling adequate surgical resection.

Mastrangelo et al. (32), treating three patients with ^{131}I-MIBG at diagnosis, demonstrated complete disappearance of the tumor in one patient, persisting for 4 years, and a significant reduction of tumor masses in the other two.

3. Therapy Using ^{125}I-MIBG

An alternative approach to the management of neuroblastoma is the use of ^{125}I-MIBG for therapy. This may have a role in the treatment of micrometastases and bone marrow infiltration, particularly as the results of ^{131}I-MIBG therapy under these circumstances are poor. Although the range of the ^{125}I Auger electrons in the storage vesicles would seem to be inadequate to deliver a lethal radiation dose to the nucleus, the finding of a considerable degree of extragranular storage in neuroblastoma (33) may provide a basis for this treatment. Preliminary experience in five patients with neuroblastoma (34,35) demonstrated tumor arrest and minor disease regression, but the efficacy of this treatment needs to be confirmed in a greater number of patients. In a Phase I dose-escalating study it was shown that, as the whole-body dose per MBq ^{125}I-MIBG is about four times lower than that of ^{131}I-MIBG, higher doses could be administered without causing serious toxicity, which led to >1-year progression-free survival in five of 10 treated patients (36). The availability of ^{125}I and the handling of radioactive waste are logistical problems for this type of treatment.

4. Toxicity

Both the ^{131}I-MIBG therapy and the isolation are generally well tolerated by children. Hematological side effects may occur, predominantly as an isolated thrombocytopenia, which may be partly due to the radiation dose to the bone marrow, but may also be explained by selective uptake of ^{131}I-MIBG into the thrombocytes (37). In patients with bone marrow involvement, ^{131}I-MIBG therapy following chemotherapy should be utilized with care, preferably when bone marrow salvage methods are available, as myelosuppression may occur. This is likely to reflect both a higher whole-body radiation burden due to impaired renal clearance of ^{131}I-MIBG, and diminished bone marrow reserve, both brought about by chemotherapy (25). The hematological toxicity varies when a fixed therapeutic dose is used, but may to some extent be predicted by tracer studies defining the dose of activity to be administered on the basis of body weight or surface (39) or maximal acceptable absorbed dose to the bone marrow (40).

Deterioration of renal function has occasionally been observed in patients whose kidneys have been compromised by intensive pretreatment with cisplatin and ifosfamide (38). Troncone et al. (26) describe a patient who had a hypertensive crisis shortly after ^{131}I-MIBG therapy requiring alpha-blocking medication.

The toxicity of ^{131}I-MIBG therapy at diagnosis is in contrast to the experience of ^{131}I-MIBG therapy after conventional therapy, as is described above. In addition, the general condition of these children improved considerably, as was demonstrated by a 10% to 15% increase in body weight during ^{131}I-MIBG treatment (30).

IV. TARGETED RADIOTHERAPY USING RADIOLABELED MONOCLONAL ANTIBODIES

A. Immunological Approaches to Neuroblastoma

Parallel to the introduction of radioiodinated MIBG in the early 1980s, several monoclonal antibodies have been developed to antigens present on the cell surface of a variety of tumors or, more specifically, neuroendocrine tumors or neural tissue. In the management of neuroblastoma monoclonal antibodies can be used in diagnosis for in vitro detection of antigen in serum and urine, for immunohistochemical staining of bone marrow aspirates and biopsies, for radioimmunoscinti-graphic localization of disease, as well as in therapy for the purging of bone marrow invaded by neuroblastoma prior to autologous bone marrow transplant (41), for immunotherapy, and for the specific targeting of radiation doses by radioimmunotherapy.

After biological characterization studies had demonstrated the selective binding of a monoclonal antibody UJ13A (of the IgG_1 subclass) to most tissues of neuroectodermal origin in 1983 (42), Goldman et al. (43) reported successful radioimmunoscintigraphic localization of primary tumors and metastases in eight patients with neuroblastoma, using 100 to 300 μg UJ13A labeled with 37–100 MBq (1 to 2.8 mCi) [123]I or [131]I. All six primary tumors and 10 of 12 meta-static sites were correctly identified, two of which had not been detected by other techniques; there were one false-positive and two false-negative findings. Al-though the uptake in the reticuloendothelial system varied, there was no brain uptake, as these antibodies generally do not cross the blood-brain barrier. Horne et al. (44) describe another case in which the primary tumor and a metastasis could not be detected by ^{123}I-UJ13A but was clearly shown by ^{123}I-MIBG scintig-raphy.

In 1985 Cheung et al. (45) developed a monoclonal antibody of the IgG_3 subclass against the oncofetal antigen ganglioside G_{D2}, which is present in high density on the cell surface of melanoma, neuroblastoma, and neural tissue. Unlike UJ13A, this 3F8 antibody does not react significantly with normal tissues other than the central nervous system. In vitro tests showed that the $3F8$-G_{D2} complex is stable and that the antigen does not undergo modulation by long incubation with 3F8. Initial results of radioimmunoscintigraphy using 111 to 185 MBq (3 to 5 mCi) [131]I-3F8 showed strong accumulation in tumor (T/NT ratios of 10:1 to 20:1) in five of six patients with neuroblastoma (46). When this series was expanded to 24 patients by 1989, an average percent administered dose of $0.082/cm^3$ tissue was reported for tumor, versus 0.021 for blood, 0.009 for kid-ney, 0.008 for liver, 0.006 for lung, and 0.002 for brain—i.e., favorable radiation dosimetry for therapeutic use. More lesions were detected by 3F8 imaging than by bone scintigraphy, plain x-ray, or CT scan (47). Both radioimmunoscintigra-phy and MRI were found to be very sensitive methods to detect bone marrow involvement, but 3F8 imaging is more specific (48).

Yeh et al. (49) compared the results of [131]I-3F8 with ^{131}I-MIBG, bone scin-tigraphy, CT scan, and MRI in 42 patients with neuroblastoma. On a patient basis there was good overall agreement (90%) between [131]I-3F8 and ^{131}I-MIBG of both scans being positive or negative, but the number of abnormal sites was greater for radioimmunoscintigraphy. Although the excellent sensitivity and specificity of [131]I-3F8 imaging was demonstrated, it should be noted that differences in the administered dose (2 mCi for [131]I-3F8 vs. 0.5 to 1 $mCi/1.7 \ m^2$ for ^{131}I-MIBG) and equipment used may have favored the immunoscintigraphic results.

In 1989 the use of a ^{99m}Tc-labeled monoclonal antibody for neuroblastoma, BW575/9, was reported (50), and in a comparative scintigraphic study using ^{99m}Tc-BW575/9 and ^{123}I-MIBG in seven neuroblastoma patients 21 of 26 lesions were detected by ^{123}I-MIBG versus 18 by ^{99m}Tc-BW575/9 (51).

More recently, a mouse/human chimeric antibody specific for a cell surface glycoprotein of human neuroblastoma, chCE7, was constructed which, in neuroblastoma-bearing nude mice, yielded high specific tumor uptakes up to 32% ID/g 1 day after administration, decreasing to 15% ID/g after 7 days (52). First results in eight patients (seven neuroblastoma, one paraganglioma) using 185 MBq (5 mCi) ^{123}I-chCE7 or 75 MBq (2 mCi) ^{131}I-chCE7 showed positive imaging of thoracic, abdominal, hepatic, and skeletal tumor sites with less contrast than by MIBG scintigraphy, but in one case revealed bone marrow infiltration not detected by MIBG imaging (53). Feine et al. (54), comparing ^{123}I-MIBG with ^{99m}Tc-ch14.18, a chimeric antisialoganglioside antibody, in 12 patients, demonstrated the complementary role of the two approaches in the detection of neuroblastoma: 11 studies were positive by both agents, four only by ^{123}I-MIBG, and three only by radioimmunoscintigraphy.

B. Therapeutic Studies in Animal Models

In experimental studies of radioimmunotherapy Jones (55) and Kemshead (56) reported the biodistribution and tumoricidal effects of ^{131}I-UJ13A in athymic nude mice bearing TR14 human neuroblastoma xenografts of about 1 cm^3. Following administration of 150 µCi of activity a 10% decrease in the tumor volume was observed, and although tumors disappeared after repeated administrations, they always recurred within 2 months. When similar doses of ^{125}I- and ^{123}I-labeled UJ13A were administered, no tumor response was observed. Etoh et al. (57) treated nude mice bearing human neuroblastoma xenografts of 15 mm diameter (2.3 g) with 300 µCi ^{131}I-CNM-5 antibody (2 mg). No decrease in volume but inhibition of growth was observed, in contrast to animals treated with equal amounts of CNM-5 or ^{131}I alone and untreated controls.

More impressive results were obtained by Cheung et al. (58), who treated athymic nude mice with 0.45 to 2 cm^3 human neuroblastoma xenografts with escalating doses of ^{131}I-3F8 antibody. Compared to controls, administered doses of 0.125 mCi of activity led to temporary growth delay only, 0.5 mCi led to a variable decrease in tumor volume, and animals treated with doses of 1 mCi showed the most pronounced tumor shrinkage. When these results were evaluated on the basis of delivered radioactivity per gram tumor, it was demonstrated that tumors receiving an absorbed radiation dose of >42 Gy were completely ablated and did not recur within 30 days, in contrast to tumors receiving <39 Gy. The total body burden for mice treated with 0.5 mCi varied between 110 and 380 cGy, which, apart from weight loss, was not associated with toxic effects; mice treated with 1 mCi ^{131}I-3F8 had bone marrow depression.

In a comparative study of external beam radiotherapy and escalating doses of ^{131}I-BW575/9 in SK-N-SH neuroblastoma in nude mice, Sautter-Bihl et al. (59) demonstrated a clear dose response relationship with complete tumor regression both after administration of 26 MBq antibody (absorbed radiation dose: 32 Gy) and 24 Gy by external beam.

C. Clinical Results

1. Therapy Using ^{131}I-UJ13A Monoclonal Antibodies

In 1987 the results of a Phase I study using therapeutic doses of ^{131}I-UJ13A in five patients with stage IV neuroblastoma who had relapsed or failed conventional therapy were reported (60). Administered doses of 1.3 to 2.0 GBq (35 to 55 mCi) resulted in one objective response, i.e., clearance of bone marrow involvement for 8 months, stabilization of disease for 5 months in one case, but no response in the other patients. The following side effects were encountered: mild pyrexia in all and nausea/vomiting in two patients, bone marrow aplasia in two patients treated at the highest dose level, and anaphylaxis in another patient despite a negative skin test. Apart from the toxicity, the problem of altered biodistribution of the antibody on second exposure was recognized. In an additional case, reported by Horne et al. (44), progression of disease followed therapy using an even higher dose (3.2 GBq/80 mCi).

Comparing the characteristics of MIBG and UJ13A for targeted radiotherapy, Lashford et al. (61) described the major limitations of UJ13A as the slower clearance from the blood leading to a higher whole-body radiation dose, the greater accumulation and retention in the liver, and the fact that both induction of human antimouse antibody response and alteration of the kinetics limit the usefulness of repeated application.

2. Therapy Using ^{131}I-3F8 Monoclonal Antibodies

Utilizing the mechanisms of specific neuroblastoma targeting, activation of human complement, and antibody-dependent cell-mediated cytotoxicity (ADCC), Cheung et al. (62) have used unlabeled murine 3F8 antibody in escalating doses of 5 to 100 mg/m^2 for immunotherapy of 17 patients, eight of whom had neuroblastoma. Complete remission was attained in two patients treated at the lowest dose levels; there was stabilization in two and progression of disease in four patients. The major side effects were severe pain, hypertension, urticaria, febrile reactions, and decrease of serum complement activity.

After a pilot study of radioimmunotherapy in three patients with bone marrow invaded by neuroblastoma receiving single doses of 3.7 GBq (100 mCi) and in whom [131]I-3F8 had shown severe myelotoxicity and subjective but no objective response (63), Cheung et al. (64) performed a Phase I study using escalating doses of [131]I-3F8 (resp. 6, 8, and 12 mCi/kg) in 10 patients with stage IV neuroblastoma. All required analgesics to control pain during infusion, four had diarrhea, all had pancytopenia, requiring autologous bone marrow transplant (ABMT) in eight patients. The following tumor response was recorded: one good partial remission, one partial remission, one mixed response, and stable disease for 1 to 11 months in 6 patients. Average tumor dose estimates of 20 to 36 rad/mCi with 0.36 to 2.2 rad/mCi to the bone marrow were reported. Larson et al. (65) demonstrated that PET using [124]I-3F8 may be an aid in selecting patients for radioimmunotherapy by a more accurate assessment of the absorbed tumor dose.

V. NEW DEVELOPMENTS/FUTURE DIRECTIONS

Several new applications of MIBG therapy are being investigated aiming to improve the therapeutic index. One is the use of other labels for MIBG, e.g., ^{125}I-MIBG and [211]At-MABG, which, due to their ultrashort pathway, may be of use in the treatment of minimal residual disease and bone marrow involvement, in which ^{131}I-MIBG is often myelotoxic. The tumor targeting may be enhanced by administration of ^{131}I-MIBG by alternative routes, e.g., the intra-arterial or intraperitoneal route.

Increasing the specific activity and the production of non-carrier-added MIBG attempted to improve tumor uptake. However, from animal studies and experience with MIBG therapy in humans it has been found that the optimal specific activity may vary with the tumor type. Excess of unlabeled MIBG was found to decrease ^{125}I-MIBG uptake in PC-12 pheochromocytoma xenografts in nude mice as well as in most normal tissues, but not to influence the uptake in SK-N-SH neuroblastoma (66).

The uptake and retention of ^{131}I-MIBG may also be increased by pharmacological interventions, such as the induction of tumor cell differentiation (e.g., by retinoic acid, interferon), the prolonging of retention (e.g., by calcium-channel blockers), the blockade of extratumoral specific uptake (e.g., by unlabeled MIBG, serotonin), or delaying its renal excretion. In carcinoid tumors not qualifying for ^{131}I-MIBG therapy because of insufficient tumor uptake, palliative treatment with high doses of unlabeled MIBG proved beneficial in 60% of cases and led to increased tumor/nontumor ratios in several patients (Fig. 4) (67). The enhancement of the antitumor effect by using the additive effects of other modalities, e.g., by combination of ^{131}I-MIBG therapy with oxygen under hyperbaric conditions, has been attempted (68). The response to ^{131}I-MIBG can be optimalized by introducing it early on in an integrated protocol of tumor therapy with curative intent, as described above.

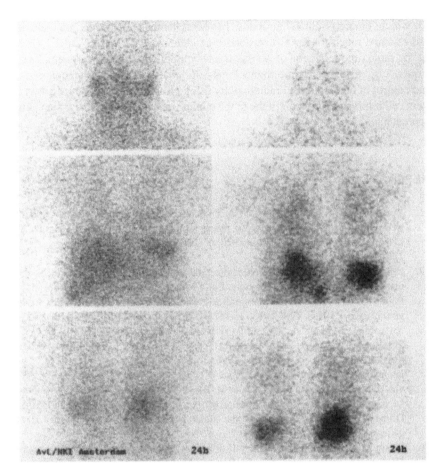

Figure 4 Diagnostic scintigrams 24 hours after 37 MBq (1 mCi) ^{131}I-MIBG in an adult patient with carcinoid metastatic to the liver. Due to minimal uptake in the liver metastases (left), the patient did not qualify for ^{131}I-MIBG therapy and subsequently received palliative treatment with a high dose of unlabeled MIBG. Repeated scintigraphy after "cold" MIBG reveals the increased tumor/nontumor ratio and the altered biodistribution, i.e., suppression of normal tissue uptake in salivary glands, heart, and normal liver (right).

New developments in radioimmunotherapy of neuroblastoma include the use of chimeric antibodies (69) to prevent antimouse Ig response limiting the effectiveness of repeated treatment that is often required; the enhancement of tumor uptake by modulation of antigen expression or by increasing the tumor perfusion/vascularity/permeability; and the use of other labels, such as copper-

67, which, bound to chCE7 antibody, has been demonstrated to be internalized and retained much longer in neuroblastoma cells than ^{125}I-labeled chCE7 (70). At the same time reduction of normal tissue activity by multistep targeting techniques, e.g., using bispecific monoclonal antibodies (71), or immunophoresis, and control of hematological radiotoxicity using growth factors, bone marrow, or stem cell reinfusion, will contribute to the clinical management of this therapeutic approach.

REFERENCES

1. Voûte PA, de Kraker J, Hoefnagel CA. Tumours of the sympathetic nervous system. Neuroblastoma, ganglioneuroma and phaeochromocytoma. In: Voûte PA, Barrett A, Lemerle J, eds. Cancer in Children: Clinical Management. Berlin: Springer, 1992: 226–243.
2. Hoefnagel CA. Metaiodobenzylguanidine and somatostatin in oncology: role in the management of neural crest tumours. Eur J Nucl Med 1994; 21:561–581.
3. Reubi JC. Neuropeptide receptors in health and disease: the molecular basis for in vivo imaging. J Nucl Med 1995; 36:1825–1835.
4. Virgolini I, Kurtaran A, Raderer M, Leimer M, Angelberger P, Havlik E, Li S, Scheithauer W, Niederle B, Valent P, Eichler H-G. Vasoactive intestinal peptide receptor scintigraphy. J Nucl Med 1995; 36:1732–1739.
5. Krenning EP, Kwekkeboom DJ, Bakker WH, Breeman WAP, Kooij PPM, Oei HY, van Hagen M, Postema PTE, de Jong M, Reubi JC, Visser TJ, Reijs AEM, Hofland LJ, Koper JW, Lamberts SWJ. Somatostatin receptor scintigraphy with [^{111}In-DTPA-D-Phe^{1}]- and [^{123}-Tyr^{3}]-octreotide: the Rotterdam experience with more than 1000 patients. Eur J Nucl Med 1993; 20:716–731.
6. Krenning EP, Kooij PPM, Bakker WH, Breeman WAP, Postema PTE, Kwekkeboom DJ, Oei HY, de Jong M, Visser TJ, Reijs AEM, Lamberts SWJ. Radiotherapy with a radiolabeled somatostatin analogue, [^{111}In-DTPA-D-Phe^{1}]-octreotide. A case history. Ann NY Acad Sci 1994; 733:496–506.
7. Ninane J, Vermylen C, Cornu G. Tumour markers for neuroblastoma. In: Sluyser M, Voûte PA, eds. Molecular Biology and Genetics of Childhood Cancer: Approaches to Neuroblastoma. Chicester: Ellis Horwood, 1988:13–25.
8. Shulkin BL, Wei Chen S, Sisson JC, Shapiro B. Iodine-131 MIBG scintigraphy of the extremities in metastatic pheochromocytoma and neuroblastoma. J Nucl Med 1987; 28:315–318.
9. Schoemaker JH, Hoefnagel CA, van der Schoot CE, van Leeuwen EF. Diagnosis of bone marrow involvement in neuroblastoma; the complementary role of 3 different methods. Med Pediatr Oncol 1992; 20:427.
10. Seeger RC, Brodeur GM, Sather H, Dalton A, Siegel SE, Wong KY, Hammond D. Association of multiple copies of the N-myc oncogene with rapid progression of neuroblastomas. N Engl J Med 1985; 313:1111–1116.
11. Caron H, van Sluis P, van Hoeve M, de Kraker J, Bras J, Slater R, Mannens M, Voûte

PA, Westerveld A, Versteeg R. Allelic loss of chromosome 1p36 in neuroblastoma is of preferential maternal origin and correlates with N-myc amplification. Nature Genet 1993; 4:187–190.

12. Pinkerton CR, Philip T, Biron P, Frapazz D, Phillipe N, Zucker JM, Bernard JL, Philip I, Kemshead J, Favrot M. High-dose melphalan, vincristine, and total body-irradiation with autologous bone marrow transplantation in children with relapsed neuroblastoma: a phase II study. Med Pediatr Oncol 1987; 15:236–240.

13. Wieland DM, Wu J-I, Brown LE, Mangner TJ, Swanson DP, Beierwaltes WH. Radiolabeled adrenergic neuron-blocking agents: adrenomedullary imaging with [^{131}I] iodobenzylguanidine. J Nucl Med 1980; 21:349–353.

14. Sisson JC, Frager MS, Valk TW, Gross MD, Swanson DP, Wieland DM, Tobes MC, Beierwaltes WH, Thompson NW. Scintigraphic localization of pheochromocytoma. N Engl J Med 1981; 305:12–17.

15. Hoefnagel CA, Voûte PA, de Kraker J, Marcuse HR. Radionuclide diagnosis and therapy of neural crest tumors using iodine-131 metaiodobenzylguanidine. J Nucl Med 1987; 28:308–314.

16. Hoefnagel CA, de Kraker J. Childhood neoplasia. In: Murray IPC, Ell PJ, eds. Nuclear Medicine in Clinical Diagnosis and Treatment. Edinburgh: Churchill Livingstone, 1994:765–777.

17. Solanki KK, Bomanji J, Moyes J, Mather SJ, Trainer PJ, Britton KE. A pharmacological guide to medicines which interfere with the biodistribution of radiolabelled meta-iodobenzylguanidine (MIBG). Nucl Med Commun 1992; 13:513–521.

18. Fielding SL, Flower MA, Ackery DM, Kemshead JT, Lashford LS, Lewis I. The dosimetry of ^{131}I mIBG for treatment of resistant neuroblastoma—results of a UK study. Eur J Nucl Med 1991; 18:308–316.

19. Hoefnagel CA, Lewington VJ. MIBG therapy. In: Murray IPC, Ell PJ, eds. Nuclear Medicine in Clinical Diagnosis and Treatment. Edinburgh: Churchill Livingstone, 1994:851–864.

20. Wafelman AR, Suchi R, Hoefnagel CA, Beijnen JH. Radiochemical purity of [^{131}I]MIBG infusion fluids; a report from the clinical practice. Eur J Nucl Med 1993; 20:614–616.

21. Bestagno M, Guerra P, Puricelli GP, Colombo L, Calculli G. Treatment of neuroblastoma with ^{131}I-metaiodobenzylguanidine: the experience of an Italian study group. Med Pediatr Oncol 1987; 15:203–205.

22. Hartmann O, Lumbroso J, Lemerle J, Schlumberger M, Ricard M, Aubert B, Coonaert S, Merline L, Olive D, De Lumley L, Parmentier C. Therapeutic use of ^{131}I-metaiodobenzylguanidine (MIBG) in neuroblastoma: a phase II study in nine patients. Med Pediatr Oncol 1987; 15:205–211.

23. Treuner J, Klingebiel T, Bruchelt G, Feine U, Niethammer D. Treatment of neuroblastoma with ^{131}I-metaiodobenzylguanidine: results and side effects. Med Pediatr Oncol 1987; 15:199–202.

24. Voûte PA, Hoefnagel CA, de Kraker J, Evans AE, Hayes A, Green A. Radionuclide therapy of neural crest tumors. Med Pediatr Oncol 1987; 15:192–195.

25. Hoefnagel CA, Voûte PA, de Kraker J, Valdés Olmos RA. [^{131}I]Metaiodobenzylguanidine therapy after conventional therapy for neuroblastoma. J Nucl Biol Med 1991; 35:202–206.

26. Troncone L, Rufini V, Montemaggi P, Danza FM, Lasorella A, Mastrangelo R. The diagnostic and therapeutic utility of radioiodinated metaiodobenzylguanidine (MIBG): 5 years experience. Eur J Nucl Med 1990; 16:325–335.
27. Klingebiel T, Berthold F, Treuner J, Schwabe D, Fischer M, Feine U, Maul FD, Waters W, Wehinger H, Niethammer D. Metaiodobenzylguanidine (mIBG) in treatment of 47 patients with neuroblastoma: results of the German neuroblastoma trial. Med Pediatr Oncol 1991; 19:84–88.
28. Troncone L, Galli G. Proceedings, International Workshop on the Role of [^{131}I]Metaiodobenzylguanidine in the Treatment of Neural Crest Tumors. J Nucl Biol Med 1991; 35:177–362.
29. Hoefnagel CA, de Kraker J, Voûte PA, Valdés Olmos RA. Preoperative [^{131}I]metaiodobenzylguanidine therapy of neuroblastoma at diagnosis ("MIBG de novo"). J Nucl Biol Med 1991; 35:248–251.
30. Hoefnagel CA, de Kraker J, Valdés Olmos RA, Voûte PA. ^{131}I-MIBG as a first-line treatment in high-risk neuroblastoma patients. Nucl Med Commun 1994; 15:712–717.
31. Hoefnagel CA, de Kraker J, Valdés Olmos RA, Caron H, Voûte PA. Survival of neuroblastoma after I-131 MIBG therapy at diagnosis. J Nucl Med 1996; 37:237P. Abstract.
32. Mastrangelo R, Lasorella A, Troncone L, Rufini V, Iavarone A, Riccardi R. [^{131}I]Metaiodobenzylguanidine in neuroblastoma patients at diagnosis. J Nucl Biol Med 1991; 35:252–254.
33. Smets L, Loesberg L, Janssen M, Metwally E, Huiskamp R. Active uptake and extravesicular storage of metaiodobenzylguanidine in human SK-N-SH cells. Cancer Res 1989; 49:2941–2944.
34. Sisson JC, Hutchinson RJ, Shapiro B, Zasadny KR, Normolle D, Wieland DM, Wahl RL, Singer DA, Malette SA, Mudgett EE. Iodine-125-MIBG to treat neuroblastoma: preliminary report. J Nucl Med 1990; 31:1479–1485.
35. Hoefnagel CA, Smets L, Voûte PA, de Kraker J. Iodine-125-MIBG therapy for neuroblastoma. J Nucl Med 1991; 31:361–362.
36. Sisson JC, Shapiro B, Hutchison RJ, Shulkin BL, Zempel S. Survival of patients with neuroblastoma treated with 125-I MIBG. Am J Clin Oncol 1996; 19:144–148.
37. Rutgers M, Tytgat GAM, Verwijs-Janssen M, Buitenhuis C, Voûte PA, Smets LA. Uptake of the neuron-blocking agent meta-iodobenzylguanidine and serotonin by human platelets and neuroadrenergic tumour cells. Int J Cancer 1993; 54:290–295.
38. Voûte PA, Hoefnagel CA, de Kraker J, Majoor M. Side effects of treatment with ^{131}I-meta-iodobenzylguanidine (^{131}I-MIBG) in neuroblastoma patients. In: Evans AE, ed. Advances in Neuroblastoma Research 2. New York: Alan R. Liss, 1988:679–687.
39. Sisson JC, Shapiro B, Hutchinson RJ, Carey JE, Zasadny KR, Zempel SA, Normolle DP. Predictors of toxicity in treating patients with neuroblastoma by radiolabeled metaiodobenzylguanidine. Eur J Nucl Med 1994; 21:46–52.
40. Lashford LS, Lewis IJ, Fielding SL, Flower MA, Meller S, Kemshead JT, Ackery D. Phase I/II study of iodine-131 metaiodobenzylguanidine in chemoresistant neuroblastoma: a United Kingdom Children's Cancer Study Group investigation. J Clin Oncol 1992; 10:1889–1896.

41. Saarinen UM, Coccia PF, Gerson SL, Pelley R, Cheung NKV. Eradication of neuro-blastoma cells in vitro by monoclonal antibody and human complement: method for purging autologous bone marrow. Cancer Res 1985; 45:5969–5975.

42. Allan PM, Garson JS, Harper EI, Asser U, Coakham HB, Brownell B, Kemshead JT. Biological characterisation and clinical application of a monoclonal antibody recognising an antigen restricted to neuroectodermal tissues. Int J Cancer 1983; 31: 591–598.

43. Goldman A, Vivian G, Gordon I, Pritchard J, Kemshead JT. Immunolocalization of neuroblastoma using radiolabeled monoclonal antibody UJ13A. J Pediatr 1984; 105: 252–256.

44. Horne T, Granowska M, Dicks-Mireaux C, Hawkins LA, Britton KE, Mather S, Bomanji J, Kemshead JT, Kingston J, Malpas JS. Neuroblastoma imaged with 123I-meta-iodo-benzylguanidine and with ^{123}I-labelled monoclonal antibody, UJ13A, against neural tissue. Br J Radiol 1985: 58:476–480.

45. Cheung NKV, Saarinen UM, Neely JE, Landmeier B, Donovan D, Coccia PF. Mono-clonal antibodies to a glycolipid antigen on human neuroblastoma cells. Cancer Res 1985; 45:2642–2649.

46. Miraldi FD, Nelson AD, Kraly C, Ellery S, Landmeier B, Coccia PF, Strandjord SE, Cheung NKV. Diagnostic imaging of human neuroblastoma with radiolabeled antibody. Radiology 1986; 161:413–418.

47. Miraldi F. Monoclonal antibodies and neuroblastoma. Semin Nucl Med 1989; 19: 282–294.

48. Fletcher BD, Miraldi FD, Cheung NKV. Comparison of radiolabeled monoclonal antibody and magnetic resonance imaging in the detection of metastatic neuro-blastoma in bone marrow. Pediatr Radiol 1989; 20:72–75.

49. Yeh SDJ, Larson SM, Burch L, Kushner BH, Laquaglia M, Finn R, Cheung NKV. Radioimmunodetection of neuroblastoma with iodine-131-3F8: correlation with bi-opsy, iodine-131-metaiodobenzylguanidine and standard diagnostic modalities. J Nucl Med 1991; 32:769–776.

50. Baum RP, Maul FD, Schwarz A, Hertel A, Bosslet K, Hör G. Diagnosis and treat-ment of stage IV neuroblastoma with Tc-99m- and I-131-labeled monoclonal anti-body BW 575/9. J Nucl Med 1989; 30:904.

51. Smolarz K, Waters W, Sieverts H, Linden A, Berthold F, Schicha H, Gladke E. Immu-noscintigraphy with Tc-99m-labeled monoclonal antibody BW 575 compared with I-123-MIBG scintigraphy in neuroblastoma. Radiology 1989; 173(p):152. Abstract.

52. Novak-Hofer I, Amstutz HP, Haldemann A, Blaser K, Morgenthaler J-J, Bläuenstein P, Schubiger PA. Radioimmunolocalization of neuroblastoma xenografts with chi-meric antibody chCE7. J Nucl Med 1992; 33:231–236.

53. Haldemann AR, Leibundgut K, Dörr U, Novak-Hofer I, Amstutz HP, Wagner HP, Bihl H, Roesler H. Radioimmunoscintigraphy with chimeric antibody chCE7: first clinical results. J Nucl Med 1994; 35:217P. Abstract.

54. Feine U, Reuland P, Geiger L, Handgretinger R, Haen B, Klingebiel T, Müller-Schauenburg W, Niethammer D. Tübinger experiences with an anti-sialoganglioside antibody for diagnosis and therapy of children suffering from neuroblastoma. Proc Int Meeting, Ten Years of Experience in Neuroblastoma. Quo Vadis MIBG? New Horizons, 1994, Westerland, Sylt, Germany.

55. Jones DH, Goldman A, Gordon I, Pritchard J, Gregory BJ, Kemshead JT. Therapeutic application of a radiolabeled monoclonal antibody in nude mice xenografted with human neuroblastoma: tumoricidal effects and biodistribution studies. Int J Cancer 1985; 35:715–720.

56. Kemshead JT, Jones DH, Lashford L, Pritchard J, Gordon I, Breatnach F, Coakham HB. 131-I coupled to monoclonal antibodies as therapeutic agents for neuroectodermally derived tumors: fact or fiction? Cancer Drug Del 1986; 3:25–43.

57. Etoh T, Takahashi H, Maie M, Ohnuma N, Tanabe M. Tumor imaging by antineuroblastoma monoclonal antibody and its application to treatment. Cancer 1988; 62: 1282–1286.

58. Cheung NKV, Landmeier B, Neely J, Nelson AD, Abramowsky C, Ellery S, Adams RB, Miraldi F. Complete tumor ablation with iodine-131-radiolabeled disialoganglioside GD2-specific monoclonal antibody against human neuroblastoma xenografted in nude mice. J Natl Cancer Inst 1986; 77:739–745.

59. Sautter-Bihl ML, Wessely R, Bihl H. Comparison of systemic radiotherapy with I-131-labeled monoclonal antibody BW575/9 to external beam radiotherapy in human neuroblastoma xenografts. Strahlenther Onkol 1993; 169:595–600.

60. Lashford L, Jones D, Pritchard J, Gordon I, Breatnach F, Kemshead JT. Therapeutic application of radiolabeled monoclonal antibody UJ13A in children with disseminated neuroblastoma. NCI Monogr 1987; 3:53–57.

61. Lashford LS, Clarke J, Kemshead JT. Systemic administration of radionuclides in neuroblastoma as planned radiotherapeutic intervention. Med Pediatr Oncol 1990; 18:30–36.

62. Cheung NKV, Lazarus H, Miraldi FD, Abramowsky CR, Kallick S, Saarinen UM, Spitzer T, Strandjord SE, Coccia PF, Berger NA. Ganglioside G_{D2} specific monoclonal antibody 3F8: a phase I study in patients with neuroblastoma and malignant melanoma. J Clin Oncol 1987; 5:1430–1440.

63. Cheung NKV, Miraldi FD. Iodine-131-labeled G_{D2} monoclonal antibody in the diagnosis and therapy of human neuroblastoma. In: Evans AE, ed. Advances in Neuroblastoma Research 2. New York: Alan R. Liss, 1988:595–604.

64. Cheung NKV, Yeh SDJ, Kushner BH, Burch L, Gulati S, Larson SM. Radioimmunotherapy using 131-I-3F8 in neuroblastoma (NB): a phase I clinical study. Med Pediatr Oncol 1990; 18:380. Abstract.

65. Larson SM, Pentlow KS, Volkow ND, Wolf AP, Finn RD, Lambrecht RM, Graham MC, Di Resta G, Bendriem B, Daghighian F, Yeh SDJ, Wang G-J, Cheung NKV. PET scanning of iodine-124-3F8 as an approach to tumor dosimetry during treatment planning for radioimmunotherapy in a child with neuroblastoma. J Nucl Med 1992; 33:2020–2023.

66. Rutgers M, Buitenhuis C, Smets LA. "Cold" MIBG pre-treatment: a way to improve the relative neuroblastoma over normal tissue exposure of ^{131}I-MIBG. Proc Int Meeting on Ten Years of Experience in Neuroblastoma. Quo Vadis MIBG? New Horizons, 1994, Westerland, Sylt, Germany.

67. Taal BG, Hoefnagel CA, Valdés Olmos RA, Boot H, Beijnen JH. Palliative effect of metaiodobenzylguanidine in metastatic carcinoid tumors. J Clin Oncol 1996; 14: 1829–1838.

68. Voûte PA, van der Kleij AJ, de Kraker J, Hoefnagel CA, Tiel–van Buul MMC, van

Gennip H. Clinical experience with radiation enhancement by hyperbaric oxygen in children with recurrent neuroblastoma stage IV. Eur J Cancer 1995; 31A:596–600.

69. Novak-Hofer I, Amstutz HP, Morgenthaler J-J, Schubiger PA. Internalization and degradation of monoclonal antibody chCE7 by human neuroblastoma cells. Int J Cancer 1994; 57:427–432.

70. Novak-Hofer I, Amstutz HP, Mäcke HR, Schwarzbach R, Zimmerman K, Morgenthaler J-J, Schubiger PA. Cellular processing of copper-67-labeled monoclonal antibody chCE7 by human neuroblastoma cells. Cancer Res 1995; 55:46–50.

71. Michon J, Perdereau B, Brixy F, Moutel S, Fridman WH, Teillaud JL. In vivo targeting of human neuroblastoma xenograft by anti-G_{D2}/anti-F_c gamma RI (CD64) bispecific antibody. Eur J Cancer 1995; 31A:631–636.

15
Targeted Radiotherapy of Squamous Head and Neck Cancer

Guus A. M. S. van Dongen, Frank B. van Gog, Ruud H. Brakenhoff, Jasper J. Quak, Remco de Bree, Gerard W. M. Visser, and Gordon B. Snow
Free University Hospital, Amsterdam, The Netherlands

I. INTRODUCTION

In this chapter the potential applications of radioimmunotherapy (RIT) for the treatment of head and neck squamous cell carcinoma (HNSCC) are outlined. A major aim in the management of head and neck cancer is the development of an effective adjuvant systemic therapy. About 30 monoclonal antibodies (Mabs) reactive with HNSCC are discussed with respect to their suitability for RIT. Only a few of these Mabs have been evaluated in animal models or in HNSCC in patients. Radioimmunoscintigraphy (RIS) and biodistribution studies in HNSCC xenograft-bearing nude mice and HNSCC patients have shown that the radiolabeled Mabs E48 and U36 might be capable of delivery of a tumoricidal dose to HNSCC in patients. On the basis of its physical properties ^{186}Re seems to be a promising radionuclide for treatment of minimal residual HNSCC. The suitability of ^{186}Re for adjuvant RIT is demonstrated in subcutaneous and metastatic tumor models in mice. Progress in the field of ^{186}Re labeling of Mabs for clinical application is described. Aforementioned attainments resulted in the design of clinical RIT studies with ^{186}Re-labeled Mabs in HNSCC patients. The use of RIT in combination with Mabs directed against the epidermal growth factor receptor is highlighted as one of the possibilities to enhance the efficacy of RIT.

II. NEED FOR EFFECTIVE ADJUVANT THERAPY

During 1995 approximately 39,500 Americans developed head and neck cancer and 12,460 died from it. Worldwide more than 500,000 new cases are projected annually, and the incidence is rising (1). Squamous cell carcinoma accounts for approximately 90% of all head and neck tumors. About one-third of patients present with early-stage (I and II) HNSCC, while two-thirds present with locoregional advanced disease (stages III and IV) (2). Although early-stage HNSCC can be cured with surgery or radiotherapy alone in the great majority of cases, the locoregional failure rate after surgery and/or radiotherapy in advanced stages is more than 50%. Moreover, about 25% of these patients develop distant metastases (3–6). Autopsy studies report on a much higher incidence, 40% to 57% (7–9). The lungs are the most frequent site of metastases (52% to 60%), followed by the skeletal system (19% to 35%). Other localizations of metastatic deposits are the liver, mediastinum, skin, and brain (4,6). It has been shown that the incidence in both local recurrences and distant metastases is directly related to the number of tumor-positive lymph nodes in the neck (3,4,10,11). For example, when four or more lymph nodes contained tumor, the risk of developing distant metastases was found to be almost 50% (6).

These data illustrate that the development of an effective systemic therapy is needed that reduces the occurrence of metastatic disease and improves the effectiveness of local therapies in obtaining locoregional control. Chemotherapy has been used in advanced head and neck cancer as induction therapy, in combination with radiation therapy, and as salvage therapy for the treatment of either locally recurrent or metastatic disease (12). The overall response rate with methotrexate, 5-fluorouracil, bleomycin, cisplatin, and carboplatin as single agents is 15% to 30%, but unfortunately these responses are partial, brief in duration, and have no effect on overall survival (12). Cisplatin followed by 5-fluorouracil infusion is the most active combination chemotherapy: responses of up to 70% with complete response rates of 20% to 27% have been reported in patients with recurrent disease, but an overall survival benefit has only been noted for those who achieve a complete response (13). Also several strategies of immunotherapy have been tried in head and neck cancer patients. Although responses have been observed as with interleukin-2, complete responses occurred infrequently, and the effects were not long-lasting (14,15). This limited efficacy may be explained by the deficiencies in cellular and humoral immune functions as has frequently been described in HNSCC patients. In these patients the degree of immunodeficiency is variable and immune function depression has been demonstrated to be hierarchical, more at the local level than on the regional level and lowest on the systemic level (16).

Just recently the use of Mabs has been considered as an alternative approach for the treatment of HNSCC patients. Especially the use of radiolabeled Mabs may be suitable for the treatment of HNSCC due to the intrinsic radiosensitivity of this tumor type (17). At this moment there are two major aims for the application of RIT in head and neck oncology. In one approach RIT is aimed to be developed to an effective adjuvant systemic therapy for the treatment of patients at high risk for developing locoregional recurrences and distant metastases (18,19). Roughly 30% of the HNSCC patients would benefit from the availability of an effective adjuvant RIT. In another approach RIT is aimed to be used in combination with external-beam irradiation to obtain locoregional control. Researchers active in this latter field are doubtful whether it will become possible to deliver a tumoricidal dose by RIT alone (20,21). They envision that when it becomes possible to achieve a 10% to 20% increase of the currently applied dose by use of combined modality radiotherapy, a significant number of patients who fail treatment due to lymph node micrometastases and/or postsurgical microscopic local tumor remnants may be cured (22). In this chapter the progress in RIT of head and neck cancer will be summarized and its feasibility will be discussed.

III. MABS FOR TARGETED RADIOTHERAPY

While in the last decade Mabs have been administered to thousands of patients with various types of tumors for both diagnostic and therapeutic purposes, the application of Mabs in head and neck oncology has not kept pace. Two of the main reasons for this slow progress have been the lack of Mabs with a high specificity for HNSCC and a restricted reaction pattern on normal tissues.

For effective RIT all tumor deposits, including tumor nodules, malignant cell clusters, and single tumor cells need to be adequately targeted. In our view a Mab should fulfil a number of criteria before clinical evaluation is considered. It is ideal that the Mab recognizes an antigen exclusively expressed in tumor tissue, but not in any normal tissue. However, this is not a strict criterion since the accessibility of the antigen can also make a Mab "operationally" selective. For example, the endothelium of skin and oral mucosa is poorly permeable for molecules with high molecular weight, while the fenestrated endothelium of HNSCC tumors is much more permeable. Moreover, these tumors frequently have a defective basement membrane thus enhancing their permeability. Thus, squamous-associated antigens which are expressed in normal squamous epithelia as well as in HNSCC can be suitable targets for Mab therapy (see later in this chapter).

So far, at least 30 Mabs directed against HNSCC have been described in literature (Table 1) (20,23–47). Some of these Mabs are reactive with squamous cell carcinoma only. Other Mabs recognize several types of tumor, the so-called pancarcinoma Mabs. Many of the Mabs and the antigens recognized by the Mabs are poorly characterized with respect to their tissue specificity. For these Mabs it is difficult to speculate about their suitability for RIT. Almost all of the more

Table 1 Monoclonal Antibodies Directed Against Squamous Cell Carcinoma

Mab	Ref.	Antigen	Specificity	Limitations
1g6	23	Unknown	Unknown	Poorly characterized
LAM-2	24	45, 125 kDa	Pancarcinoma	Poorly characterized, IgM
A1 16	25	Unknown	Unknown	Poorly characterized
LuCa2	26	Unknown	Pancarcinoma	Poorly characterized, reactive with various normal tissues including thyroid, kidney, colon, and other epithelia
SQM1	27	48 kDa	Pancarcinoma	IgM; reactive with normal blood vessels
KM-32, KM-34	28	Unknown	Unknown	Poorly characterized
PF1/A to PF1/E	29	38, 80, 180 kDa	Squamous	Poorly characterized; reactive with normal epidermis; heterogeneous reactivity with HNSCC
A9	30	Integrin $\alpha^6\beta_4$	Pancarcinoma	Reactive with normal blood vessels and basal cells of squamous epithelia in association with the basement membrane
17.13	31	Unknown	Squamous	IgM; reactive with basal cells of normal squamous epithelia; cytoplasmic antigen
B10	32	Various keratins	Pancarcinoma	IgM; reactive with various normal tissues; cytoplasmic antigen
1H5	32	Various keratins	Pancarcinoma	IgM; heterogeneous reactivity with HNSCC; preferentially reactive with well-differentiated HNSCC; reactive with various normal tissues; cytoplasmic antigen
425	33	170 kDa, EGFR	Pancarcinoma	Reactive with various normal tissues
3F8E3	34	71, 124 kDa	Squamous	Poorly characterized; reactive with basal cells of normal squamous epithelia; low affinity
174H.64	35	48 and 57 kDa	Squamous	Reactive with basal cells of normal squamous epithelia; cytoplasmic antigen

E48	36	16–20 kDa	Squamous	Reactive with basal and suprabasal cells of normal squamous epithelia
K931	37	40 kDa, Ep-CAM	Pancarcinoma	Heterogeneous antigen expression
INS-2	38	40 kDa	Squamous	IgM; reactive with normal squamous epithelia; cytoplasmic antigen
1/A to 1/E	39	Unknown	Squamous	Poorly characterized; reactive with normal squamous epithelia
3H-1	40	55 kDa	Pancarcinoma	Poorly characterized; IgM; heterogeneous and cytoplasmic antigen expression in a proportion of HNSCC
225	41	170 kDa, EGFR	Pancarcinoma	Reactive with various normal tissues
K984	42	125 kDa	Pancarcinoma	Reactive with basal cells of normal squamous epithelia and various other normal tissues
K928	42	50–55 kDa	Pancarcinoma	Reactive with suprabasal cells of normal squamous epithelia and various other normal tissues
175F4, 175F11	43	45–50 kDa	Pancarcinoma	Reactive with normal squamous epithelia
CAK1	44	40 kDa	Pancarcinoma	Reactive with normal mesothelium and basal epithelium of trachea; heterogeneous antigen expression
U36	45	200 kDa, epican	Squamous	Reactive with basal and suprabasal cells of normal squamous epithelia; soluble antigen present in blood
BM2	46	52 kDa	Squamous	IgM; reactive with basal cells of normal squamous epithelia
HMFG1	20	>400 kDa, polymorphic epithelial mucin	Pancarcinoma	Heterogeneous antigen expression
VFF18	47	200 kDa, epican	Squamous	Reactive with basal and suprabasal cells of normal squamous epithelia; soluble antigen present in blood

extensively described Mabs have drawbacks for tumor targeting in patients, as indicated in Table 1. Therefore, most Mabs have been used for immunohisto-chemistry only.

IV. CLINICAL RADIOIMMUNOSCINTIGRAPHY AND BIODISTRIBUTION STUDIES

Because of the drawbacks indicated in Table 1, only a few Mabs have been administered to HNSCC patients (Table 2) (20,41,48–63). Among these are the pancarcinoma Mabs K984 and K928 as well as anti-CEA Mabs and anti-Ep-CAM Mab 323/A3, which in clinical RIS studies showed extensive accumulation at nontumor sites, thus hampering their applicability for RIT (20,48–51,61). The same seems also to be true for Mabs directed against the epidermal growth factor receptor (EGFR) like Mabs 225, RG 83852, and 425 (41,52–54). An interesting aspect of the latter Mabs, however, is their capacity to inhibit the growth of squamous tumor cells in vitro and in vivo (64–66). The Mabs are able to block

Table 2 Monoclonal Antibodies Used for Targeting of Squamous Cell Carcinoma in Patients[a]

Antibody	No of patients	Ref.
Anti-CEA	5	48
	13	49
	29	50
	7	51
Anti-EGFR	11	52
Mab 225/anti-EGFR	19	41
Mab RG 83852/anti-EGFR	10	53
Mab 425/anti-EGFR	12	54
Mab 174H.64	21	55–57
	11	58
Mab E48	21	59, 60
Mab SF-25	1	61
Mab 323/A3/anti-Ep-CAM	3	61
Mab K928	6	61
Mab HMFG1/anti-MUC-1	29	20
Mab U36/anti-CD44v6	20	62, 63

[a] All studies were performed with head and neck cancer patients (except the study with Mab 225 in which patients with lung cancer were imaged) and included radioimmunoscintigraphy (except the study with Mab 425).

the binding of EGF and TGF-α without stimulating tyrosine kinase activity. Despite the crossreactivity with normal tissues, anti-EGFR Mabs are well tolerated by patients. Patients with non-small-cell lung cancer were shown to tolerate a dose of 600 mg/m^2 cold Mab RG 83852, while patients with head and neck cancer tolerated 400 mg cold Mab 425, resulting in EGFR saturation in both studies (53,54). The possibility to incorporate anti-EGFR Mabs in RIT strategies in head and neck cancer patients will be outlined later in this chapter.

With respect to tumor selectivity, Mabs directed against squamous-associated antigens such as Mabs 174H.64, E48, and U36 may have a better potential for RIT (55–60,62,63,67). Preoperative RIS with ^{99m}Tc-labeled MAb 174H.64 in 21 HNSCC patients revealed visualization of all 18 primary tumors, while 15 out of 18 locoregional lymph node metastases and two out of three distant metastases were identified (55). No Mab accumulation at nontumor sites was found. Unfortunately, no tissue uptake levels of the Mab were determined. Mab 174H.64 recognizes a 57,000-Da cytoskeletal protein, most probably a cytokeratin. The internal localization of the 174H.64 antigen may be a serious problem for adjuvant RIT (35).

The most extensively studied Mab for targeting head and neck cancer is Mab E48. Mab E48 recognizes a 16- to 20-kDa glycosylphosphatidylinositol (GPI)-anchored membrane bound surface antigen located on desmosomes and along the cell membrane and apparently involved in cell-cell adhesion (68,69). The capacity of ^{99m}Tc-, ^{131}I-, and ^{125}I-labeled Mab E48 IgG and F(ab')$_2$ to target primary HNSCC and lymph node metastases in the neck was evaluated in RIS/biodistribution studies in 32 patients who underwent neck dissection (59,60). The studies with Mab E48 had four objectives of importance for ranking its suitability for RIT: (a) to assess the sensitivity and specificity for tumor detection by RIS; (b) to assess the uptake levels of the Mab in primary tumors, lymph node metastases, and normal tissues; (c) to compare the imaging/biodistribution results obtained with E48 IgG with those obtained with E48 F(ab')$_2$; and (d) to assess the spatial distribution of the Mab throughout primary tumors and lymph node metastases. For this purpose, preoperative findings on the status of the lymph nodes in the neck obtained by RIS and assessed per level and per side were compared with CT, MRI, palpation, and the histopathological outcome of the neck dissection specimens. From surgical specimens obtained 2 to 7 days after simultaneous injection of ^{99m}Tc-labeled E48 IgG, ^{131}I-labeled E48 IgG, or ^{125}I-labeled E48 F(ab')$_2$, biopsies were taken to obtain quantitative data on Mab accumulation in the tumor. Cryosections of these tumors were made to assess the spatial distribution of the injected Mab throughout the tumor by use of immunohistochemistry.

In 32 HNSCC patients imaged with either radiolabeled E48 IgG or E48 F(ab')$_2$, all 31 tumors at the primary site were visualized. RIS was correct in 201 of 221 levels (accuracy 91%) and in 38 of 47 sides (accuracy 81%) (59). Sensitivity and specificity of RIS were similar to those of palpation, CT, and MRI. The diagnostic value of RIS with E48 IgG or E48 F(ab')$_2$ appeared to be similar. Tumors not detected by RIS appeared to be small positive lymph nodes (<1 cm diameter), containing a large proportion of necrosis, keratin, or fibrin.

Tumor uptake of ^{131}I-labeled E48 IgG 2 days after injection ranged from 7.2% to 82.3% of the injected dose per kilogram (ID/kg), with a mean of 27.8 ± 18.5% ID/kg (Table 3). This uptake level was higher than in normal tissues, as indicated by the tumor/nontumor ratio of 2.8 for mucosa, 4.6 for bone marrow aspirate, 4.1 for blood, 20.3 for fat, and 21.0 for muscle. Activity uptake in tumor-positive nodes was 4.7 times higher than in negative lymph nodes. Tumor uptake levels were on average 49% higher for IgG than for coadministered F(ab')$_2$, while tumor/nontumor ratios were in general just slightly lower for IgG.

For tumor biopsies taken 7 days after injection E48 IgG uptake levels were 8.9 ± 8.9% ID/kg. Tumor/nontumor ratios for oral mucosa, muscle, blood, and bone marrow aspirate were at that time point 2.5, 25.2, 4.7 and 4.0, respectively. Tumor uptake of E48 IgG is high when compared to other Mabs in other tumor types (Table 3).

The distribution of Mab E48 throughout the tumors was heterogeneous when administered at a dose of 2 to 12 mg, and homogeneous when administered at a dose of 52 mg (63). Moreover, from this immunohistochemical analysis it appeared that Mab E48 had targeted all tumor deposits including the small deposits which were not detected by RIS. One of the main conclusions from these

Table 3 Tumor Uptake Levels of Monoclonal Antibodies in Patients

Disease	Mab	Days postinjection	% ID/kg	Ref.
Head and neck	E48	2	27.8	61
Head and neck	E48	7	8.9	63
Head and neck	U36	2	20.4	62
Head and neck	U36	7	8.2	63
Head and neck	HMFG1	1–3	5.0	20
Colon	B72.3	4–14	7.5	70
Colon	BW 431	4–14	7.7	71
Colon	F19	7	16.5	72
Colon	16.88	8–9	0.2	73
Ovary	OC125	2	3.1	74
Ovary	MOv18	2	8.7	75
Ovary	CTMO1	6	9.1	76
Intracranial	81C6	1–3	1.6	77
Renal	G250	8	14.0	78
Non-Hodgkin lymphoma	OKB7	3–5	1.8	79

studies is that Mab E48, when administered to HNSCC patients, is able to accumulate selectively and to a high level in all antigen-positive tumors.

A limitation of Mab E48 is the heterogenicity of the E48 antigen expression in 30% of HNSCC tumors (61). As a consequence, not all HNSCC patients will be eligible for RIT with Mab E48. For this reason our group recently developed a new Mab, designated U36. Mab U36 recognizes the v6 region of the 200-kDa squamous-specific CD44 splice variant epican (80). Expression of CD44v6 in HNSCC was found to be abundant and homogeneous in 96% of all primary HNSCC

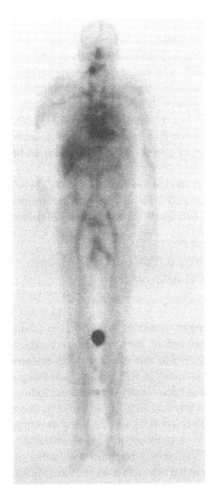

Figure 1   Anterior whole-body image of a patient with a carcinoma of the right alveolar processus 16 h after injection of ^{99m}Tc-labeled U36 IgG. Note the clear visualization of the primary tumor (From Ref. 62.)

and HNSCC lymph node metastases (61). A matter of debate regarding the suitability of anti-CD44v6 Mabs for tumor targeting is their crossreactivity with in vitro activated T-lymphocytes (81), and the presence of soluble antigen in the blood (82). In our immunohistochemical analyses with Mab U36, however, we did not find reactivity with lymphoid organs (45). Furthermore, upon administration of 2 mg Mab U36 to patients, < 10% of the Mab formed a high-molecular-weight complex. CD44v6 expression has also been described for several other tumor types like colon, breast, lung, cervix, and bladder carcinoma as well as for non-Hogdkin's lymphoma. For these tumor types the expression of CD44v6 splice variants is sometimes low and heterogeneous (45,80).

Until now Mab U36 IgG has been administered to 20 HNSCC patients and evaluated in the same way as described for Mab E48 (62,63). From these studies it appeared that E48 IgG and U36 IgG are equally well suited for targeting antigen-positive HNSCC tumors. The capacity of MAb U36 for selective tumor targeting is illustrated by the whole-body image in Figure 1. Tumor biopsies taken 2 days after injection showed a mean uptake of $20.4 \pm 12.4\%$ ID/kg (Table 3), while tumor/nontumor ratios were similar to those for E48 IgG. Because of its more homogeneous reactivity pattern on sections of HNSCC, Mab U36 seems to be better qualified for RIT than Mab E48.

Most recently, the characteristics of a second Mab directed against CD44v6 have been described (47). This Mab, designated VFF18, has a higher affinity than Mab U36, and is currently evaluated in RIS/biodistribution studies in HNSCC patients.

V. RADIOIMMUNOCONJUGATES FOR ADJUVANT SYSTEMIC THERAPY

Knowing that the Mabs for selective targeting of HNSCC are available, and taking into account the advantages of RIT as outlined before, the next question is which radionuclide should be coupled to the Mab. Up to this moment the β-emitters ^{131}I and ^{90}Y are the most widely used radionuclides in RIT studies. Advantages and disadvantages of these radionuclides have been clearly documented. Iodine-131 is easy to label and has an appropriate physical half-life (8 days), particle energy (β; E_{max}, = 0.6 MeV), and path length (r_{90} = 0.83 mm, r_{90} being the range in which 90% of the energy is released) (83). A problem of ^{131}I is the instability of the radioimmunoconjugate at the tumor site, as will be illustrated further on in this chapter. This problem may be solved in the near future by the introduction of new labeling techniques as are outline in Chapter 5 of this book (84). A problem that cannot be solved is the γ-emission, which represents 65% of the released energy and poses hazard to the patient and the medical personnel. ^{90}Y has a high particle energy (β; E_{max}, 2.2 MeV) and comparable long path length (r_{90} = 5.34

mm), which may be an advantage when RIT is used in combination with external-beam irradiation for the treatment of large HNSCC tumors, but not for treatment of minimal residual disease as aimed for by our group. For binding of ^{90}Y to an antibody the chelate DTPA has been used for a long time. The antibody-chelate conjugate appeared instable, resulting in sequestering of ^{90}Y in nontarget organs like spleen, liver, and especially bone marrow (85). This resulted in dose-limiting myelotoxicity (86). Strategies to overcome this problem include the use of better chelators like DOTA, as is outlined in Chapter 4 this book (87).

Wessels and Rogus (88) have suggested that ^{186}Re would be an excellent radionuclide for adjuvant RIT. With its half-life of 3.7 days, its 9% γ-emission

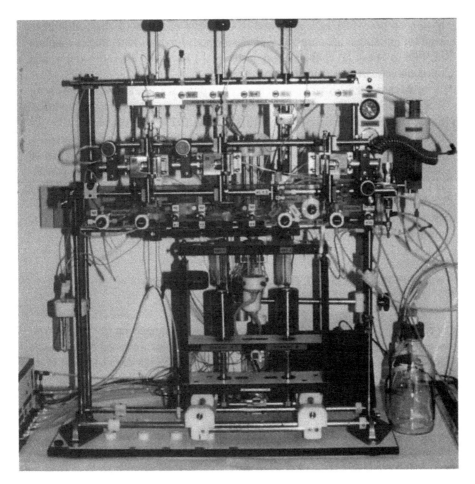

Figure 2 Unshielded semiautomated device for labeling of Mabs with up to 1 Ci ^{186}Re.

which has an ideal energy (137 KeV) for imaging, and its 71% β-emission of 1.07 MeV and 21% β-emission of 0.94 MeV, theoretically ^{186}Re seems to be better suited for adjuvant RIT than ^{131}I and ^{90}Y. The physical properties of ^{99m}Tc and ^{186}Re seem to be ideal for RIS and RIT, respectively, and the chemical properties of ^{99m}Tc and ^{186}Re are considered to be similar. This gives the opportunity to use ^{99m}Tc imaging to identify ^{186}Re candidates. However, for this we also consider the use of zirconium-89-labeled Mabs in PET imaging a realistic option. At our university methods have been developed for the production of ^{89}Zr and its coupling to Mabs (89,90). Such conjugates will be evaluated for their value in tumor diagnosis and dosimetry in head and neck cancer patients shortly (see Chapter 3 of this book).

Recently, several methods for direct and indirect coupling of ^{186}Re to Mabs have been described, as is reviewed in Chapter 4 of this book. Basically, three kinds of limitations are observed with the methods for direct and indirect coupling of ^{186}Re to Mabs: (a) conjugates are instable; (b) Re:Mab ratios are too low; and (c) conjugates accumulate at nontumor sites.

Because of the limitations of these procedures we developed suitable chemical protocols for the coupling of ^{186}Re to Mabs by introducing some modifications to the procedure described by Fritzberg et al. (91,92). Moreover, we adjusted these protocols for high-dose ^{186}Re coupling (up to 1 Ci) for clinical purposes, and developed a "kit" procedure for the coupling of ^{186}Re to Mabs that can be used at any medical center (93,94). To minimize radiation exposure of the personnel caused by the handling of such high activities, a semiautomated labeling device has been developed (Fig. 2). With respect to clinical application it should be noted that the availability of ^{186}Re with sufficiently high specific activity is not a problem any longer.

VI. EFFICACY OF RIT IN SUBCUTANEOUS AND METASTATIC TUMOR MODELS

What about the efficacy of ^{186}Re-Mab conjugates in comparison to ^{131}I-Mab conjugates? In previous studies in HNSCC-bearing nude mice we found evidence that RIT with ^{186}Re-labeled Mabs is more effective than RIT with ^{131}I-labeled Mabs (95,96). This observation was confirmed by animal experiments in which the therapeutic efficacies of equal (suboptimal) doses of ^{186}Re-Mab U36 and ^{131}I-Mab U36 were directly compared. As shown in Figure 3A, ^{186}Re-Mab U36 caused a much longer growth delay than ^{131}I-Mab U36. These results are promising in view of the fact that patients seem to tolerate a higher dose of ^{186}Re-labeled IgG than ^{131}I-labeled IgG (97).

The different efficacy of ^{186}Re-Mab U36 and ^{131}I-Mab U36 can be at least partly explained by the difference in biodistribution of these conjugates. While

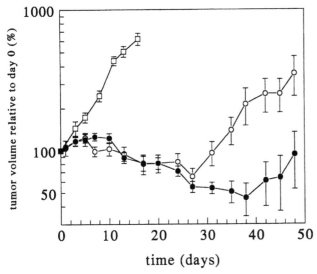

(A)

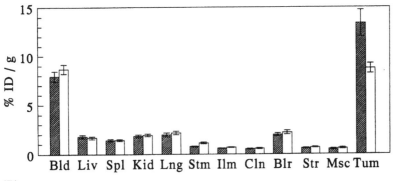

(B)

Figure 3 Comparison of the antitumor effect and the biodistribution of [186]Re-labeled Mab U36 IgG and ^{131}I-labeled Mab U36 IgG in nude mice bearing HNX-OE xenografts. (A) Tumor growth in (-□-) control group injected with saline; (-●-), group injected with 400 μCi [186]Rc-labeled Mab U36; and (○), group injected with 400 μCi ^{131}I-labeled Mab U36. (B) Biodistribution of tracer doses coadministered [186]Re-labeled Mab U36 IgG (hatched bars) and ^{131}I-labeled Mab U36 IgG (open bars), 3 days after injection (n = 6). Bld = blood; Liv = liver; Spl = spleen; Kid = kidney; Lng = lung; Stm = stomach; Ilm = ileum; Cln = colon; Blr = bladder; Str = sternum; Msc = muscle; Tum = tumor. Note the lower levels of ^{131}I in comparison to [186]Re in the tumor.

^{186}Re and ^{131}I levels were found to be similar in normal tissues, a much higher level of ^{186}Re in comparison to ^{131}I was found in the tumor as illustrated by Figure 3B at 3 days after injection. This latter phenomenon may be due to dehalogenation of ^{131}I-labeled Mab U36.

What about the therapeutic efficacy of ^{186}Re-Mab conjugates at increasing radioactivity dose? We evaluated the therapeutic efficacy of RIT with ^{186}Re-labeled Mab E48 preclinically in HNSCC-bearing nude mice. When mice with xenografts of 75 mm^3 were treated at the MTD with a single injection of 600 µCi ^{186}Re-labeled E48 IgG, 100% complete remissions were observed (98). In the same animal model, RIT was shown to be more effective than the clinically used and experimental chemotherapeutic agents doxorubicin, 5-fluorouracil, cisplatin, bleomycin, methotrexate, or 2'2'-difluorodeoxycytidine. No cures were observed with any of these chemotherapeutic agents (95).

Curative treatment can be more difficult in an adjuvant setting when smaller and larger tumor nodules also have to be eradicated. That eradication of larger tumors is a problem was demonstrated in the same animal model as described before. When mice bearing HNSCC of 140 mm^3 (instead of 75 mm^3) were treated with 600 µCi ^{186}Re-labeled E48, only 33% of the tumors demonstrated complete remission (96). This lower efficacy could be explained by the decreased Mab uptake in the larger tumors as compared to the smaller tumors.

Also eradication of very small tumors (<1 mm) is expected to be difficult since in that case a significant portion of the dose delivered by ^{186}Re will be lost outside the tumor (99–102). Whether the decreased energy absorption in such small tumors is compensated by the higher tumor uptake of Mabs in the in vivo situation needed further investigation. To this end, we assessed the efficacy of ^{186}Re-Mab E48 in an in vivo metastatic model. Due to the lack of a suitable metastatic model for HNSCC we used the melanoma cell line BLM which after IV injection into nude mice grows out to lung metastases of variable size (103). Upon stable transfection with either the E48 cDNA, the U36/epican cDNA, or both cDNAs, this cell line can be used in an animal model for systemic tumor targeting with the ^{186}Re-labeled Mabs E48 and U36. Here we will present preliminary data obtained with E48 cDNA transfected BLM cells (BLM-E48 cells). Ten million BLM-E48 cells were injected in the tail vein and after 7 days groups of 11 mice received either 300 µCi ^{186}Re-labeled Mab E48 or saline only. Body weights were measured daily and mice were inspected for breathing difficulties. Toxicity was considered unacceptable when weight loss was >10% within 2 days, or >5% within 1 day accompanied by severe breathing difficulties. When unacceptable toxicity was reached mice were sacrificed and checked for the presence of tumor deposits in the lungs and other organs. Lungs were removed, frozen, sectioned, and stained with hematoxylin/eosin to assess the tumor load and the viability of the tumor nodules.

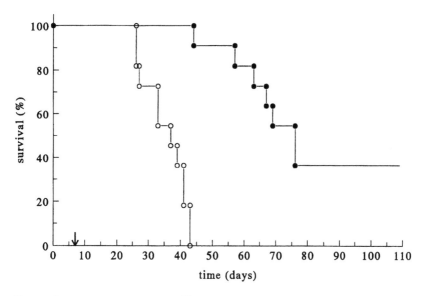

Figure 4 Therapeutic efficacy of [186]Re-labeled Mab E48 in a metastatic tumor model. Mice were injected with BLM-E48 cells and treated with 300 µCi [186]Re-Mab E48 (-●-) or saline (-○-). At day 7 after injection of tumor cells, [186]Re-labeled Mab E48 was administered (arrow).

Figure 4 shows the therapeutic efficacy of [186]Re-labeled Mab E48 in this metastatic tumor model. From the untreated group the first mice were sacrificed at 26 days after injection of the tumor cells, and after 43 days all mice had unacceptable toxicity. From the group that received [186]Re-labeled Mab E48 the first mouse was sacrificed 44 days after tumor cell injection. Four out of 11 mice of the treatment group were still living without any sign of toxicity at 100 days after the start of RIT. Histochemical analysis revealed that all sacrificed mice had tumor nodules in the lungs. In contrast, no viable microscopic tumor deposits were found in the lungs of the surviving mice, which were sacrificed at 100 days after the start of RIT. These data indicate that RIT with [186]Re-labeled Mabs might be suitable for eradication of very small tumor deposits.

The potential of RIT for eradication of minimal residual disease was also demonstrated by Goldenberg and colleagues (104,105). They used a micrometastatic model of a human colonic carcinoma cell line in the nude mouse lung. Also, clinical studies showed that RIT may be particularly effective in eradicating minimal residual disease due to the higher Mab uptake in small tumor deposits (74,106–109).

VII. CLINICAL RIT STUDIES IN HEAD AND NECK CANCER PATIENTS

Until now, no clinical RIT studies have been performed with head and neck cancer patients and therefore no pertinent data exist on the feasibility of RIT. However, by combining the biodistribution data on E48 IgG and U36 IgG in patients with data obtained from animal studies, we are able to speculate about such feasibility.

The use of radiolabeled Mabs in combination with external-beam radiotherapy to improve locoregional control of head and neck cancer as proposed by Maraveyas *et al.* (20,21) seems to be one of the options. They reconstructed a theoretical phantom of the larynx and derived local dosimetric data for the selection of β-emitting radionuclides. With such combined irradiation approach they expect the greatest acute local toxicity in the oral mucosa. Toxicity can be expected at 10 Gy. This toxicity is of particular concern when using radiolabeled MAbs E48 and U36, since these Mabs were shown to accumulate in the oral mucosa. Tumor-to-normal mucosa ratios 2 days after injection are for Mab E48 and Mab U36 2.8 and 2.3, respectively. In their dosimetric calculations the authors take into account that some of the disintegration energy dissipates outside the distribution volume of the tissue. For ^{186}Re the absorbed fraction in tumors will be about 1.6 times larger than in normal mucosa, which leads to a greater tumor/mucosa dose advantage. Despite this, radiation toxicity of the mucosa is expected to become a dose-limiting factor, and a compensatory decrease to the external-beam radiotherapy may be needed when combined with RIT.

The use of ^{186}Re-labeled Mabs E48 and U36 in RIT in an adjuvant setting is a second option. When using previously mentioned biodistribution values of, e.g., U36 IgG, an approximate dosimetry calculation can be made for large tumors (diameter > 1 cm). Assuming that patients tolerate a dose of 200 mCi ^{186}Re, as was the case in a first Phase I clinical trial with ^{186}Re-labeled NR-LU-10 IgG described by Breitz et al. (97), and assuming an energy per transition of 0.73 g.cGy/(µCi.h) for ^{186}Re (110), one may expect an absorbed tumor dose of approximately 20 Gy. In our animal studies with HNSCC-bearing nude mice we observed complete remissions with such an absorbed tumor dose (96). Moreover, in these animal studies we showed that RIT with ^{186}Re-labeled Mabs was particularly effective in eradicating small tumors, due to the higher uptake of Mabs in small tumors. When a similar size correlation applies for head and neck tumors in patients, and assuming that patients indeed tolerate a dose of 200 mCi ^{186}Re, achieving radiation doses in tumor tissue enabling elimination of minimal residual disease lies within reach.

At our department, after a Phase I trial in HNSCC patients with advanced disease, priority will be given to an adjuvant RIT trial with ^{186}Re-labeled Mabs in patients at high risk of developing distant metastases and locoregional recurrences.

VIII. ENHANCEMENT OF THE EFFICACY OF RADIOIMMUNOTHERAPY

A variety of methods have been investigated to improve the therapeutic efficacy of RIT. These include the use of fragments (59,75), targeting with genetically engineered single-chain antibodies (111), administration of agents to increase tumor blood flow (112) or antigen expression (113), the use of two- or three-step delivery methods (114), and the combination with external-beam irradiation (115). An alternative approach is to potentiate the therapeutic action of radioimmunoconjugates at the tumor site and thus improve the efficacy of RIT by decreasing the effective dose required for antitumor activity. This can be done by drugs that have no antitumor activity of their own, the so-called radiosensitizers (116). Besides that, several anticancer drugs have been examined for synergistic effects with radiation including cyclophosphamide, cisplatin, mitomycin C, 5-fluorouracil, doxorubicin, taxol, and topoisomerase I inhibitors (117–119).

An approach that may be of particular interest for the improvement of the efficacy of adjuvant RIT in HNSCC patients is the combination of RIT with a Mab directed against EGFR (see previously in this chapter). The motivation for such an approach comes from animal studies in which Mabs directed against EGFR effectively enhanced the therapeutic efficacy of chemotherapy (119,120). This beneficial effect of anti-EGFR Mab is thought to result from an increase of the sensitivity of tumor cells to DNA damage. It has been speculated that the combination of anti-EGFR Mabs and chemotherapy leads to synergistic effects by acting upon common biochemical pathways involving apoptosis (120). Because radiation also leads to DNA damage and apoptosis of tumor cells, the combination of RIT and anti-EGFR Mabs might have an increased therapeutic effect in comparison with the single treatments.

At our laboratory we recently started studies to assess the efficacy of combination therapy with RIT and anti-EGFR Mab 425 in HNSCC-bearing nude mice. Figure 5 shows one of the first experiments in this field. Nude mice bearing HNX-OE xenografts were randomized and treated when tumors reached a mean volume of 100 to 150 mm^3. Treatment groups received a single injection of 200 µCi ^{186}Re-labeled Mab U36 (day 0), or multiple injections (days 0, 7, 14, and 21) of 1.1 mg Mab 425 or a combination of the two. In Figure 5 the tumor volume during therapy relative to the tumor volume at day 0 for the control group and the four treatment groups is plotted against time.

Tumors of mice in the untreated group showed exponential growth with a tumor volume doubling time of 11 days. In all treatment groups tumors stopped growing shortly after the start of treatment. Tumors of the single-modality treatment groups became smaller until day 11 to 15 days postinjection and started regrowth shortly thereafter. Antitumor effects were much more pronounced in

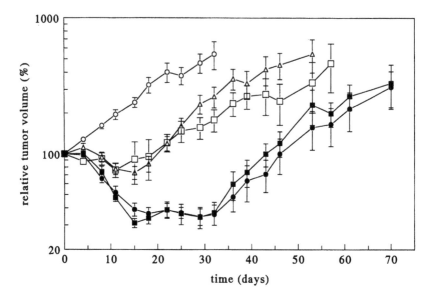

Figure 5 Therapeutic efficacy of [186]Re-labeled Mab U36 in combination with anti-EGFR Mab 425 in nude mice bearing HNX-OE xenografts. Mice were treated with: (-△-), 200 μCi [186]Re-labeled MAb U36; (-□-), four injections of 1.1 mg Mab 425 at day 0, 7, 14, and 21 PI; (-■-), 200 μCi [186]Re-labeled Mab U36 in combination with a single injection of 1.1 mg Mab 425 at day 0; (-●-), 200 μCi [186]Re-labeled Mab U36 in combination with four injections of 1.1 mg Mab 425 at days 0, 7, 14, and 21 PI; or (-○-), saline. The tumor size is expressed as the average tumor volume (±SEM) during therapy relative to the average tumor volume at the start of therapy.

the combination treatment groups. In these groups the mean tumor size was further reduced, and tumor growth was delayed for a much longer time period. The growth curves of the two combination treatment groups did not differ significantly. These initial results indicate that it might be attractive to combine the selective antitumor activity of RIT with [186]Re-labeled Mabs E48 or U36 with the potentiating effect of anti-EGFR Mabs.

REFERENCES

1. Wingo PA, Tong T, Bolden S. Cancer statistics 1995. CA Cancer J Clin 1995; 45: 8–30.
2. Vernham GA, Crowther JA. Head and neck carcinoma—stage at presentation. Clin Otolaryngol 1994; 19:120–124.

3. Berger DS, Fletcher GH. Distant metastases following local control of squamous cell carcinoma of the nasopharynx, tonsillar fossa and the base of the tongue. Radiology 1971; 100:141–143.

4. Merino OR, Lindberg RD, Fletcher GH. An analysis of distant metastases from squamous cell cancer of the upper respiratory and digestive tracts. Cancer 1977; 40:145–151.

5. Vikram B, Strong EW, Shah JP, Spiro R. Failure at distant sites following multimodality treatment for advanced head and neck cancer. Head Neck Surg 1984; 6:730–733.

6. Leemans CR, Tiwari R, Nauta JJP, Van der Waal I, Snow GB. Regional lymph node involvement and its significance in the development of distant metastases in head and neck cancer. Cancer 1993; 71:452–456.

7. Dennington ML, Carter DR, Meijers AD. Distant metastases in head and neck carcinoma. Laryngoscope 1980; 90:196–201.

8. Zbären P, Lehmann W. Frequency and sites of distant metastases in head and neck squamous cell carcinoma. An analysis of 101 cases at autopsy. Arch Otolaryngol Head Neck Surg 1987; 113:762–764.

9. Nishijima W, Takooda S, Tokita N, Takayama S, Sakura M. Analyses of distant metastases in squamous cell carcinoma of the head and neck and lesions above the clavicle at autopsy. Arch Otolaryngol Head Neck Surg 1993; 119:65–68.

10. Cerezo L, Millan I, Torre A, Aragon G, Otero J. Prognostic factors for survival and tumor control in cervical lymph node metastases from head and neck cancer. A multivariate study of 492 cases. Cancer 1992; 69:1224–1234.

11. Ellis ER, Mendelhall WM, Rao PV, Parsons JT, Sprangler AE, Million RR. Does node location affect the incidence of distant metastases in head and neck squamous cell carcinoma? Int J Radiat Oncol Biol Phys 1989; 17:293–297.

12. Hong WK, Bromer R. Chemotherapy in head and neck cancer. N Engl J Med 1983; 308:75–78.

13. Al-Sarraf M. Head and neck cancer: chemotherapy concepts. Semin Oncol 1988; 15:70–75.

14. Cortesina G, De Stefani A, Sacchi M, Rosso S, Galeazzi E. Immunomodulation therapy for sqamous cell carcinoma of the head and neck. Head Neck 1993; 15: 266–270.

15. Cortesina G, De Stefani A, Galeazzi E, Cavallo GP, Badellino F, Margarino G, Jemma C, Forni G. Temporary regression of recurrent squamous cell carcinoma of the head and neck is achieved with a low but not with a high dose of recombinant interleukin 2 injected perilymphatically. Br J Cancer 1994; 69:572–576.

16. Wang MB, Lichtenstein A, Mickel RA. Hierarchical immunosuppression of regional lymph nodes in patients with head and neck squamous cell carcinoma. Otolaryngol Head Neck Surg 1991; 105:517–527.

17. Wessels BW, Harisiadis L, Carabell SC. Dosimetry and radiobiological efficacy of clinical radioimmunotherapy. J Nucl Med 1989; 30:827.

18. Van Dongen GAMS, Brakenhoff RH, De Bree R, Gerretsen M, Quak JJ, Snow GB. Progress in radioimmunotherapy of head and neck cancer. Oncol Rep 1994; 1:259–264.

19. Gerretsen M, Quak JJ, Brakenhoff RH, Snow GB, Van Dongen GAMS. The feasibility of radioimmunotherapy in head and neck cancer. Eur J Cancer Part B; Oral Oncol 1994; 30B:82–87.
20. Maraveyas A, Stafford N, Rowlinson-Busza G, Stewart JSW, Epenetos AA. Pharmacokinetics, biodistribution, and dosimetry of specific and control radiolabeled monoclonal antibodies in patients with primary head and neck squamous cell carcinoma. Cancer Res 1995; 55:1060–1069.
21. Maraveyas A, Myers M, Stafford N, Rowlinson-Busza G, Stewart JSW, Epenetos AA. Radiolabeled antibody combined with external radiotherapy for the treatment of head and neck cancer: reconstruction of a theoretical phantom of the larynx for radiation dose calculation to local tissues. Cancer Res 1995; 55:1020–1027.
22. Keane TJ, Cummings BJ. Radiotherapy of head and neck cancer. Clin Oncol 1986; 5:557–573.
23. Zenner HP. Monoklonale antikörper zur Erkennung von Larynxkarzinomenzellen. Arch Otorhinolaryngol 1981; 233:161–172.
24. Stahel RA, Speak JA, Bernal SD. Murine monoclonal antibody LAM2 defines cell membrane determinant with preferential expression on human lung small-cell carcinomas. Int J Cancer 1985; 35:11–17.
25. Prat M, Bussolita G, Spinatto MR, Comoglio PM. Monoclonal antibodies against the human epidermoid carcinoma A431. Cancer Detect Prev 1985; 8:169–179.
26. Kyoizumi S, Akiyama M, Kouno N, Kobuke K, Hakoda M, Jones SL, Yamakido M. Monoclonal antibodies to human squamous cell carcinoma of the lung and their application to tumor diagnosis. Cancer Res 1985; 45:3274–3281.
27. Boeheim K, Speak JA, Frei E, Bernal SD. SQM1 antibody defines a surface membrane antigen in squamous carcinoma of the head and neck. Int J Cancer 1985; 36: 137–142.
28. Hanai N, Shitara K, Yoshida H. Generation of monoclonal antibodies against human lung squamous cell carcinoma and adenocarcinoma using mice rendered tolerant to normal human lung. Cancer Res 1986; 46:4438–4443.
29. Fernsten PD, Pekny KW, Reisfeld RA, Walker LE. Antigens associated with human squamous cell lung carcinoma defined by murine monoclonal antibodies. Cancer Res 1986; 46:2970–2977.
30. Kimmel KA, Carey TE. Altered expression in squamous cells of an orientation restricted epithelial antigen detected by monoclonal antibody A9. Cancer Res 1986; 46:3614–3623.
31. Ranken R, White CF, Gottfried TG, Yonkovich SJ, Blazek BE, Moss MS, Fee WE, Liu Y-SV. Reactivity of monoclonal antibody 17.13 with human squamous cell carcinoma and its application to tumor diagnosis. Cancer Res 1987; 47:5684–5690.
32. Myoken Y, Moroyama T, Miyauchi S, Takada K, Namba M. Monoclonal antibodies against human oral squamous cell carcinoma reacting with keratin proteins. Cancer 1987; 60:2927–2937.
33. Murthy U, Basu A, Rodeck U, Herlyn M, Ross AH, Das M. Binding of an antagonistic monoclonal antibody to an intact and fragmented EGF-receptor polypeptide. Arch Biochem Biophys 1987; 252:549–560.
34. Tatake RJ, Amin KM, Maniar HS, Jambhekar NA, Srikhande SS, Gangal SG.

Monoclonal antibody against human sqaumous-cell-carcinoma-associated antigen. Int J Cancer 1989; 44:840–845.

35. Samuel J, Noujaim AA, Willans DJ, Brzezinska GS, Haines DM, Longenecker BM. A novel marker for basal (stem) cells of mammalian stratified squamous epithelia and squamous cell carcinoma. Cancer Res 1989; 49:2465–2470.

36. Quak JJ, Van Dongen GAMS, Balm AJM, Brakkee JPG, Scheper RJ, Snow GB, Meijer CJLM. A 22-kDa surface antigen detected by monoclonal antibody E48 is exclusively expressed in stratified squamous and transitional epithelia. Am J Pathol 1990; 136:191–197.

37. Quak JJ, Van Dongen GAMS, Gerretsen M, Hayashida D, Balm AJM, Brakkee JPG, Snow GB, Meijer CJLM. Production of monoclonal antibody (K931) to a squamous cell carcinoma antigen identified as the 17-1A antigen. Hybridoma 1990; 9:377–387.

38. Inoue M, Nakanishi K, Sasagawa T, Tanizawa O, Inoue H, Hakura A. A novel monoclonal antibody against squamous cell carcinoma. Jpn J Cancer Res 1990; 81:176–182.

39. Fantozzi RD. Development of monoclonal antibodies with specificity to oral squamous cell carcinoma. Laryngoscope 1991; 101:1076–1080.

40. Parsons PG, Leonard JH, Kearsley JH, Takahashi H, Lin-Jian X, Moss DJ. Characterization of a novel monoclonal antibody, 3H-1, reactive with squamoproliferative lesions and squamous-cell cancers. Int J Cancer 1991; 47:847–852.

41. Divgi CR, Welt S, Kris M, Real FX, Yeh SDJ, Gralla R, Merchant B, Schweighart S, Unger M, Larson SM, Mendelsohn J. Phase I and imaging trial of indium-111-labeled anti-epidermal growth factor receptor monoclonal antibody 225 in patients with squamous cell lung carcinoma. J Natl Cancer Inst 1991; 83:97–104.

42. Quak JJ, Schrijvers AHGJ, Brakkee JGP, Davis HD, Scheper RJ, Balm AJM, Meijer CJLM, Snow GB, Van Dongen GAMS. Expression and characterization of two differentiation antigens in stratified squamous epithelia and carcinomas. Int J Cancer 1992; 50:507–513.

43. Balm AJM, Hageman PC, Mulder CJ, Hilkens J. Carcinoma-associated monoclonal antibodies in head and neck carcinoma: immunohistochemistry and biodistribution of monoclonal antibodies 175F4 and 175F11. Eur Arch Otorhinolaryngol 1992; 249:237–242.

44. Chang K, Pastan I, Willingham MC. Frequent expression of the tumor antigen CAK1 in squamous-cell carcinomas. Int J Cancer 1992; 51:548–554.

45. Schrijvers AHGJ, Quak JJ, Uyterlinde AM, Van Walsum M, Meijer CJLM, Snow GB, Van Dongen GAMS. MAb U36, a novel monoclonal antibody successful in immunotargeting of squamous cell carcinoma of the head and neck. Cancer Res 1993; 53:4383–4390.

46. Yoshiura M, Murakami H, Tashiro H, Kurisu K. Production of a human monoclonal antibody to normal basal and squamous cell carcinoma-associated antigen. J Oral Pathol Med 1993; 22:451–458.

47. Heider K-H, Sproll M, Susani S, Patzelt E, Beaumier P, Ostermann E, Ahorn H, Adolf GR. Characterization of a high-affinity monoclonal antibody specific for CD44v6 as candidate for immunotherapy of squamous cell carcinomas. Cancer Immunol Immunother 1996; 43:245–253.

48. Tranter RMD, Fairwheather DS, Bradwell AR, Dykes PW, Watson-James S, Chandler S. The detection of squamous cell tumours of the head and neck using radiolabelled antibodies. J Laryngol Otol 1984; 98:71–74.

49. Kairemo KJA, Hopsu EVM. Imaging of tumours in the parotid region with indium-111 labelled monoclonal antibody reacting with carcinoembryonic antigen. Acta Oncol 1990; 29:539–543.

50. Kairemo KJA, Hopsu EVM. Imaging of pharyngeal and laryngeal carcinomas with indium-111-labeled monoclonal anti-CEA antibodies. Laryngoscope 1990; 100: 1077–1082.

51. Timon CI, McShane D, Hamilton D, Walsh MA. Head and neck cancer localization with indium labelled carcinoembryonic antigen: a pilot project. J Otolaryngol 1991; 20:283–287.

52. Soo KC, Ward M, Roberts KR, Keeling F, Carter RL, McCready VR, Ott RJ, Powell E, Ozanne B, Westwood JH, Gusterson BA. Radioimmunoscintigraphy of squamous carcinomas of the head and neck. Head Neck Surg 1987; 9:349–352.

53. Perez-Soler R, Donato NJ, Shin DM, Rosenblum MG, Zhang H-Z, Tornos C, Brewer H, Chan JC, Lee JS, Hong WK, Murray JL. Tumor epidermal growth factor receptor studies in patients with non-small-cell lung cancer or head and neck cancer treated with monoclonal antibody RG 83852. J Clin Oncol 1994; 12:730–739.

54. Bier H, Reiffen KA, Haas I, Stasiecki P. Dose-dependent access of murine anti–epidermal growth factor receptor monoclonal antibody to tumor cells in patients with advanced laryngeal and hypopharyngeal carcinoma. Eur Arch Otorhinolaryngol 1995; 252:433–439.

55. Baum RP, Adams S, Kiefer J, Niesen A, Knecht R, Howaldt H-P, Hertel A, Adamietz IA, Sykes T, Boniface GR, Noujaim AA, Hör G. A novel technetium-99m labeled monoclonal antibody (174H.64) for staging head and neck cancer by immuno-SPECT. Acta Oncol 1993; 32:747–751.

56. Heissler E, Grünert B, Barzen G, Fritsche L, Hell B, Felix R, Bier J. Radioimmunoscintigraphy of squamous cell carcinoma in the head and neck region. Int J Oral Maxillofac Surg 1994; 23:149–152.

57. Kiefer J, Baum RP, Knecht R, Hertel A, Niesen A, Von Iiberg C, Hör G. Immunszintigraphie von Karzinomen im Kopf-Hals-Bereich mit Technetium-99m-markiertem monoklonalem Antikörper 174H.64. HNO 1994; 42:546–552.

58. Adamietz IA, Baum RP, Schemman F, Niesen A, Knecht R, Saran F, Tieku S, Boniface GR, Hör G, Böttcher HD. Improvement of radiation treatment planning in squamous-cell head and neck cancer by immuno-SPECT. J Nucl Med 1996; 37: 1942–1946.

59. De Bree R, Roos JC, Quak JJ, Den Hollander W, Van den Brekel MWM, Van de Wal JE, Snow GB, Van Dongen GAMS. Clinical imaging of head and neck cancer with ^{99m}Tc-labeled monoclonal antibody E48 IgG or F(ab')$_2$. J Nucl Med 1994; 35: 775–783.

60. De Bree R, Roos JC, Quak JJ, Den Hollander W, Wilhelm AJ, Van Lingen A, Snow GB, Van Dongen GAMS. Biodistribution of radiolabeled monoclonal antibody E48 IgG and (F(ab')$_2$ in patients with head and neck cancer. Clin Cancer Res 1995; 1: 277–286.

61. De Bree R, Roos JC, Quak JJ, Den Hollander W, Snow GB, Van Dongen GAMS.

Clinical screening of monoclonal antibodies 323/A3, cSF-25, and K928 for suit-ability of targeting tumors in the upper-aerodigestive and respiratory tract. Nucl Med Commun 1994; 15:613–627.

62. De Bree R, Roos JC, Quak JJ, Den Hollander W, Snow GB, Van Dongen GAMS. Radioimmunoscintigraphy with ^{99m}Tc-labeled monoclonal antibody U36 and its bi-odistribution in patients with head and neck cancer. Clin Cancer Res 1995b; 1: 591–598.

63. De Bree R, Roos JC, Plaizier MABD, Quak JJ, Van Kamp GJ, Den Hollander W, Snow GB, Van Dongen GAMS. Selection of monoclonal antibody E48 IgG or U36 IgG for adjuvant radioimmunotherapy in head and neck cancer patients. Br J Cancer 1997; 75:1049–1060.

64. Masui H, Morayama T, Mendelsohn J. Mechanisms of antitumor activity in mice for anti-EGF-receptor monoclonal antibodies with different isotypes. Cancer Res 1986; 46:5592–5598.

65. Aboud Pirak E, Hurwitz E, Pirak ME, Bellot F, Schlessinger J, Sela M. Efficacy of antibodies to epidermal growth factor receptor against KB carcinoma in vitro and nude mice. J Natl Cancer Inst 1988; 80:1605–1611.

66. Schnürch H-G, Stegmüller M, Vering A, Beckmann MW, Bender HG. Growth inhibition of xenotransplanted human carcinomas by a monoclonal antibody di-rected against the epidermal growth factor receptor. Eur J Cancer 1994; 30A:491–496.

67. Van Dongen GAMS, Leverstein H, Roos JC, Quak JJ, Van den Brekel MWM, Van Lingen A, Martens HJM, Castelijns J, Visser GWM, Meijer CJLM, Teule JJ, Snow GB. Radioimmunoscintigraphy of head and neck tumors using ^{99m}Tc-labeled monoclonal antibody E48 F(ab')$_2$. Cancer Res 1992; 52:2569–2574.

68. Schrijvers AHGJ, Gerretsen M, Fritz J, Van Walsum M, Quak JJ, Snow GB, Van Dongen GAMS. Evidence for a role of the monoclonal antibody E48 defined anti-gen in cell-cell adhesion in squamous epithelia and head and neck squamous cell carcinomas. Exp Cell Res 1991; 196:264–269.

69. Brakenhoff RH, Gerretsen M, Knippels ECM,Van Dijk M,Van Essen H, Olde Weghuis D, Sinke R, Snow GB, Van Dongen GAMS. The human E48 antigen, highly homologous to the murine Ly-6 antigen ThB, is a GPI-anchored molecule apparently involved in keratinocyte cell-cell adhesion. J Cell Biol 1995; 129:1677–1689.

70. Larson SM, Carrasquillo JA, Colcher DC, Yokoyama K, Reynolds JC, Bacharach A, Raubitheck A, Pace L, Finn RD, Rotman M, Stabin M, Neumann RD, Sug-arbaker P, Schlom J. Estimates of radiation absorbed dose for intraperitoneally ad-ministered iodine-131 radiolabeled B72.3 monoclonal antibody in patients with peritoneal carcinomatoses. J Nucl Med 1991; 32:1661–1667.

71. Bares R, Fass J, Hauptmann S, Braun J, Grehl O, Reinartz R, Buell U, Schupelick V, Mittmayer C. Quantitative analysis of anti-CEA antibody accumulation in hu-man colorectal carcinomas. J Nucl Med 1993; 32:65–72.

72. Welt S, Divgi CR, Scott AM, Garin-Chesa P, Finn RD, Graham M, Carswell EA, Cohen A, Larson SM, Old LJ, Rettig WJ. Antibody targeting in metastatic colon cancer: a phase I study of monoclonal antibody F19 against a cell-surface protein of reactive tumor stromal fibroblasts. J Clin Oncol 1994; 12:1193–1203.

73. Rosenblum MG, Levin B, Roh M, Hohn D, McCabe R, Thompson L, Cheung L, Murray JL. Clinical pharmacology and tissue disposition studies of ^{131}I-labeled anticolorectal carcinoma human antibody LiCO 16.88. Cancer Immunol Immunother 1994; 39:397–400.

74. Chatal, J-F, Saccavini J-C, Gestin J-F, Thrédez P, Curtet C, Kremer M, Guerreau D, Nobilé D, Fumoleau P, Guillard Y. Biodistribution of indium-111-labeled OC 125 monoclonal antibody intraperitoneally injected into patients operated on for ovarian carcinomas. Cancer Res 1989; 49:3087–3094.

75. Buist MR, Kenemans P, Den Hollander W, Vermorken JB, Molthoff CJM, Burger CW, Helmerhorst TJM, Baak JPA, Roos JC. Kinetics and tissue distribution of the radiolabeled chimeric monoclonal antibody MOv18 IgG and F(ab')$_2$ fragments in ovarian cancer patients. Cancer Res 1993; 53:5413–5418.

76. Van Hof AC, Molthoff CFM, Davies Q, Perkins AC, Verheijen RHM, Kenemans P, Den Hollander W, Wilhelm AJ, Baker TS, Sopwith M, Frier M, Symonds EM, Roos JC. Biodistribution of ^{111}indium-labeled engineered human antibody CTMO1 in ovarian cancer patients: influence of protein dose. Cancer Res 1996; 56:5179–5185.

77. Zalutsky MR, Mosely RP, Coakham HB, Coleman RE, Bigner DD. Pharmacokinetics and tumor localization of ^{131}I-labeled anti-tenascin monoclonal antibody 81C6 in patients with gliomas and other intracranial malignancies. Cancer Res 1989; 49:2807–2813.

78. Oosterwijk E, Bander NH, Divgi CR, Welt S, Wakka JC, Finn RD, Carswell EA, Larson SM, Warnaar SO, Fleuren GJ, Oettgen HF, Old LJ. Antibody localization in human renal cell carcinoma: a phase I study of monoclonal antibody G250. J Clin Oncol 1993; 11:738–750.

79. Scheinberg DA, Straus DJ, Yeh SD, Divgi C, Garin-Chesa P, Graham M, Pentlow K, Coit D, Oettgen HF, Old LJ. A phase I toxicity, pharmacology, and dosimetry trial of monoclonal antibody OKB7 in patients with non-Hodgkin's lymphoma: effects of tumor burden and antigen expression. J Clin Oncol 1990; 8:792–803.

80. Van Hal NLW, Van Dongen GAMS, Rood-Knippels EMC, Van der Valk P, Snow GB, Brakenhoff RH. Monoclonal antibody U36, a suitable candidate for clinical immunotherapy of squamous cell carcinoma, recognizes a CD44 isoform. Int J Cancer 1996; 69:520–527.

81. Koopman G, Heider K-H, Horst E, Adolf GR, Van den Berg F, Ponta H, Herrlich P, Pals ST. Activated human lymphocytes and aggressive non-Hodgkin's lymphomas express a homologue of the rat metastasis-associated variant CD44. J Exp Med 1993; 177:897–904.

82. Jung K, Lein M, Weiss S, Schnorr D, Henke W, Loening S. Soluble CD44 molecules in serum of patients with prostate cancer and benign prostatic hyperplasia. Eur J Cancer 1996; 32A:627–630.

83. Simpkin DJ, Mackie TR. EGS4 Monte Carlo determination of the beta dose kernel in water. Med Phys 1990; 17:179–186.

84. Zalutsky MR, Noska MA, Colapinto EV, Garg PK, Bigner DD. Enhanced tumor localization and in vivo stability of a monoclonal antibody radioiodinated using N-succimidyl 3-(tri-n-butylstannyl)benzoate. Cancer Res 1989; 49:5543–5549.

85. Vaughan ATM, Keeling A, Yankuba SCS. The production and biological distribution of yttrium-90-labeled antibodies. Int J Appl Radiat Isot 1985; 36:800–805.

86. Sharkey RM, Kaltovich FA, Shih LB, Fand I, Govelitz G, Goldenberg DM. Radioimmunotherapy of human colonic cancer xenografts with ^{90}Y-labeled monoclonal antibodies to carcinoembryonic antigen. Cancer Res 1988; 48:3270–3275.

87. Meares CF, Moi MK, Diril H, Kubis DL, McCall MJ, Deshpande SV, DeNardo SJ, Snook D, Epenetos AA. Macrocyclic chelates of radiometals for diagnosis and therapy. Br J Cancer 1990; 62:21–26.

88. Wessels BW, Rogus RD. Radionuclide selection and model absorbed dose calculations for radiolabeled tumor associated antibodies. Med Phys 1984; 11:638–645.

89. Meijs WE, Herscheid JDM, Haisma HJ, Wijbrandts R, Van Langevelde F, Van Leuffen PJ, Mooy R, Pinedo HM. Production of highly pure no-carrier-added zirconium-89 for the labelling of antibodies with a positron emitter. Appl Radiat Isot 1994; 45:1143–1147.

90. Meijs WE, Haisma HJ, Klok RP, Van Gog FB, Kievit E, Pinedo HM, Herscheid JDM. Zirconium 88/89 labeled monoclonal antibodies: distribution in tumor-bearing nude mice. J Nucl Med 1997; 38:112–118.

91. Fritzberg AR, Abrams PG, Beaumier PL, Kasina S, Morgan AC, Rao TN, Reno JM, Sanderson JA, Srinivasan A, Wilbur DS, Vanderheyden J-L. Specific and stable labeling of antibodies with technetium-99m with a diamide dithiolate chelating agent. Proc Natl Acad Sci USA 1988; 85:4025–4029.

92. Visser GWM, Gerretsen M, Herscheid J, Snow GB, Van Dongen GAMS. Labeling of monoclonal antibodies with [186]Re using the MAG3 chelate for radioimmunotherapy of cancer: a technical protocol. J Nucl Med 1993; 34:1953–1963.

93. Van Gog FB, Visser GWM, Klok R, Van der Schors R, Snow GB, Van Dongen GAMS. Monoclonal antibodies labeled with rhenium-186 using the MAG3 chelate for clinical application: relationship between the number of chelated groups and biodistribution characteristics. J Nucl Med 1996; 37:352–362.

94. Van Gog FB, Visser GWM, Stroomer JWG, Roos JC, Snow GB, Van Dongen GAMS. High dose [186]Re-labeling of monoclonal antibodies for clinical application: pitfalls and solutions. Cancer 1997. In press.

95. Gerretsen M, Schrijvers AHGJ, Van Walsum M, Braakhuis BJM, Snow GB, Van Dongen GAMS. Radioimmunotherapy of head and neck squamous cell carcinoma with ^{131}I-labeled monoclonal antibody E48. Br J Cancer 1992; 66:496–502.

96. Gerretsen M, Visser GWM, Van Walsum M, Meijer CJLM, Snow GB, Van Dongen GAMS. [186]Re-labeled monoclonal antibody E48 IgG mediated therapy of human head and neck squamous cell carcinoma xenografts. Cancer Res 1993; 53:3524–3529.

97. Breitz HB, Weiden PL, Vanderheyden J-L, Appelbaum JW, Bjorn MJ, Fer MF, Wolf SB, Ratliff BA, Seiler CA, Foisie DC, Fisher DR, Schroff RW, Fritzberg AR, Abrams PG. Clinical experience with rhenium-186-labeled monoclonal antibodies for radioimmunotherapy: results of phase I trials. J Nucl Med 1992; 33:1099–1109.

98. Gerretsen M, Visser GWM, Brakenhoff RH, Van Walsum M, Snow GB, Van Dongen GAMS. Complete ablation of small head and neck cancer xenografts with [186]Re-labeled MAb E48 IgG. Cell Biophys 1994; 24:135–142.

99. Langmuir VK, Mendonca HL, Vanderheyden J-L, Su FM. Comparison of the efficacy of [186]Re- and ^{131}I-labeled antibody in multicell spheroids. Int J Radiat Oncol Biol Phys 1992; 24:127–132.

100. Bardiès M, Thredez P, Gestin J-F, Marcille B-M, Guerreau D, Faivre-Chauvet A, Mahé M, Sai-Maurel C, Chatal J-F. Use of multi-cell spheroids of ovarian carcinoma as an intraperitoneal radio-immunotherapy model: uptake, retention kinetics and dosimetric evaluation. Int J Cancer 1992; 50:984–991.

101. O'Donoghue JA, Bardiès M, Wheldon TE. Relationships between tumor size and curability for uniformly targeted therapy with beta-emitting radionuclides. J Nucl Med 1995; 36:1902–1909.

102. Sgouros G. Radioimmunotherapy of micrometastases: sidestepping the solid-tumor hurdle. J Nucl Med 1995; 36:1910–1911.

103. Van Muijen GNP, Cornelissen LMHA, Jansen CFJ, Figdor CG, Johnson JP, Bröckner EB, Ruiter DJ. Antigen expression of metastasizing and non-metastasizing human melanoma cells xenografted into nude mice. Clin Exp Metastasis 1991; 9: 259–272.

104. Sharkey RM, Weadock KS, Natale A, Haywood L, Aninipot R, Blumenthal RD, Goldenberg DM. Successful radioimmunotherapy for lung metastasis of human colonic cancer in nude mice. J Natl Cancer Inst 1991; 83:627–632.

105. Blumenthal RD, Sharkey RM, Haywood L, Natale AM, Wong GY, Siegel JA, Kennel SJ, Goldenberg DM. Targeted therapy of athymic mice bearing GW-39 human colonic cancer micrometastases with ^{131}I-labeled monoclonal antibodies. Cancer Res 1992; 52:6036–6044.

106. Williams LE, Bares RB, Fass J, Hauptmann S, Schumpelick V, Buell U. Uptake of radiolabeled anti-CEA antibodies in human colorectal primary tumors as a function of tumor mass. Eur J Nucl Med 1993; 20:345–347.

107. Hird V, Maraveyas A, Snook D, Dhokia B, Soutter WP, Meares C, Stewart JSW, Mason P, Lambert HE, Epenetos AA. Adjuvant therapy of ovarian cancer with radioactive monoclonal antibody. Br J Cancer 1993; 68:403–406.

108. Jacobs AJ, Fer M, Su F-U, Breitz H, Thompson J, Goodgold H, Cain J, Heaps J, Weiden P. A phase I trial of a rhenium-186-labeled monoclonal antibody administered intraperitoneally in ovarian carcinoma: toxicity and clinical response. Obstet Gynecol 1993; 82:586–593.

109. Crippa F, Bolis G, Seregni E, Gavoni N, Scarfone G, Ferraris C, Buraggi GL, Bombardieri E. Single-dose intraperitoneal radioimmunotherapy with the murine monoclonal antibody I-131 MOv18: clinical results in patients with minimal residual disease of ovarian cancer. Eur J Cancer 1995; 31A:686–690.

110. Weber DA, Eckerman KF, Dillman LT, Ryman JC, eds. MIRD: Radionuclide Data and Decay Schemes. New York: Society of Nuclear Medicine, 1989.

111. Colcher D, Bird R, Roselli M, Hardman KD, Johnson S, Pope S, Dodd SW, Pantoliano, MW, Milenic DE, Schlom J. In vivo tumor targeting of a recombinant single-chain antigen-binding protein. J Natl Cancer Inst 1990; 82:1191–1197.

112. Smyth MJ, Pietersz GA, McKenzie IF. Use of vasoactive agents to increase tumor perfusion and the antitumor efficacy of drug–monoclonal antibody conjugates. J Natl Cancer Inst 1987; 79:1367–1373.

113. Greiner JW, Guadagni F, Goldstein D, Smalley RV, Borden EC, Simpson JF, Moli-

nolo A, Schlom J. Intraperitoneal administration of interferon-y to carcinoma patients enhances expression of tumor-associated glycoprotein-72 and carcinoembryonic antigen on malignant ascites cells. J Clin Oncol 1992; 10:735–746.

114. Goodwin DA. Tumor pretargeting: almost the bottom line. J Nucl Med 1995; 36: 876–879.

115. Pedley RB, Begent RHJ, Boden JA, Adam T, Bagshawe KD. The effect of radio-sensitizers on radio-immunotherapy, using ^{131}I-labeled anti-CEA antibodies in a human colonic xenograft model. Int J Cancer 1991; 47:597–602.

116. Vokes EE, Weichselbaum RR. Concomitant chemoradiotherapy: rationale and clinical experience in patients with solid tumors. J Clin Oncol 1990; 8:911–934.

117. Vokes EE. Interaction of chemotherapy and radiation. Semin Oncol 1993; 20:70–79.

118. Roffler SR, Chan J, Yeh M-Y. Potentiation of radioimmunotherapy by inhibition of topoisomerase I. Cancer Res 1994; 54:1276–1285.

119. Baselga J, Norton L, Masui H, Pandiella A, Coplan K, Miller WH Jr, Mendelsohn J. Antitumor effects of doxorubicin in combination with anti–epidermal growth factor receptor monoclonal antibodies. J Natl Cancer Inst 1993; 85:1327–1333.

120. Fan Z, Baselga J, Masui H, Mendelsohn J. Antitumor effect of anti–epidermal growth factor receptor monoclonal antibodies plus cis-diamminedichloroplatinum on well established A431 cell xenografts. Cancer Res 1993; 53:4637–4642.

Index

9 780367 398361